G000065387

Improving Patient Safety Through Teamwork and Team Training

Improving Patient Safety Through Teamwork and Team Training

Edited by

Eduardo Salas, PhD
Pegasus & Trustee Chair Professor
Department of Psychology
Institute for Simulation & Training
University of Central Florida
Orlando, Florida

Karen Frush, MD
Chief Patient Safety Officer
Professor of Pediatrics
Duke University School of Medicine
Clinical Professor
Duke University School of Nursing
Durham, North Carolina
With

David P. Baker, PhD
Vice President, Health Practice Research
IMPAQ International, LLC
Columbia, Maryland

James B. Battles, PhD
Social Science Analyst
US Agency for Healthcare
Research and Quality
Rockville, Maryland

**Heidi B. King, MS,
FACHE, BCC, CPPS**
Director, Patient Safety Solutions Center
Office of the Assistant Secretary
of Defense (Health Affairs):
TRICARE Management Activity
Falls Church, Virginia

**Robert L. Wears, MD,
MS, PhD**
Professor of Emergency Medicine
University of Florida
Jacksonville, Florida
and
Visiting Professor
Imperial College, London

OXFORD
UNIVERSITY PRESS

Oxford University Press is a department of the University of Oxford. It furthers the
University's objective of excellence in research, scholarship, and education by publishing
worldwide.

Oxford   New York
Auckland   Cape Town   Dar es Salaam   Hong Kong   Karachi
Kuala Lumpur   Madrid   Melbourne   Mexico City   Nairobi
New Delhi   Shanghai   Taipei   Toronto

With offices in
Argentina   Austria   Brazil   Chile   Czech Republic   France   Greece
Guatemala   Hungary   Italy   Japan   Poland   Portugal   Singapore
South Korea   Switzerland   Thailand   Turkey   Ukraine   Vietnam

Oxford is a registered trademark of Oxford University Press in the UK and certain other countries.

Published in the United States of America by
Oxford University Press
198 Madison Avenue, New York, NY 10016

Copyright © 2013 by Oxford University Press

All rights reserved. No part of this publication may be reproduced, stored in a retrieval
system, or transmitted, in any form or by any means, without the prior permission in writing
of Oxford University Press, or as expressly permitted by law, by license, or under terms agreed
with the appropriate reproduction rights organization. Inquiries concerning reproduction
outside the scope of the above should be sent to the Rights Department, Oxford University
Press, at the address above.

You must not circulate this work in any other form
and you must impose this same condition on any acquirer.

Library of Congress Cataloging-in-Publication

Data Improving patient safety through teamwork and team training / edited by Eduardo Salas, Karen Frush.
  p. ; cm.
  Includes bibliographical references and index.
  ISBN 978-0-19-539909-7
  I. Salas, Eduardo. II. Frush, Karen.
  [DNLM: 1. Patient Care Team--United States.   2. Inservice Training--United States.   3. Organizational Case
  Studies—United States.   4. Patient Safety—United States.   5. Safety Management—United States.   6. Staff
  Development—United States. WX 162.5] LC Classification not assigned
  362.1068—dc23
  2012006852

Printed in the United States of America on acid-free paper

PREFACE

We know that patient care is a team sport. We know that patient safety is about people doing the right thing. It's about people in teams coordinating, communicating, cooperating with each other and making quick decisions in a flawless and fluid manner. We know that patient safety is about the attitudes, behaviors, and cognitive processes that people in teams engage in to ensure proper care. We also know that human performance interactions can better minimize errors and, of course, improve safety. And team training can be one of these interventions.

Team training has been around for decades. It started in aviation and now has transitioned to healthcare—a much welcomed event. Team training, when designed systematically and based on science, can produce significant results in clinical outcomes—the data are coming in now! The data are very encouraging. And, it is safe to say a science of teamwork and team training is emerging. A science that is robust and practical. Not perfect, but reliable enough to yield positive outcomes. This volume is motivated by that goal—keeping the science moving.

This volume represents one forum aimed at promoting the science of team training in health-care. We hope that the readers of this volume get a glimpse of what this science is all about. We hope readers are motivated by the thoughts, ideas, and practical insights offered by the authors. There is something here for all, we hope, from those in the front line to those in the lab. This is one of many forums that highlight the science and practice of medical team training now and in the future.

Eduardo Salas, PhD
Pegasus & Trustee Chair Professor
University of Central Florida

CONTENTS

CONTRIBUTORS

Alexander Alonso, PhD
Senior Research Scientist
American Institutes for Research
Society for Human Resource Management
Washington, DC

Shilo H. Anders, PhD
Assistant Research Professor of Anesthesiology
Center for Research and Innovation in Systems
 Safety
Vanderbilt University Medicine Center
Nashville, TN

Jeffrey Augenstein, MD, PhD
Director, Medical Computer Systems Laboratory
Director, William Lehman Injury Research Center
Medical Director, Trauma Intensive Care Unit
Professor of Surgery
University of Miami School of Medicine
Miami, FL

James B. Battles, PhD
Social Science Analyst
US Agency for Healthcare Research and Quality
Rockville, MD
and
Adjunct Professor of Bioinformatics
Department of Bioinformatics
Uniformed Services University of the Health
 Sciences
Bethesda, MD

David J. Birnbach, MD, MPH
Professor of Anesthesiology and Public Health
Director, UM-JMH Center for Patient Safety
University of Miami Miller School of Medicine
Miami, FL

Nana E. Coleman, MD, EdM
Assistant Professor of Pediatrics
Weill Cornell Medical College
New York, NY

Tripp Driskell, MS
Graduate Research Assistant
Institute for Simulation and Training
University of Central Florida
Orlando, FL

Dana M. Dunleavy, PhD
Manager, Admissions Research
Association of American Medical Colleges
Washington, DC

Walter J. Eppich, MD, MEd
Assistant Professor of Pediatrics and Medical
 Education
Northwestern University Feinberg School of
 Medicine
Ann & Robert H. Lurie Children's Hospital of
 Chicago
Division of Emergency Medicine
Chicago, IL

Jennifer Feitosa, BS
I/O Psychology Doctoral Student
Institute for Simulation and Training
University of Central Florida
Orlando, FL

Daniel J. France, PhD, MPH
Research Associate Professor of Anesthesiology &
   Medicine
Center for Research and Innovation in
   Systems Safety
Vanderbilt University School of Medicine
Nashville, TN

Allan S. Frankel, MD
Co-Chief Medical Officer
Pascal Metrics Inc.
Washington, DC

Jonathan Gallo
Duke University
Durham, NC

George D. Garcia, MD, FACS
Lieutenant Colonel, Medical Corps
US Army Director, US Army Trauma
   Training Center
Assistant Professor of Surgery
University of Miami Miller School of Medicine
Miami, FL

Sara N. Goldhaber-Fiebert, MD
Clinical Assistant Professor of Anesthesia
Co-Director of Evolve simulation program
Stanford University School of Medicine
Stanford, CA

Stephen W. Harden, BS, ATP
Chairman and CEO
LifeWings Partners LLC
Collierville, TN

Heidi B. King, MS, FACHE, BCC, CPPS
Deputy Director, Department of Defense Patient
   Safety Program Director, Patient Safety Solutions
   Center
Office of the Assistant Secretary of Defense (Health
   Affairs)
TRICARE Management Activity Falls Church, VA

and
Adjunct Assistant Professor of Biomedical
   Informatics School of Medicine Uniformed
   Services
University of the Health Sciences Bethesda, MD

Andrew P. Knight, PhD
Assistant Professor of Organizational Behavior
Faculty Scholar, Institute for Public Health
Washington University in St. Louis
St. Louis, MO

Carol Koeble, MD, MS, CPE
Executive Director
NC Center for Hospital Quality and Patient Safety
Cary, NC

Sheila K. Lambert, RN, MSN
Senior Director, Pediatric Services
Carilion Clinic Children's Hospital
Roanoke, VA

Elizabeth H. Lazzara, MA
Doctoral Candidate & Graduate Research Associate
Institute for Simulation & Training
Department of Psychology
University of Central Florida
Orlando, FL

Michael W. Leonard, MD
Co-Chief Medical Officer, Pascal Metrics
Adjunct Professor of Medicine, Duke University
Washington, DC

Susan C. Mann, MD
Director of Simulation and Team Training
Department of Obstetrics and Gynecology
Assistant Professor, Harvard Medical School
Boston, MA

Jill A. Marsteller, PhD, MPP
Associate Professor of Health Policy and
   Management
Johns Hopkins Bloomberg School of Public Health
and
Member, Executive Committee
Armstrong Institute for Patient Safety and Quality
Johns Hopkins School of Medicine
Baltimore, MD

Sara E. Massie, MPH
Program Director
Quality Improvement Research Partnership
University of North Carolina School of Medicine
Chapel Hill, NC

Celeste M. Mayer, PhD
Patient Safety Officer
University of North Carolina Health
    Care System
Chapel Hill, NC

Laura Maynard, MDiv
Director of Collaborative Learning
North Carolina Center for Hospital Quality and
    Patient Safety
North Carolina Hospital Association
Cary, NC

Lisa M. Mazzia, MD
Physician Educator, Medical Team Training
National Center for Patient Safety
Department of Veterans Affairs
Ann Arbor, MI

Sandra S. McDonald, MSN, RN
Patient Safety Officer
Shands Jacksonville
Jacksonville, FL

William C. McGaghie, PhD
Jacob R. Suker, MD, Professor of Medical
    Education
Professor of Preventive Medicine
Northwestern University Feinberg School of
    Medicine
Chicago, IL

Kevin J. O'Leary, MD, MS
Associate Professor of Medicine
Northwestern University Feinberg School of
    Medicine
Chicago, IL

Douglas E. Paull, MD, FACS, FCCP
Director Patient Safety Curriculum
National Center for Patient Safety
Department of Veterans Affairs
Ann Arbor, MI

Priyadarshini R. Pennathur, PhD
Post-doctoral Research Fellow
Armstrong Institute for Patient Safety and Quality
Department of Anesthesiology and Critical Care
    Medicine
Johns Hopkins University School of Medicine
Baltimore, MD

Shawna J. Perry, MD
Director for Patient Safety Systems Engineering
Associate Professor, Associate Chair
Department of Emergency Medicine
Virginia Commonwealth University
Richmond, VA

Stephen D. Pratt, MD
Chief, Division of Quality and Safety
Department of Anesthesia, Critical Care and Pain
    Medicine
Beth Israel Deaconess Medical Center
Boston, MA

Peter J. Pronovost, MD, PhD, FCCM
Professor of Anesthesiology and Critical Care
    Medicine
Director, Armstrong Institute for Patient
    Safety and Quality
Johns Hopkins Medicine Senior Vice-President
    for Patient Safety and Quality
Johns Hopkins University School of Medicine
Baltimore, MD

Michael A. Rosen, PhD
Assistant Professor
Armstrong Institute for Patient Safety and Quality, and
Department of Anesthesiology & Critical
    Care Medicine
Johns Hopkins University School of Medicine
Baltimore, MD

Mary L. Salisbury MS, RN
President
The Cedar Institute, Inc.
North Kingstown, RI

Nicola Schiebel, MD
Assistant Professor of Emergency Medicine
Mayo Clinic College of Medicine
Rochester, MN

René Schwendimann, PhD, RN
Director of Education
Institute of Nursing Science (INS)
University of Basel, Switzerland
and
Consulting Professor
Duke University School of Nursing
Durham, NC

Rhea Seddon, MD
Partner
LifeWings Partners, LLC
Memphis, TN

Noa Segall, PhD
Assistant Professor
Department of Anesthesiology
Duke University Medical Center
Durham, NC

Gwen Sherwood, PhD, RN, FAAN
Professor and Associate Dean for Academic
    Affairs
University of North Carolina at Chapel Hill
School of Nursing
Chapel Hill, NC

Salvatore Silvestri, MD, FACEP
Program Director
Orlando Regional Medical Center
and
Emergency Medicine Residency
Associate EMS Medical Director
Orange County EMS System
and
Clinical Associate Professor of Emergency
    Medicine,
University of Central Florida College of Medicine
Orlando, FL

Anthony D. Slonim, MD, DrPH
Executive Vice President/Chief Medical Officer
Barnabas Health
West Orange, NJ
and
Professor, Basic Sciences, Medicine,
    and Pediatrics
Virginia Tech-Carilion School of Medicine
Roanoke, VA

Renae E. Stafford, MD, MPH, FACS
Chief, Surgical Critical Care
Assistant Professor of Surgery
Division of Trauma, Critical Care Surgery and
    Acute Care Surgery
University of North Carolina School of Medicine
Chapel Hill, NC

Kenneth Stahl, MD, FACS
Associate Prof of Surgery and Director of Patient
    Safety
The DeWitt Daughtry Family Department of Surgery
Division of Trauma and Surgical Critical Care
The University of Miami Miller School
    of Medicine
Director of Patient Safety Research
William Lehman Injury Research Center
Medical Director, Ryder Trauma PSO
Miami, FL

Scott I. Tannenbaum, PhD
President
The Group for Organizational Effectiveness, Inc.
Albany, NY

David A. Thompson, DNSc, RN
Department of Anesthesiology and Critical Care
    Medicine
Johns Hopkins University School of Medicine
Associate Professor
Johns Hopkins School of Nursing
Baltimore, MD

John A. Vozenilek, MD
Associate Professor of Emergency Medicine
Medical Education, and Healthcare Studies
and
Director, Center for Simulation Technology and
    Immersive Learning
Feinberg School of Medicine
Northwestern University
Chicago, IL

Robert L. Wears, MD, MS
Professor of Emergency Medicine
University of Florida
Jacksonville, Florida
and
Visiting Professor
Imperial College, London

Sallie J. Weaver, PhD
Assistant Professor
Armstrong Institute for Patient Safety and Quality *and*
Department of Anesthesiology & Critical Care
   Medicine
Johns Hopkins University School of Medicine
Baltimore, MD

Matthew B. Weinger, MD
Norman Ty Smith Chair of Patient Safety and
   Medical Simulation
Professor of Anesthesiology, Biomedical
   Informatics, and Medical Education
Vice Chair for Faculty Affairs, Department of
   Anesthesiology
Director, Center for Research and Innovation in
   Systems Safety
Vanderbilt University School of Medicine
and
Staff Physician and Senior Scientist
Geriatric Research Education and Clinical Center
Tennessee Valley VA Healthcare System
Nashville, TN

Tina M. Schade Willis, MD
Associate Professor
Department of Anesthesiology
Department of Pediatrics
University of North Carolina School
   of Medicine
Chapel Hill, NC

Melanie C. Wright, PhD
Program Director, Patient Safety Research
Trinity Health System and Saint Alphonsus Health
   System
Boise, ID

Teresa S. Wu, MD, FACEP
Director, EM Ultrasound Program &
   Fellowship
Co-Director, Simulation Based
   Training Program
Assistant Program Director
Maricopa Integrated Health System
Phoenix, AZ

PART ONE

THE SCIENTIFIC FOUNDATIONS OF TEAMWORK AND
TEAM TRAINING

1

THE THEORETICAL DRIVERS AND MODELS OF TEAM PERFORMANCE AND EFFECTIVENESS FOR PATIENT SAFETY

Sallie J. Weaver, Jennifer Feitosa, Eduardo Salas, Rhea Seddon, and John A. Vozenilek

Teamwork is an integral component of healthcare today—embraced as a value, norm, and requirement for high-quality care as disease processes grow in complexity, diagnostic capabilities become increasingly specialized, and treatment options diversify. In the last decade the concept of teamwork has been integrated into the language of providers, administrators, patients, and regulators, into national patient safety goals,[1] and into models of provider education.[2,3] Thanks to seminal reports such as *Crossing the Quality Chasm*[4] coupled with significant effort on the part of champion providers, administrators, and educators, the culture of healthcare is changing. Teamwork is now recognized and embraced as a critical component of the healthcare vocabulary and as an integral part of the continuum of care.

Despite these gains, however, evidence suggests that the daily practice environment remains characterized by a notable lack of cooperation, coordination, and communication[5-7] Although the 2009 benchmarking database for the Agency for Healthcare Quality and Research's Hospital Survey on Patient Safety Culture indicates that 79% of providers ($N = 196,462$) felt positively about the teamwork within their units, only 62% felt positively about

the communication openness, and only 44% felt positively about handoffs and transitions.[8] Furthermore, Joint Commission statistics continue to cite communication—an essential teamwork component—as a primary root cause in the majority of sentinel events. Specifically, communication was identified as the primary root cause in 533 of 843 analyzed sentinel events occurring between 1995 and July 2006.[9] Greater than 65% of these 533 events involved problems with communication among staff and greater than 45% involved communication between staff and physicians. Additionally, a survey of more than 1,700 providers conducted by The American Association of Critical Care Nurses and VitalSmarts[10] found that nearly 53% of nurses and other clinical care providers characterized 10% or more of their coworkers as reluctant to help, impatient, or refusing to answer questions.

Such evidence demonstrates that the culture of teamwork within healthcare is still developing. The translation of teamwork into daily care practices is limited by the fact that a definition of healthcare teamwork has not been uniformly adopted, and conceptually well-developed, yet practically relevant models of healthcare teamwork delineating critical antecedents, processes, and outcomes across the care continuum are still rare.[11] Clinical treatment algorithms rely on a firm evidence-based foundation, and we argue that the same rigor should be applied to the conceptual development, training, and use of vital nontechnical skills such as teamwork.[12] High-quality clinical practices are the product of expert communication, cooperation, coordination, and leadership, which reflect the context and culture in which they are embedded. In short, a firm foundation in the science of team performance and effectiveness matters for patient safety.

Still, no single definition or model of teamwork can be expected to capture every aspect of teamwork within a specific specialty or service line.[13] Arguably, the term *teamwork* means different things to different specialties, across the various levels of care leadership, and across different care settings.[14] Emergency resuscitation teams differ from procedural-based surgical teams, who differ from nursing unit teams (e.g., progressive care units) and ambulatory care teams, yet all must work collaboratively to reach shared goals across disjointed performance episodes and disparate performance contexts. The same can be said about more "traditional" organizational teams. Empirical evidence demonstrates that expert teams working on such apparently dissimilar tasks within diverse contexts share several key commonalities in how they collectively think, feel, and act.

One way to develop a theoretically sound understanding of phenomena within complex and diverse contexts is to develop an overarching model capturing the key components and mechanisms of the phenomena. To this end, the purpose of this chapter is to summarize and synthesize the existing team performance literature so as to outline the critical cognitive, behavioral, and attitudinal foundations of patient safety–focused teamwork. This review is organized around a framework for healthcare teamwork that specifies core team behaviors, attitudes, and cognitions, and that can be further contextualized to capture practice, specialty, or profession-specific teamwork competencies. Such a model was highlighted as a critical research need in an Agency for Healthcare Research and Quality (AHRQ) report dedicated to medical teamwork and patient safety[15] in order to provide a common language for labeling and defining essential components of healthcare

team performance, as well as a common frame for describing and testing hypotheses.

To this end, we begin by defining the core constructs of teams, teamwork, and team performance. We then review the existing science of team performance and highlight healthcare-specific models offered to date. Next, we present a framework for describing teamwork in healthcare that synthesizes essential antecedents, processes, and outcomes in order to organize a review of the cognitive, behavioral, and attitudinal foundations of patient safety–focused teamwork. This work is designed to reflect not only within-team performance, but also inter-team collaboration, considering that overall patient health is a function of multiple teams and individuals interacting over time. Throughout, the chapter focuses on distilling the core processes and mechanisms of team performance, with an explicit focus on available empirical evidence that has examined teamwork in healthcare.

DEFINING TEAMS AND TEAMWORK

Traditional definitions of teams conceptualize them as identifiable groups of two or more individuals working interdependently toward a shared goal that requires the coordination of effort and resources to achieve mutually desired outcomes.[16] Importantly, teams see themselves and are seen by others as distinctive social entities working within a larger organization[17] and are, therefore, differentiated from groups. Teamwork refers to the actual behaviors (e.g., information exchange), cognitions (e.g., shared mental models), and attitudes (e.g., cohesion) that make interdependent performance possible.[18] At a minimum, effective teamwork requires: (1) multiple opportunities for members to interact (*task interdependence*), (2) that team members share in the consequences of their collective efforts (*outcome interdependence*), and (3) that members share in the belief that the team collectively has the skills and resources necessary to accomplished team goals (*team potency*).[19]

Specific definitions of teamwork within the healthcare context have also been developed. The Medical Subject Headings (MeSH), the vocabulary used by the National Library of Medicine catalogue, first introduced a definition for the term *patient care team* in 1968:

> Care of patients by a multidisciplinary team usually organized under the leadership of a physician; each member of the team has specific responsibilities and the whole team contributes to the care of the patient. (http://www.nlm.nih.gov/mesh/)

Teamwork has also been defined as "the interaction or relationship of two or more healthcare professionals who work interdependently to provide care for patients."[20]

Defining Teams in Healthcare

Two salient, interrelated issues are commonly cited in the definitions of teams and teamwork in healthcare: (1) who is part of a given "team" (i.e., how is the team construct defined? what are the boundaries that define a given team?), and (2) what are the differences and commonalities between teamwork and related constructs such as collaboration? For example, care delivery teams can be defined in terms of patient population (e.g., pediatric care teams), disease types (e.g., cardiac care teams), care delivery settings (e.g., hospital, ambulatory care clinic, long-term care), professional identity (e.g., nursing care teams), and crisis scenarios (e.g., rapid response teams).[21] Trauma teams have, for example, been described as extreme action teams:

> ...teams whose highly skilled members cooperate to perform urgent, unpredictable, interdependent, and high consequential tasks while simultaneously coping with frequent changes in team composition and training their teams' novice members.[22]

Teamwork versus Collaboration

As pinpointed in a recent review of the healthcare team literature,[23] teamwork is not synonymous with the concept of collaboration—although the terms are often used interchangeably. Although theoretical arguments regarding the boundaries of the terms abound, collaboration is commonly conceptualized as a prerequisite for teamwork; that is, collaboration is a necessary, but not sufficient, condition of teamwork.[24] The definition of teamwork goes beyond collaboration to specifically require shared, predefined collective goals.

Team Performance versus Team Effectiveness

Team performance and team effectiveness may also erroneously be used as interchangeable terms. *Performance* is defined specifically as "what employees do" in striving to complete daily work, whereas *effectiveness* refers to an evaluative statement regarding the degree to which employee behaviors contribute to organizational goals.[25] In this sense, *performance* refers to those behaviors, cognitions, and affect in which team members engage in working collaboratively toward shared goals. Conversely, *effectiveness* refers to evaluative judgments regarding the results of performance. Effectiveness generally represents a subjective assessment, although some indicators of effectiveness (e.g., adverse events, patient outcome data) fall arguably more on the objective end of the continuum. It is important to note, however, that all indicators of effectiveness are colored by contextual, organizational, and system-level factors other than performance.

The actual behaviors, feelings, and thoughts that team members engage in (i.e., performance) are the product of declarative knowledge, procedural knowledge, and motivation.[25] *Declarative knowledge* (i.e., fact-based knowledge) refers to one's understanding of what is required by the task, whereas *procedural knowledge* emphasizes one's understanding of how the task should be executed. *Motivation* refers to the forces driving the allocation of effort toward a given action. It refers to the combination of (1) whether one chooses to expend effort, (2) how much effort is expended, and (3) how long one persists in this expenditure of effort. These factors directly underlie both individual and team performance.

Several models of team performance elaborate on the aforementioned conceptualizations of performance and effectiveness so as to delineate key team processes, the mechanisms underlying these processes, and their relationship to outcomes. The subsequent section summarizes several such conceptual models to facilitate an understanding of the core mechanisms of effective teamwork in healthcare.

Providers, administrators, and patients striving to optimize teamwork benefit from a conceptual understanding of teamwork because it directly facilitates the insight necessary for development and testing of team strategies and interventions targeting healthcare professionals. These conceptual models shed light on the "black box" of teamwork to operationally define how expert teams function, the competencies effective team members demonstrate, critical antecedents, outcomes, and the reciprocal relationships among them, as well as the impact of time and levels of analysis.

How Teams Function: Theoretical Foundations of Team Performance and Effectiveness

The scientific understanding of how teams function has grown exponentially over the past 30 years.[26–29] Although this is in no way an exhaustive review, we briefly summarize a sampling of conceptual teamwork models to provide a foundational background for the discussion of teamwork in healthcare. More comprehensive reviews can be found by Mathieu et al.[30] and Cannon-Bowers and Bowers.[31]

Team Effectiveness: Models and Frameworks

Early social psychology produced a significant body of work dedicated to understanding groups (e.g., impact of group stimuli on individual group members, social processes of affiliation, group cognition and decision making) that formed a foundation for much of the initial thinking about teams and their functioning.[32–37] Building from this school of thought, teams were conceptualized in terms of classic systems models; thus, teamwork was traditionally conceptualized in terms of a linear input-process-output (IPO) framework.[37,38] In this basic IPO framework, inputs including organizational characteristics, individual team member characteristics, and characteristics of the broader environmental context were conceptualized as antecedents that influenced team affective (i.e., emotional, attitudinal), behavioral, and cognitive processes that, in turn, influenced team outcomes such as achievement of team goals and ratings of effectiveness.

For example, Tannenbaum et al.[39] combined several previous teamwork models to develop an integrated framework of team effectiveness. Inputs, including characteristics of the environment, task, and individual team members themselves affect not only team processes, but also interact with each other to affect team processes. For example, the heterogeneity of team member expertise can influence how power is distributed within the team and can also interact with task type. In support of this notion, evidence to date across a variety of settings and team types indicates that it is best to have heterogeneous teams working on creative tasks, but not routine tasks.[40,41] Thus, interdisciplinary care teams may demonstrate the greatest effectiveness in complex care tasks.

Team processes identified in the Tannenbaum et al.[39] model included coordination, communication, conflict resolution, decision making, problem solving, and boundary spanning (i.e., interactions with other teams and non–team members). Outputs included team performance and more proximal outcomes such as changes in the team (e.g., formation of new roles, changes in cohesion, collective efficacy) and individual team members (e.g., changes in attitude or motivation). This model also underscores that organizational and situational characteristics influence team effectiveness at several points—not only in their role as inputs. For example, organizational reward structures and culture can moderate how conflict resolution affects team performance; such as reward structures that reinforce individual performance over cooperative team performance or an organizational climate that is unsupportive of cross-unit collaboration may diminish quality of team performance, even when the team is effective in their conflict resolution processes.

In addition to broaching issues related to both interactions among immediate team members and interactions between different teams, this model incorporates team interventions (e.g., training and team building) as moderators that can potentially affect team processes. It also incorporates feedback loops among the various model components—an important step in the transition from identifying teams as relatively static entities to conceptualizing teams as dynamic, adaptive systems.[42]

Teams as Adaptive Systems: Taxonomies of Teamwork Processes and the Impact of Time

Complex adaptive systems are characterized by both a network of interdependent components and the capacity to learn and change over time.[42–44] In line with such thinking, team theorists explored more thoroughly the aspects of team development and the notion of collective emergent states—the affective and cognitive components of team performance. For example, collective efficacy, motivation, team values, team mental models, transactive memory systems, and other phenomena emerge as a function of social interaction, making them greater or quantifiably different than the sum or average of individual team members. Marks, Mathieu, and Zaccaro[45] developed taxonomy of team processes that helped clarify the distinction between processes and emergent states. Processes are those team activities that actually change inputs into outputs. For instance, consider a team that has a certain mix of specialized expertise (input) and needs to accomplish a complex procedure safely and effectively (output). The coordination activities (i.e., the actual behaviors the team engages in to determine who does what, when) used by the team to transform such skills into the determined outcome is an illustration of process. Emergent states, on the other hand, are dynamic—less tangible aspects of the team's performance that influence team processes, and in turn, can be reciprocally influenced by team processes. For example, as the team engages in coordination processes, this may trigger a representation of the team's beliefs in their competence to accomplish the given procedure (i.e., collective efficacy) and/or how they trust in their teammates, which in turn will affect how they will coordinate in future performance episodes.

Similarly, Ilgen et al.[46] expand the traditional IPO model that they argue implies linearity and ignore the fact that many of the factors affecting how team inputs get turned into outputs are not processes at all, but rather cognitive and affective states that emerge over time and through interaction among team members. The Ilgen et al.[46] IMOI (input-mediator-output-input) model clarifies that team outputs feedback to affect future team performance. The model also explicitly addresses interactions among inputs and processes, processes and other processes, and

processes and emergent states. For example, a study of anesthesia teams during induction found that these teams adapt their coordination strategies based on variations in situational demands (e.g., nonroutine events such as equipment failure or unusual patient response).[47]

Marks et al.[45] also integrates the influence of time on teamwork and accounts for the fact that teams often carry out multiple tasks simultaneously by distinguishing team processes into three reoccurring phases: *transitional phase processes, action phase processes,* and *interpersonal processes.* In the *transitional phase,* team processes mainly focus on planning activities such as mission analysis, goal specification, and strategy formulation. *Action phase* processes, on the other hand, describe activities such as monitoring progress toward goal, monitoring team and environmental systems, backup behavior (i.e., assisting fellow team members), and coordination. Alternatively, *interpersonal processes* such as conflict management, affect management (i.e., emotion regulation), motivation, and confidence building could happen concurrently during the transitional phase and/or action phase. As the most sensitive category, interpersonal processes can greatly affect the effectiveness of activities carried out in transition or action phases. For example, if a surgical team does not use effective methods to work through disagreements that arise between members, such as a surgeon and the anesthesia provider, both coordination (i.e., action process) and planning (i.e., transition processes) may be negatively impacted in the future and, in turn, may thus negatively impact overall team effectiveness (i.e., patient care). Figure 1.1 exemplifies how the processes described in the preceding manifest across theses phases.

Similarly, Salas, Sims, and Burke[48] developed a practical framework known as the "Big Five" model of teamwork to distill the large number of team processes described in the literature down into five core components of effective team performance and three coordinating mechanisms that affect how the five core components work in synchrony. The big five include: team leadership, mutual performance monitoring, backup behavior, adaptability, and team orientation. *Team leadership* describes transition processes such as direction and coordination of team member effort, organization, and planning, action processes such as assessment of team performance,

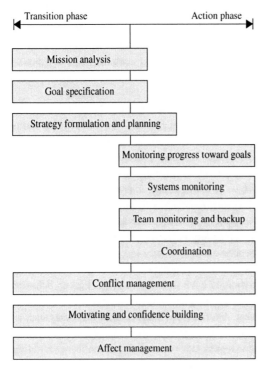

Figure 1.1
Examples of processes across transition and action phases given by Marks et al.[45] Reprinted with permission from Marks, M. A., Mathieu, J. E., & Zaccaro, S. J. (2001). A temporally based framework and taxonomy of team processes. *The Academy of Management Review, 26*(3), 356–376.

workload distribution, and the development of team knowledge, and interpersonal processes such as motivation of team members and establishing a positive atmosphere. *Mutual performance monitoring* refers to action processes dedicated to developing a common awareness regarding the environmental and situational context in which the team is operating and strategies used to maintain awareness of fellow teammate performance. This component is especially important when a team is under stress or when there is an increased susceptibility to slips or serious mistakes (e.g., if various team members have been working long hours and are likely to be fatigued). The third component of the big five, *backup behavior*, refers to action processes such as anticipation of team member needs and assisting fellow team members that are facilitated by transition processes dedicated to ensuring all team members have an

accurate understanding of team roles, responsibilities, task strategies, and interdependencies among these roles. *Adaptability* refers to action processes associated with identification of cues signaling environmental or situational changes that warrant a change in team action or strategy, as well as efforts to maintain awareness of these cues and the outcomes of new strategies. Finally, *team orientation* describes interpersonal processes reflective of the propensity for team members to consider others, beliefs regarding the importance of team goals, and collective orientation.

These five elements are coordinated through three mechanisms: (1) *shared mental models* (i.e., shared or complementary cognitive knowledge structures representing the strengths and weaknesses of each team member, team task strategies, the environment/context, team strategy, and the relationships among these elements), (2) *closed-loop communication* (i.e., a systematic, behavioral communication strategy in which information transmitted between sender and receiver is fully verified as accurate by both parties), and (3) *mutual trust* (i.e., shared affective belief that team members will perform their roles to the best of their ability, share information, admit to mistakes, accept feedback, and protect team interests). These coordinating mechanisms are not viewed as actual inputs, but as facilitators to the functioning of the big five components.

Within healthcare, the big five framework has served as the backbone for the TeamSTEPPS® program developed by the Department of Defense and Agency for Healthcare Research and Quality.[49] Additionally, it has been used to identify effective and ineffective examples of teamwork among nursing teams working in patient care units.[50]

Team Adaptation: The Nuts and Bolts

Continuous adaptation is necessary to achieve highly reliable, safe outcomes in the context of complex care systems and relatively unpredictable circumstances.[51] The concept of team adaptation is vital across the healthcare continuum, from trauma resuscitation teams to nursing care teams working in general medical units, primary care, and long-term care settings. Adaptation refers to a change in team behaviors, attitudes, or knowledge in response to salient contextual cues that indicate that current team strategies are not obtaining desired outcomes or could be producing better outcomes if performed differently.[52,53] But how do teams actually do this?

Burke et al.[54] offered a conceptualization of team adaptation (Fig. 1.2) looking both across multiple levels of analysis and also various phases of team performance.

An environmental cue triggers a cyclic adaptive process comprised of four phases: (1) *situation assessment* (i.e., cue recognition and meaning ascription), (2) *plan formulation* (i.e., generating ideas, setting goals, clarifying roles), (3) *plan execution* (i.e., mutual monitoring, communication, back-up behavior, leadership), and (4) *team learning* (i.e., collective development of knowledge). Shared mental models, team situation awareness, and psychological safety (i.e., a feeling that the team is supportive of interpersonal risk taking such as speaking up or raising concerns) are three critical emergent phenomena that help the team move through these four phases.

Additionally, this model highlights the role of feedback as a critical aspect of this adaptive cycle—to learn continuously and optimize effectiveness, teams must incorporate lessons learned into future performance episodes and individual team members must take these lessons with them when working with new team members.

Healthcare Specific Models of Teamwork

Building on some the general organizational literature about teams and groups, similar IPO models of healthcare teamwork have been developed, such as the *Integrated (Healthcare) Team Effectiveness Model* (ITEM).[21] This model identifies organizational contextual factors such as information and training systems as essential inputs that influence elements of task design including task type (e.g., project versus patient care), task features (e.g.,

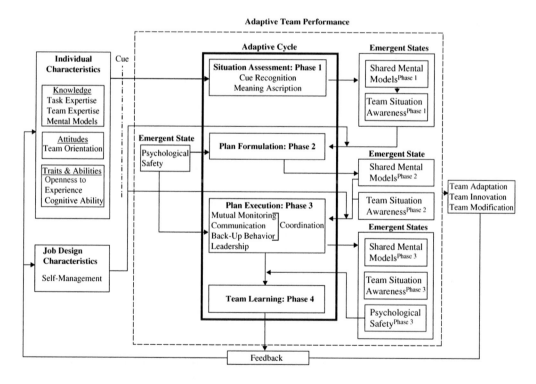

Figure 1.2
Input-throughput-output model of team adaptation from Burke et al.[54] Reprinted with permission from Burke, C. S., Stagl, K. C., Salas, E., Pierce, L., & Kendall, D. (2006). Understanding team adaptation: A conceptual analysis and model. *Journal of Applied Psychology, 91*(6), 1189–1207.

level of interdependence, need for specialized expertise), and team composition (e.g., diversity in age, gender, discipline). In turn, these task characteristics are depicted as drivers of team processes and psychosocial traits (i.e., emergent states) such as cohesion and collective efficacy. Although the ITEM model is linear, it includes some unique elements. For example, few models of team performance integrate the nature of forces external to the organization that influence team behavior, such as social, regulatory, and policy factors or highlight the potential for interaction between team processes and emergent states. Furthermore, the multidisciplinary nature of team outcomes is broken down in a 3 × 2 framework that addresses level of analysis (e.g., patient, team, organizational) and the nature of the outcome measure itself (e.g., objective versus subjective).

On the other hand, the model does not show the same dynamism regarding certain constructs, such as cohesion and efficacy. By operationalizing them as team psychosocial traits, the fluidity and flexibility associated with emerging states is absent.[45] Also, this model lacks the continuity of IMOI models.[46] A feedback loop from the output to the input might have solved this issue. Furthermore, certain characteristics of task design may not be influenced by the organizational, social, and policy context. For instance, supervision is unlikely to directly affect members' ages. Instead, supervision can moderate the relationship between members' ages and their communication. For instance, transformational leadership can diminish age differences by improving members' interaction.

Reflecting some of the difficulties in identifying general teamwork processes across the wide range of healthcare teams or even really viewing some types of teams in healthcare as similar enough for comparison, several models of teamwork in healthcare have limited their focus to specific care settings. For example, Reader et al.[55] reviewed 35 referred articles investigating teamwork within the intensive care unit (ICU) to develop a framework to describe ICU team performance

The framework focuses on team processes, including communication, leadership, coordination, and decision making, and breaks team outputs down into patient- and team-focused outputs. The authors note that there are likely other factors

beyond processes that affect team outcomes (e.g., shared mental models, team adaptability, organizational culture influences) and include a feedback loop between outcomes and inputs similar to the IMOI model discussed earlier.

Given the importance of teamwork in action teams such as trauma resuscitation teams and emergency medical teams, and so forth, Fernandez et al.[56] developed a teamwork model specific to emergency medicine (Fig. 1.3). This model is unique in its simultaneous consideration of (1) variation in the phases of teamwork (planning, action, reflection) and specific processes/supporting mechanisms that are most relevant during each phase, (2) overarching team processes and supporting mechanisms that occur across phases, and (3) time. Additionally, it is one of the only models of healthcare teamwork to address interactions among multiple teams by explicitly modeling interactions with external teams such as emergency medical services (EMS).

Overall, much work is being done to integrate what we know about teams and effective teamwork from other complex, dynamic industries into the science of teamwork in healthcare. However, there are several aspects that are in need of consideration when conceptualizing teamwork for patient safety, including: (1) collective efforts that may not fit the traditional definition of teamwork, such as interactions among multiple teams or collaborations between teams and external individuals, (2) the interactions among various input factors, (3) the moderation effects of professional, team, unit, and organizational climate for patient safety, (4) the dense network of feedback loops among core concepts that contributes to the evolution of team functioning over time, and (5) issues associated with simultaneous, ad hoc team membership. To spur more in-depth consideration of these factors in both the science and practice of teamwork in healthcare, we outline a synthesized framework of team effectiveness for patient safety in healthcare. Although parsimony in such conceptual models is desirable, reluctance to simplify a complex system such as healthcare is a hallmark of high reliability systems thinking.[51] Therefore, this framework is an attempt to be as comprehensive as possible given the constraints of two-dimensional illustration. Our hope is that methods for depicting and analyzing collective interactions such as three-dimensional computer modeling and network analysis[57,58] will further our

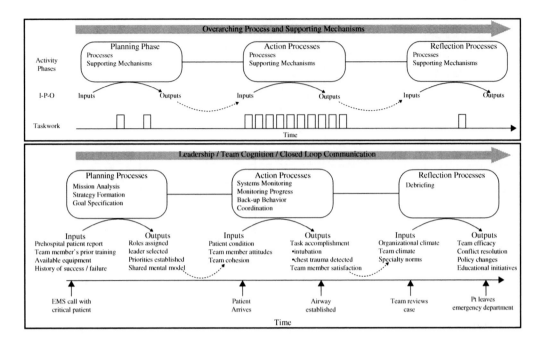

Figure 1.3
A model of teamwork in Emergency Medicine. Reprinted with permission from Fernandez, R., Kozlowski, S. W. J., Shapiro, M. J., & Salas, E. (2008). Toward a definition of teamwork in emergency medicine. *Academic Emergency Medicine, 15*(11), 1104–1112.

conceptualizations of teamwork in complex environments as well.

A Synthesized Model of Team Effectiveness for Patient Safety in Healthcare

As depicted in Figure 1.4, we have attempted to integrate aspects of both within-team and between-team interactions, as well as the dynamic, cyclical nature of performance underlying team effectiveness for patient safety in healthcare. In line with previous models we also incorporate social policy and regulatory characteristics as important influences on both model inputs and actual team performance processes. For example, when the Joint Commission introduced surgical timeouts before incision as an accreditation criterion, organizational characteristics such as organizational documentation requirements were affected, as were daily team processes before each case. Teams had to determine how to most effectively and efficiently integrate this timeout and the

associated organizational documentation requirements into their team roles and case workflow.

In addition to macro level inputs such as general social policy, the model also addresses meso (e.g., organizational, unit) and micro (e.g., individual) level inputs affecting both within and between team processes, including: organizational characteristics (e.g., documentation protocols, technology, physical layout, management hierarchy), patient characteristics (e.g., comorbidities, trust in care system, knowledge, attitudes, behaviors), task characteristics (e.g., procedural aspects of care, documentation, interdependence), and individual team member characteristics (e.g., personality, previous experiences). For parsimony, these characteristics are depicted as individual boxes; however, it is critical to think of them not in singularity, *but as a constellation of factors that create the context in which teamwork occurs.* The literature shows the pattern among these factors has a stronger impact than any one of them alone. For example, an ad-hoc team (team characteristic) may have no problem coordinating (intrateam process)

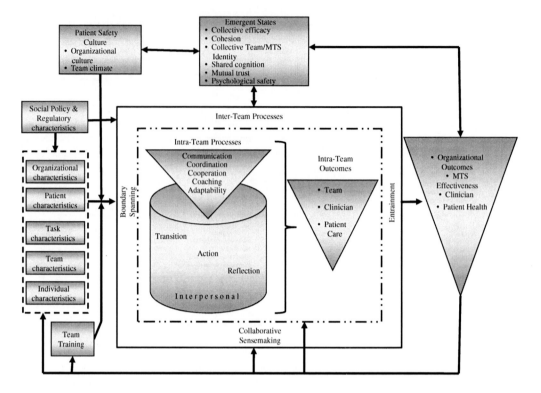

Figure 1.4
An integrated model of team effectiveness for patient safety in healthcare.

during a highly routine procedure (task characteristic); however, their coordination may breakdown during novel or time critical procedures. Effective teams tend to rely on implicit coordination strategies (i.e., nonverbalized) during times of high stress and ad hoc teams may not have the capacity to effectively engage in such implicit strategies.[59]

Moderators such as team training and patient safety culture, however, can influence the relationship between these inputs and team processes. Continuing our previous example, team training can provide ad hoc team members with standardized communication protocols (e.g., the SBAR protocol for patient handovers) and other tools that can be generalized across a range of team types, tasks, and patients. Using transferable teamwork competencies and generalizable teamwork tools can help ad hoc teams mitigate the lack of (or limited) previous experience working together.[60] Similarly, a strong organizational and unit culture/climate of patient safety can promote swift development of a

patient safety–oriented team climate and provide cues for team members regarding goal priorities and behavior–outcome contingencies. Patient safety climate refers to shared, multidimensional perceptions of the work environment emerging from collective sensemaking processes regarding the priority of patient safety and the degree to which actions related to patient safety will be reinforced.[61] Organizational culture is a broader term that refers to:

> shared values (what is important) and beliefs (how things work) that interact with a company's people, organizational structures and control systems to produce behavioral norms (the way we do things around here).[62]

Generally, climate tends to be measured using surveys of healthcare employees, whereas culture tends to be measured using a more qualitative, anthropological style.[63] However, many researchers and practitioners today use the terms interchangeably.

Empirical evidence has also demonstrated that alignment between organizational climate and unit or group/team climate predicts the degree to which employees engage in safe behavior and safety audit scores.[64,65]

Team Processes and Emergent States

The processes and emergent states that characterize team performance lay the foundation for identification of the teamwork competencies underlying effective teamwork; that is, the knowledge, skills, and attitudes team members need to effectively contribute to team efforts. The team processes and emergent states included in our model reflect those identified in previously discussed models; however, they are packaged in a slightly more user friendly way, as the "Eight Cs" of team performance. As depicted in Figure 1.4 these include four core processes—communication, coordination, cooperation, coaching—and four supporting emergent phenomena—cognition, cohesion, collective efficacy, collective identity. Mutual trust and psychological safety are also included as core affective emergent states. For parsimony, we discuss these team processes, emergent states, and related teamwork competencies included in our model at the team level of analysis in subsequent sections. However, patient care is the product of both interactions among immediate team members and interactions among multiple teams. Therefore, our model depicts both within (intra) and between (inter) team processes and emergent states. Although the evidence regarding interactions between multiple teams is still developing, the literature to date suggests that many of the processes that occur between teams are similar to those that occur among immediate team members.[66] The dashed box in Figure 1.4 is designed to depict this notion that the Eight Cs, mutual trust, and psychological safety are critical for both within team and between team interactions. Outside of the dashed box, several additional processes appear that have been suggested to be critical components of interactions between multiple teams. These processes are discussed in more detail in a subsequent section on multi-team systems. Before discussing these, however, we provide more detail regarding the Eight Cs and the underlying knowledge, skills, and attitudes team members must possess to effectively engage in them.

The Eight Cs: Processes

As indicated in the review of existing models of team effectiveness, *Communication*—defined as the exchange and sharing of information—is a crucial component of teamwork. More precisely, standardized forms of communication such as closed-loop communication are vital mechanisms through which team tasks are completed. Effective communication also facilitates the emergence of team cohesion, collective identity, shared cognition, and other emergent states. To be effective communicators, team members must first have knowledge of effective information exchange strategies, be able to effectively engage in these strategies, identify cues that indicate when these strategies should be used, and believe that the team supports the use of these strategies.

Coordination refers to the processes of interaction that "integrate a collective set of interdependent tasks"[67] and critically influence the execution of team goals. Fernandez et al.[56] gave an example of a patient whose condition was more critical than reported, so the team had to quickly recompose, change roles, and make more rapid decisions. Coordination is necessary, but insufficient without good communication, adaptation and other competencies. Third, *Cooperation* is described as a collaborative behavior that is task related.[18] Cooperation usually is paired with coordination to synchronize team dynamics.

Fourth, *Coaching* is often referred as team leadership. According to Salas and colleagues,[18] the functional approach to leadership (i.e., leader as a team facilitator to define and accomplish goals) and also shared leadership (i.e., transferring leadership role to enhance members' skills) play an important role promoting team effectiveness. Fifth, *Cognition* usually refers to shared mental models and shared situational awareness. Shared mental models are shared cognitive representations of the task, situation/environment, team, or other factors that enable team members to anticipate one another's actions, provide backup when needed, and facilitate group effectiveness. Burke and colleagues[54] suggest that shared mental models guide team members' actions relative to the original plan when teams must adapt.

For example, in long cardiac surgeries, it is beneficial to the team to have frequent updates from the surgeon so all members will be aware of the progress of the case and difficulties for the team to reestablish a shared mental model. To develop and support of shared mental models, team must have shared situational awareness. Shared situation awareness exists when team members have a common understanding of their roles in relation to internal and external cues.[68] Thus, it can be acquired by members' scanning of the situations that surround them. It is also considered an essential process facilitating team adaptation when situational conditions change (e.g., the patient's blood pressure drops suddenly after induction).[54]

Specifically in healthcare scenarios, critical thinking is a significant interpersonal responsibility that should exist across all phases. Critical thinking is relevant to team performance, as well as the development of a better team. It refers to skills ranging from recognizing the need for care and reflection on practice to evaluating and taking responsibility for one's own performance.[69]

Emergent States

Emergent states are defined as "constructs that characterize properties of the team that are typically dynamic in nature and vary as a function of team context, inputs, processes, and outcomes."[45] It is important to differentiate emergent states, more mutable conditions, from the actual team processes, inputs, and outputs. For instance, members of a certain hospital may have high psychological safety, which allows them to coordinate better with each other. In turn, the good coordination among team members leads to an increase in psychological safety. Thus, team processes influence emerging states and vice versa, leading to a double arrow between these two constructs.

Collective efficacy and cohesion fall into the category of emergent states along with mutual trust and psychological safety. Collective efficacy is among the best predictors of team performance. Bandura[70] defines *collective efficacy* as the team's belief in their ability as a unit to accomplish their goals. High levels of confidence in the team ability can positively influence other factors, such as members' commitment to the team. Likewise, the existence of mutual trust within a team is highly important. Mutual trust

is defined by Cannon-Bowers et al.[68] as "an attitude held by team members regarding the aura or mood of the team's internal environment". It reflects the degree that members believe that they can rely on one another.[48,71] In the case of a shift change, for example, an oncoming nurse manager may assume the departing nurse has relayed information to the other team members about their patients' condition if these team members have built mutual trust and there are clear role responsibilities for relaying such information as part of shift handovers.

Equally important to the team is psychological safety. Burke et al.[54] defined psychological safety as "shared belief reflecting interpersonal trust, mutual respect, and a comfortableness with interpersonal risk taking". In other words, members do not feel threatened by others, who thus will be more willing to share information. Edmonson[72] empirically showed that psychological safety is associated with team learning. Another important aspect of teamwork is how cohesive the team is. *Cohesion* refers to team bonding among members and the desire to maintain ties within the team.[73] It is part of attitude competencies,[68] and helps during time critical situations.[73] For instance, if the team encounters a scenario that requires rapid help for other team members, team bonding promotes a better response to the new situation. Thus, collective efficacy, mutual trust, psychological safety, and cohesion are all important emergent states that can significantly influence other team actions and vice versa. Table 1.1 also summarizes each of the core team concepts.

Phases of Team Performance Processes

As suggested by Marks et al.,[55] our model underscores the dynamic, cyclical nature of team functioning. The Eight Cs unfold across transition, action, and reflection phases associated with each team task. For teams working on multiple tasks simultaneously, these phases may unfold in parallel. For example, a surgical team on the cusp of completing a case is still in the action phase for their current case, but may be simultaneously in the transition phase for their next case—completing some of the planning processes during this time. Additionally, some teams or team members may be able to spend a greater amount of time defining roles and strategizing their plan before

Table 1.1   The Eight Cs of Team Performance

	Definition	**Citation**
Communication	Exchange of information that teams use to perform such tasks as negotiating their goals, making decisions, and providing one another task status information	Fussel, Kraut, Lerch, Scherlis, McNally, & Caduz[74]
Cooperation	Motivation and desire to engage in coordinative and adaptive behavior	Fiore, Salas, Cuevas, & Bowers[75]
Coordination	The process of orchestrating the sequence and timing of interdependent actions	Marks, Mathieu, & Zaccaro[45]
Coaching	Direct interaction with a team intended to help members make coordinated and task-appropriate use of their collective resources in accomplishing the team's work	Hackman & Wageman[76]
Cognition	Detecting and recognize pertinent cues, make decisions, problem solving, storing and remembering relevant information, planning, and seeking and acquiring necessary knowledge	Orasanu[77]
Cohesion	Affective attraction to the team, team goals, and desire to remain part of the team	Zaccaro & Lowe[78]; Beal et al.[79]
Collective Efficacy	Belief in the ability of the team as a unit to accomplish shared goals	Bandura[70]
Collective Identity	Perceptions of oneness with a particular group of others	Ashforth & Mael[80]

acting. By contrast, in an emergency room disaster scenario, there is an immediate need for action for multiple patients simultaneously, so that planning and reflection phases may be compressed or may overlap to a greater extent with action phases.

The evidence to date suggests that the reflection and transition phases of team performance may play an even more significant role in healthcare team outcomes compared with teams working in less complex task environments.[81] Using mechanisms such as debriefing to help team members reflect on what they actually did, felt, and thought during the action and transition phases has been found to be an important component of team learning, and affects the ability of the team to adapt and self-correct in subsequent performance episodes.[82,83] Interpersonal processes, processes that help teams manage conflicts and also influence team process effectiveness, matter across all phases of performance.[45,84] For example, conflict management, motivation and confidence building, and affect management must occur throughout

transition, action, and reflection phases of performance in order to facilitate the Eight Cs.

Teamwork Processes in Teams versus Multi-team Systems

Although most models of teamwork to date have focused on "the team" as a single level of analysis, patient safety is the product of both interactions among both team members and various teams. Therefore, both intra-team (i.e., within a single, identifiable team) processes and inter-team (i.e., between teams) processes are included in this model. Although much is known about the processes and emergent phenomena that occur within identifiable teams, less is known to date about the interactions among various teams working in what is known as a multi-team system (MTS).

An MTS is defined as "two or more teams that interface directly and interdependently ... toward the accomplishment of collective goals."[85] For example, surgical care team members must communicate, cooperate, and coordinate with one another to achieve safe patient care. However, to achieve the ultimate system goal—patient health—they must do so in concert with other teams such as the hospital's pharmacy team, the preoperative and postoperative nursing teams, and the patient's primary care team. There is ongoing debate regarding the extent to which the teamwork processes occurring between multiple teams are similar to or different from the well-researched processes we know occur among immediate team members.[86] For example, leadership processes such as goal prioritization and clarification have been found to affect coordination both within teams and between teams working in an MTS.[66] It is likely that effective interactions between teams require many of the same basic processes as effective within team functioning. However, several additional processes may be needed to navigate added complexity and the geographic distribution of multiple teams. Therefore, the hashed line surrounding the intra-team processes depicted in Figure 1.4 signifies that these same processes and cycles of performance characterize inter-team processes and the processes surrounding this hashed line denote some of the additional processes necessary for effective MTS functioning.

Therefore, our model suggests that effective collaboration among multiple teams requires boundary spanning, collaborative sensemaking, and entrainment among the various teams involved in achieving system goals.[87] *Boundary spanning* refers to leadership and attentional processes of the team that are explicitly directed toward external relationships. It has been identified as a critically important element for healthcare teams,[88,89] and has been positively related to perceived team performance when focused on by team leaders.[90] Boundary spanning roles are critical for both information processing and external representation of the team.[88] Team members in such roles are important filters and synthesizers of external information. It is critical that they funnel necessary information about the system to the team, while simultaneously preventing information overload and ambiguity.

Collaborative sensemaking is defined as an iterative, continuous process in which shared meaning is assigned to stimuli.[91] It is the active process underlying the formation of shared mental models of the

multi-team system itself, the tasks the system must collectively complete, and the roles, strengths and weaknesses, and strategies enacted by each component team within the system. Collective sensemaking occurs both among individual team members and between teams in a multi-team system. However, we know very little to date about the way in which this process unfolds among multiple teams and the role boundary spanners play in facilitating this process.

Entrainment refers to temporal coordination—the rhythm and patterns of interactions among team members or between multiple teams.[92] Ancona and Chong[93] defined entrainment in organizations as "the adjustment of the pace or cycle of an activity to match or synchronize with that of another activity" (p. 253). However, as a confounding factor at the team level of analysis, it has been found that when teams perform the same procedure over time, they develop highly normative interaction patterns or "habits" that can sometimes persist even in the face of clear evidence that these patterns are no longer effective for task completion.[94] This suggests one reason why integrating new clinical evidence into daily practice has been estimated to take a significant period of time.[95,96] This issue becomes even more complex when considering how to align the interacting rhythms of multiple teams over time.

Inter-team processes and intra-team processes are likely to reciprocally affect one another.[20] For example, if a cardiovascular specialty team effectively shares their specific knowledge with the patient's primary care team and nutritionist and vice versa, this information and boundary spanning can trigger greater information exchange among members within the patient's primary care team (inter-team processes affecting intra-team processes). On the other hand, if the imaging team does not coordinate well enough to get a STAT pulmonary magnetic resonance image (MRI) read and the results back to the patient's cardiovascular care team (a breakdown in entrainment or the rhythm of task completion between teams), then the overall system goal of safe patient care and patient health suffers.

Additionally, if these teams do not actively engage each other in collaborative sensemaking processes it is possible that interpretations and recommendations may vary significantly among teams and potentially negatively affect care. For example, if the primary care team does not consider the results of the MRI scan as posing the same level of risk as the cardiovascular team, there may be a delay in care. Similarly, little evidence is currently available regarding how to most effectively engage patients and their families as active care team members—although several projects are underway to examine such questions.

Given such complexities, it is vital that we continue to expand our understanding of how intra-team processes and inter-team collaboration are interdependent with one another. For example, one national demonstration project funded by the Foundation for Informed Medical Decision Making (http://www.informedmedicaldecisions.org) is dedicated to ensuring that patients share in clinical decision-making responsibilities by investigating how to most effectively provide patients with information regarding the existing evidence for various treatment options, probabilities of various outcomes, and remaining uncertainties regarding various treatment options.[47] On a global scale, the WHO investigated collaborative practice and results suggested that shared clinical pathways and a common patient record are critical aspects of multi-team collaboration.[97]

Outcomes

There are outputs directly influenced by intra-team processes, but also outputs derived from inter-team processes. For example, after a healthcare team completes a surgical procedure, the resident could be evaluated on his or her communication skills by the attending surgeon (individual outcome), and a team debriefing might reveal that there were processes that could have been performed better (a team outcome) and the patient's condition would improve (a patient care outcome). In healthcare practices, the goal of the operating team is to take immediate care of the patients and leave them in a stable condition. Thus, patient care is at the sharp end of intra-team outcomes.

In the case of a motor vehicle accident, more than one team will be involved in care of the injured. For example, a team of first responders may hand off the patient to an ambulance transport team, who may hand the patient off to a triage nurse on arriving at the emergency department of the hospital who, in turn, hands off the patient to a care team. For example, first

responders may begin CPR on the driver of the blue car, but as soon as the ambulance arrives on scene the transporting paramedics take over CPR of this patient. The driver of the red car is successfully extricated from the damaged vehicle and resuscitated on scene by the first responders, but his blood pressure begins to fall on the way to the hospital. When the transport team arrives at the hospital, the paramedics must accurately describe both patient histories, the course of care on scene and on the way to the hospital, and current patient status to a team of waiting physicians and nurses. Incomplete or inaccurate communication between the first responder team and paramedic team or between the paramedic team and the hospital team can lead to undesirable or fatal outcomes. The hospital could face a lawsuit (organizational outcome), the emergency department team might delay definitive care because of incomplete understanding of the case histories (team outcome), a paramedic could be reprimanded for failure to pass on important information (individual outcome), and either patient might have serious complications secondary to errors in his or her care (patient health outcome). Once again, the patient is at the sharp end of care, but in this case there is a failure in the inter-team processes.

IMPLICATIONS AND FUTURE RESEARCH NEEDS FOR THE STUDY OF TEAMS IN HEALTHCARE

This synthesized model emphasizes the view of patient safety and the ultimate goal, patient health, as the product of teamwork both within and between teams. This raises several issues important for future studies of healthcare teams.

Network features within and between teams. Much of the work on teams to date has been approached from a relatively linear perspective. However, research using advanced network analysis and computer modeling of team processes underscore that future work must examine network features both within and between teams. For example, analyses of communication network density among team members could provide insight about how teams learn from near misses and adverse events. Similar analyses of communication networks between multiple teams could shed light on boundary-spanning processes and the team members who fulfill such roles.

Faultlines and subgroups. Examining network features would also provide insight regarding the formation and impact of subgroups and faultlines within and between multiple teams. Faultlines are defined as any characteristic or attribute that has the potential to divide a group into identifiable subgroups. For example, gender faultlines can divide a team into male or female subgroups.[98] Although such faultlines lie dormant in all teams, evidence to date suggests that when such faultlines become activated (i.e., team members are actively aware of demographic subgroups), they can spur the formation of coalitions, increase team conflict, and negatively affect team satisfaction and performance.[99] For example, professional identity is an important attribute in healthcare teams that is likely to affect team interactions.[100] It would be worthwhile to investigate potential professional identity faultlines as well as their impact on conflict, psychological safety, information sharing, and patient safety. Evidence to date also suggests that a strong team identity can decrease the likelihood that activated faultlines will lead to conflict and decrease team performance.[99] Thus, examining the interaction between team identification versus professional identity would contribute to our understanding of interdisciplinary team functioning.

Patient safety culture. Lingard, Reznick, DeVito, and Espin[101] asserted that healthcare professionals often have dissonant perceptions of the roles, values, and motivations of their fellow teammates. This can affect shared mental models and coordination strategies. To cope with such diversity, the focus on patient safety culture and team training could serve as a common ground for creating shared mental models of safe care among interdisciplinary healthcare professionals. Although much has been written about the importance of patient safety culture, relatively little empirical research to date links patient safety culture and its sister construct, patient safety climate, to team functioning and outcomes. This limits the information available to practitioners, administrators, and regulators about the best way to create a functional patient safety culture.[102] Thus, additional empirical studies investigating the role of culture and climate in shaping the teamwork processes underlying safe care are needed.

Practical Implications

Several practical considerations are also relevant for consideration. First, interdisciplinary approaches to training must continue to evolve and teamwork concepts should be thoroughly integrated into early clinician education, as well as continuing education opportunities. The healthcare system has a long history of enhancing clinical knowledge and skills throughout a professional's developmental career. However, opportunities to develop interpersonal and teamwork skills, particularly inter-team skills, remain relatively lacking in healthcare education. Despite the fact that care structures today increasingly require healthcare professionals to function as part of an interdisciplinary team, training curricula are only beginning to more earnestly stress the importance of interdisciplinary collaboration and the value of effective teamwork skills in achieving the most important outcomes, patient safety, and ultimately, patient health. Segregation of clinical trainees within disciplinary silos leaves critical teamwork skills as a competency area to be developed in situ, if at all.[101] Providing the opportunity to develop the critical knowledge, skills, and attitudes underlying effective teamwork in both schoolhouse and continuing education venues is a critical practical need, especially given recent evidence examining the negative effects of disruptive behavior on information flow, collaboration, and patient safety.[103,104] There is a clear need to ensure that providers are not only equipped with the competencies necessary for working effectively in a team-based care environment, but are also reinforced for these skills in daily practice.

In one of the most prominent examples tackling this issue, the World Health Organization (WHO) directly integrated the competencies of effective teamwork into its Patient Safety Curriculum Guide for Medical Schools.[105] Additionally, areas of competence related to communication and other aspects of teamwork have been integrated as core elements of the Accreditation Council for Graduate Medical Education (ACGME)–required training competencies for medical education,[106] and discussions regarding how teamwork concepts can be more fully integrated into traditional and continuing education venues are occurring.[82,107,108] However, important questions remain regarding: (1) how and when to optimally integrate team training concepts into clinical programs of instruction, (2) what strategies are most effective for facilitating the development of these competencies during experiential learning opportunities such as internship and residency, (3) how to best prepare practicing faculty clinicians to support and reinforce the development of such skills in trainees, and (4) how to refine and reinforce the use of these skills by practicing clinicians in daily care processes.

Second, there is a clear need for more in-depth understanding of cultural diversity, its impact on team functioning in healthcare, and practical methods for developing cultural competence. As pinpointed by Helmreich and Merritt,[109] culture is multifaceted and can reflect national, organizational, and professional influences on clinician behaviors, attitudes, and cognitions. Differences in shared values, beliefs, traditions, and patterns of thought can lead to very distinct perceptions and varied behavior responses to similar stimuli.[110–112] For example, the evidence to date on cultural diversity brings important differentiation in perspective necessary for innovation and creativity.[113,114] Evidence to date also suggests that diversity in communication styles, attitudes toward hierarchy and individuation, and conflicting decision-making norms can affect essential teamwork processes,[115–118] performance outcomes,[119] and affective team outcomes such as cohesion and willingness to work together in the future.[120] From a patient safety perspective, working with dissimilar others also can increase anxiety, which in turn can limit collaborative behavior, such as voicing one's opinion and sharing.[121] Thus, understanding cultural diversity and methods for developing interdisciplinary cultural competence should be considered an important element of developing expert teamwork skills.

Furthermore, we must also continue to build our understanding of culture from the patient perspective—investigating how culture can color patient information sharing, experience of disease processes and preferences for care, interpretations of clinician bedside manner, and personal health strategies.[122–124] For example, cultural attitudes can impact the patient–clinician relationship and the degree to which patients participate in the processes of diagnosis, treatment, follow-up, and necessary self-care.[118] Additionally, national cultural values such as power distance have been suggested as explanatory

mechanisms helpful in understanding antibiotic consumption and attitudes toward disease.[125,126] For example, asking patients to choose from a pool of treatment options may be considered a desirable approach by patients from low power distance cultures. Conversely, the same approach could lead patients from high power distance culture to question the healthcare provider's competency. Furthermore, continuing to build a more comprehensive understanding of cultural influences on care processes will help to elucidate disparities in care access and usage among various cultural minority populations.[127]

Research has started to dedicate more attention toward resolving this dilemma, and the spotlight on disparities in care among cultural groups will continue to spur further understanding of these issues. For instance, Smedley, Stith, and Nelson[128] highlight the need to include cultural competency training early in clinical programs of instruction and various approaches for developing cultural competence and cultural humility within healthcare are being examined.[129–131] Furthermore, Betancourt, Green, Carrillo, and Ananeh-Firempong[127] developed a cultural competence framework that can serve as guiding point for theoretical and applied exploration of this issue. Overall, we must continue to further our understanding regarding the potential impact of national, organizational, and professional culture on (1) teamwork among healthcare professionals; (2) the patient–professional relationship, patient preferences, and role in care decisions; and (3) the effectiveness of interventions designed to enhance care safety and quality.

Further, evaluation of team-based approaches may require additional and more sensitive measures. Team and patient outcomes have been discussed extensively throughout this chapter. However, outcomes-driven research surrounding efforts designed to improve healthcare team performance can be described as sparse to date, but growing. For example, a recent landmark study conducted within the Veteran's Administration (VA) healthcare system reported an 18% decrease among a sample of 74 VA facilities that implemented a team training initiative that included precase and postcase briefings and checklists, compared with a 7% decrease in untrained facilities.[132] Untangling the amount of variance in patient outcomes that can be tied to team performance is tricky given that healthcare teams operate in highly complex environments characterized by multiple interdependencies. Within this context, highly effective teamwork might be undermined by ineffective or unreliable systems that surround the team. For example, a patient cared for by the most highly performing surgical team may still suffer an adverse event because of an improperly functioning pharmacy system or vice versa.

Additionally, adverse events and other indicators that have been traditionally leveraged to identify actual patient harm are low frequency events—which limits the power of traditional statistical methods to identify potential relationships with team processes and interventions designed to improve these processes. Thus, the institutional measures that are commonly reported to accrediting agencies may fail to detect improvements attributable to teamwork interventions. Thus, we echo recent call and efforts by the Institute for Healthcare Improvement and the Office of the Inspector General to identify new methodologies to quantify actual and potential patient harm, as well as positive health outcomes. Future investigations into team performance might thus think about recasting their hypotheses to investigate the effects of team processes and teamwork interventions on criteria such as risk reduction or improvements in reliability. The complex and interconnected networks of teams in healthcare will likely continue to frustrate these investigations without a more narrow focus and clearly defined set of criteria. For example, our example surgical team might have successfully alleviated multiple risks to the patient because of proper situational awareness, mutual trust, and proper coordination, yet appear to have only minimal impact on global clinical outcomes at the aggregate level such as mortality.

In pursuit of increased efficiency, in an environment of lean management principles, proper team functioning will require resources from within the system, resources that are in limited supply in most cases. The case can be made for properly resourcing interventions designed to enhance effective team performance in healthcare, but the unit of measurement may need to change. In this environment, proper measurement of team behaviors and the impact of these behaviors on risk reduction is more likely to provide demonstrable and, therefore, actionable impacts.

IN CLOSING

Overall, this chapter has presented an integrated model of team performance in healthcare based on current theory and fed by practical experience. In addition to summarizing the model we have also outlined several theoretical and practical implications designed to spur both future research and practical integration of this conceptual understanding of teamwork into the development, implementation, and evaluation of team-based approaches to care and quality improvement initiatives designed to optimize care quality and patient safety.

REFERENCES

1. Joint Commission. (2010, July 1). 2010 National Patient Safety Goals (NPSGs). Retrieved July 30, 2010 from: http://www.jointcommission.org/patientsafety/nationalpatientsafetygoals/

2. Birnbach, D. J., & Salas, E. (2009). Patient safety and team training. In D. H. Chestnut, L. S. Polly, L.C. Tsen, & C. A. Wong (Eds.), *Chestnut's obstetric anesthesia: principles and practice,* 4th ed. (pp. 211–21). Philadelphia: Elsevier.

3. Institute of Medicine. (2004). *Educating Health Professionals in Teams: Current Reality, Barriers, and Related Actions.* Washington, DC: National Academy Press.

4. Institute of Medicine Committee on Quality of Healthcare in America (2001). *Crossing the quality chasm: A new health system for the 21st century.* Washington, DC: National Academy Press.

5. Baldwin, D. C., & Daugherty, S. R. (2008). Interprofessional conflict and medical errors: Results of a national multi-specialty survey of hospital residents in the U.S. *Journal of Interprofessional Care, 22* (6), 573–86.

6. Danjoux Meth, N., Lawless, B., & Hawryluck, L. (2009). Conflicts in the ICU: Perspectives of administrators and clinicians. *Intensive Care Medicine, 35* (12), 2068–77.

7. Johnson, C. (2009). Bad blood: Doctor-nurse behavior problems impact patient care. *Physician Executive Journal, 35(6),* 6–11.

8. Sorra, J., Famolaro, T., Dyer, N., Nelson, D., & Khana, K. (2009, March). *Hospital survey on patient safety culture: 2009 comparative database report* (AHRQ publication No.

09–0030). Washington, DC: Agency for Healthcare Research and Quality.

9.   Cordero, C. L. (2009, March 31). *Developing hospital standards for culturally competent patient-centered care*. Presentation at the Wisconsin Literacy, Health Literacy Summit, Madison, WI. Retrieved November 12, 2009 from: http://www.wisconsinliteracy.org/HealthLiteracySummit.php

10. VitalSmarts. (2005). *Silence kills: The seven crucial conversations for healthcare*. Retrieved July 30, 2009 from: http://www.silencekills.com/

11. Baker, D. P., Salas, E., & Barach, P. (2003). *Medical teamwork and patient safety: the evidence-based relation* (AHRQ 06–0053). Rockville, MD: Agency for Healthcare Research & Quality.

12. Flin, R., O'Connor, P., & Crichton, M. (2008). *Safety at the sharp end: A guide to non-technical skills*. Aldershot, England: Ashgate,

13. Baker, D. P., Salas, E., Barach, P., Battles, J., & King, H. (2007). The relation between teamwork and patient safety. In P. Carayon (Ed.), *Handbook of human factors and ergonomics in healthcare and patient safety* (pp. 259–71). Mahwah, NJ: LEA.

14. Manser, T. (2009). Teamwork and patient safety in dynamic domains of healthcare: A review of the literature. *Acta Anaesthesiological Scandinavica, 53,* 143–51.

15. Baker, D. P., Gustafson, S., Beaubien, J., Salas, E., & Barach, P. (2005). *Medical teamwork and patient safety: The evidence-based relation* (AHRQ Publication No. 05–0053). Retrieved from: http://www.ahrq.gov/qual/medteam/

16. Salas, E., Dickinson, T. L., Converse, S. A., & Tannenbaum, S. I. (1992). Toward an understanding of team performance and training. In R. W. Swezey & E. Salas (Eds.), *Teams: Their training and performance* (pp. 3–29). Norwood, NJ: Ablex.

17. Cohen, S. G., & Bailey, D. R. (1997). What makes teams work: Group effectiveness research from the shop floor to the executive suite. *Journal of Management, 23* (4), 238–90.

18. Salas, E., Rosen, M. A., Burke, C. S., & Goodwin, G. F. (2008). The wisdom of collectives in organizations: An update of the teamwork competencies. In E. Salas, G. F. Goodwin, & C. S. Burke (Eds.), *Team effectiveness in complex organizations: Cross-disciplinary perspectives and approaches* (pp. 39–79). New York: Psychology Press.

19. Shea, G. P., & Guzzo, R. A. (1987). Group effectiveness: What really matters? *Sloan Management Review, 28* (3), 25–31.

20. Oandasan, I., Baker, G. R., Barker, K., Bosco, C., D'Amour, D., et al. (2006, June). *Teamwork in healthcare: Promoting effective teamwork in healthcare in Canada*. Canadian Health Services Research Foundation, Ottawa, Ontario. Retrieved October 10, 2009 from: http://www.fcrss.ca/ research_themes/pdf/teamwork-synthesisreport_E.pdf

21. Lemieux-Charles, L., & McGuire, W. L. (2006). What do we know about healthcare team effectiveness? A review of the literature. *Medical Care Research and Review, 63* (3), 263–300.

22. Klein, K., Ziegert, J. C., Knight, A. P., & Xiao, Y. (2006). Dynamic delegation: Shared, hierarchical and deindividualized leadership in extreme action teams. *Administrative Science Quarterly, 51,* 590–621.

23. Bosch, M., Faber, M. J., Cruijsberg, J., Voerman, G. E., Letherman, S., et al. (2009). Effectiveness of patient care teams and the role of clinical expertise and coordination: A literature review. *Medical Care Research Review, 66,* 5S–34S.

24. Bedwell, W. L., Wildman, J. L., DiazGranados, D., Lazzara, E. H., Shuffler, M. L., Xavier, L., et al. (2009, July). *What is collaboration? A multidisciplinary review*. Poster presented at the 4th Annual Conference of the Interdisciplinary Network for Group Research, Colorado Springs, CO.

25. Campbell, J. P., McCloy, R. A., Oppler, S. H., & Sagar, C. E. (1993). A theory of performance. In N. Schmitt and W. C. Borman et al. (Eds.), *Personnel selection in organizations* (pp. 35–70). San Francisco: Jossey-Bass.

26. DeChurch, L. A., & Mesmer-Magnus, J. R. (2010). The cognitive underpinnings of effective teamwork: A meta-analysis. *Journal of Applied Psychology, 95* (1), 32–53.

27. Goodwin, G. F., Burke, C. S., Wildman, J. L., & Salas E. (2008). Team effectiveness in complex organizations: An overview. In E. Salas, G. F. Goodwin, & C. S. Burke (Eds.), *Team effectiveness in complex organizations: Cross-disciplinary perspectives and approaches* (SIOP Frontiers Series). (pp. 3–16). New York: Routledge.

28. Gully, S. M., Incalcaterra, K. A., Joshi, A., Beaubien, J. M. (2002). A meta-analysis of team-efficacy, potency, and performance: Interdependence and level of analysis

asmoderators of observed relationships. *Journal of Applied Psychology, 87* (5), 819–32.

29. LePine, J. A., Piccolo, R. F., Jackson, C. L., Mathieu, J. E., & Saul, J. R. (2008). A Meta-Analysis of teamwork processes: Tests of a multidimensional model and relationships with team effectiveness criteria. *Personnel Psychology, 61,* 273–307.

30. Mathieu, J., Maynard, M. T., Rapp, T., & Gilson, L. (2008). Team effectiveness 1997–2007: A review of recent advancements and a glimpse into the future. *Journal of Management, 34,* 410–76.

31. Cannon-Bowers, J. A., & Bowers, C. (2010). Team development and functioning. In S. Zedeck (Ed.), APA Handbook of Industrial and Organizational Psychology, Vol. 1 (pp. 597–50). Washington, DC: American Psychological Association.

32. Argyris, C. (1962). *Interpersonal competence and organizational behavior* . Homewood, IL: Irwin.

33. Hackman, J. R. (1992). Group influences on individuals in organizations. In M. D. Dunnette & L. M. Hough (Eds.), *Handbook of industrial and organizational psychology,* Vol. 3 (pp. 199–267). Palo Alto, CA: Consulting Psychologists Press.

34. Hackman, J. R., & Katz, N. (2010). Group behavior and performance. In S. T. Fiske, D. T. Gilbert, & G. Lindzey (Eds.), *Handbook of social psychology,* 5th ed. (pp. 1208–51). New York: Wiley.

35. Kozlowski, S. W. J., & Bell, B. S. (2003). Work groups and teams in organizations. In W. C. Borman, D. R. Ilgen, & R. J. Klimoski (Eds.), *Handbook of psychology,* Vol. 12). *Industrial and Organizational Psychology* (pp. 333–75). New York: Wiley.

36. Leary, M. R. (2010). Affi liation, acceptance, and belonging: The pursuit of interpersonal connection. In S. T. Fiske, D. T. Gilbert, & G. Lindzey (Eds.), *Handbook of social psychology,* 5th ed. (pp. 864–97). New York: Wiley.

37. McGrath, J. E. (1984). *Groups: Interaction and performance* . Englewood Cliffs, NJ: Prentice-Hall.

38. Steiner, I. D. (1972). *Group process and productivity* . New York: Academic.

39. Tannenbaum, S. I., Beard, R. L., & Salas, E. (1992). Team building and its influence on team effectiveness: An examination of conceptual and empirical developments. In K. Kelley (Ed.), *Issues, theory, and research in industrial/ organizational psychology* (pp. 117–53). Oxford, England: North-Holland.

40. Guzzo, R. A., & Dickson, M. W. (1996). Teams in organizations: Recent research on performance and effectiveness. In J. T. Spence (Ed.), *Annual review of psychology,* Vol. 47 (pp. 307–38). Palo Alto, CA: Annual Reviews.

41. Stewart, G. L. (2006). A meta-analytic review of relationships between team design features and team performance. *Journal of Management, 32,* 29–55.

42. Arrow, H., McGrath, J. E., & Berdahl, J. L. (2000). *Small groups as complex systems: Formation, coordination, development, and adaptation* . Thousand Oaks, CA: Sage.

43. Gell-Mann, M. (1999). Complex adaptive systems. In G. A. Cowan, D. Pines, & D. Meltzer (Eds.), *Complexity: Metaphors, models, and reality* (pp. 17–46). Cambridge, MA: Perseus Books.

44. Holland, J. H. (1962). Outline for a logical theory of adaptive systems. *Journal of the Association for Computing Machinery, 9* (3), 297–314.

45. Marks, M. A., Mathieu, J. E., Zaccaro, S. J. (2001). A temporally based framework and taxonomy of team processes. *The Academy of Management Review, 26* (3), 356–76.

46. Ilgen, D. R., Hollenbeck, J. R., Johnson, M., & Jundt, D. (2005). Teams in organizations: From input-process-output models to IMOI models. *Annual Review of Psychology, 56,* 517–43. doi: 10.1146/annurev.psych.56.091103.070250

47. Burtscher, M. J., Wacker, J., Grote, G., & Manser, T. (2010). Managing nonroutine events in anesthesia: The role of adaptive coordination. Human Factors, 52(2), 282–294.

48. Salas, E., Sims, D. E., & Burke, C. S. (2005). Is there a "big fi ve" in teamwork? *Small Group Research, 36* (5), 555–99. doi: 10.1177/1046496405277134

49. Clancy, C.M. (2007). TeamSTEPPS: Optimizing teamwork in the perioperative setting. *AORN Journal, 86* (1), 18–22.

50. Kalisch, B. J., Weaver, S. J., & Salas, E. (2009). What does nursing teamwork look like? A qualitative study. *Journal of Nursing Care Quality, 24* (4), 293–307.

51. Weick, K. E., & Sutcliffe, K. M. (2007). *Managing the unexpected: Resilient performance in an age of uncertainty* . San Francisco: Wiley.

52. Stagl, K. C., Burke, C. S., Salas, L., & Pierce, L. G. (2006). Team adaptation: Realizing team synergy. In C. S. Burke, L. G. & E. Salas (Eds.), Understanding adaptability: A prerequisite for effective performance within complex environments (pp. 117–42). Oxford, UK: Elsevier.

53. Salas, E., Stagl, K. C., Burke, C. S., & Goodwin, G. F. (2007). Fostering team effectiveness in organizations: Toward an integrative theoretical framework. In B. Shuart, W. Spaulding, & J. Polland (Eds.), *Modeling complex systems: Motivation, cognition, and social processes* (pp. 185–231). New York: Nebraska Press.

54. Burke, C. S., Stagl, K. C., Salas, E., Pierce, L., & Kendall, D. (2006). Understanding team adaptation: A conceptual analysis and model. *Journal of Applied Psychology, 91* (6), 1189–207. doi: 10.1037/0021-9010.91.6.1189.

55. Reader, T. W., Flin, R., Mearns, K., & Cuthbertson, B. H. (2009). Developing a team performance framework for the intensive care unit. *Critical Care Medicine, 37* (5), 1787–93.

56. Fernandez, R., Kozlowski, S. W. J., Shapiro, M. J., & Salas, E. (2008). Toward a definition of teamwork in emergency medicine. *Academic Emergency Medicine, 15* (11), 1104–12. doi: 10.1111/j.1553-2712.2008.00250.x

57. Bhattacharyya S., & Ohlsson, S. (2010). Social creativity as a function of agent cognition and network properties: A computer model. *Social Networks*, e-pub ahead of print. doi:10.1016/j.socnet.2010.04.001.

58. Larson, J. R., Jr. (2007). Deep diversity and strong synergy: Modeling the impact of variability on members' problem-solving strategies on group problem-solving performance. *Small Group Research, 38,* 413, 36.

59. Serfaty, D., & Kleinmann, D. L. (1990). Adaptation processes in team decision making and coordination. In *Proceedings of the IEEE international conference on systems, man and cybernetic s* (pp. 394–5). Piscataway, NJ: IEEE.

60. Salas, E., DiazGranados, D., Klein, C., Burke, C. S., Stagl, K. C., et al. (2008). Does team training improve team performance? A meta-analysis. *Human Factors, 50,* 903–33.

61. Reichers, A. E., & Schneider, B. (1990). Climate and culture: An evolution of constructs. In B. Schneider (Ed.), *Organizational climate and culture* (pp. 5–39). San Francisco: Jossey-Bass

62. Uttal, B. (1983). The corporate culture vultures. *Fortune, 17,* 66–72.

63. Choudhry, R. M., Fang, D., & Mohamed, S.(2007) The nature of safety culture: A survey of the state-of-the-art. *Journal of Safety Science, 45* (10), 993–1012.

64. Zohar, D., & Luria, G. (2005). A multilevel model of safety climate: Cross-level relationships between organization and group-level climates. *Journal of Applied Psychology, 90* (4), 616–28.

65. Zohar, D., Livne, Y., Tenne-Gazit, O., Admi, H., & Donchin, Y. (2007). Healthcare climate: A framework for measuring and improving patient safety. *Critical Care Medicine, 35* (5), 1312–7.

66. DeChurch, L. A., & Marks, M. (2006). Leadership in multiteam systems. *Journal of Applied Psychology, 91* (2), 311–29.

67. Okhuysen, G. A., & Bechky, B. A. (2009). Coordination in organizations: An integrative perspective. *The Academy of Management Annals, 3* (1), 463–502.

68. Cannon-Bowers, J. A., Tannenbaum, S. I., Salas, E., & Volpe, C. E. (1995). Defining competencies and establishing team training requirements. In R. Guzzo & E. Salas (Eds.), *Team effectiveness and decision making in organizations* (pp. 333–79). San Francisco: Jossey-Bass.

69. Cashin, A., Chiarella, M., Water, D., & Potter, E. (2008). Assessing nursing competency in the correctional environment: The creation of a self-reflection and development tool. *Journal for Nurses in Staff Development, 24* (6), 267–73.

70. Bandura, A. (1986). *Social foundations of thought and action: A social cognitive theory.* Englewood Cliffs, NJ: Prentice-Hall.

71. Mayer, R. C., Davis, J. H., & Schoorman, D. (1995). An integrative model of organizational trust. *Academy of Management Journal, 20* (3), 709–34.

72. Edmonson, A. (1999). Psychological safety and learning behavior in work teams. *Administrative Science Quarterly, 44* (2), 350–83.

73. Zaccaro, S. J., Gualtieri, J., & Minionis, D. (1995). Task cohesion as a facilitator of team decision making under temporal urgency. *Military Psychology, 7* (2), 77–93.

74. Hackman, J. R., & Wageman, R. (2005). A theory of team coaching. *The Academy of Management Review,* 30(2), 269–287.

75. Fussel, S. R., Kraut, R. E., Lerch, F. J., Scherlis, W. L., McNally, M., & Cadiz, J. J. (1998) Coordination, overload and team performance: Effects of team communication strategies. Proceedings of CSCW 1998 (pp. 275–284). NY: ACM Press.

76. Fiore, S. M., Salas, E., Cuevas, H. M. & Bowers, C. A. (2003). Distributed coordination space:Toward a theory of distributed team process and performance. Theoretical Issues in Ergonomic Science, 4(4), 340–63.

77. Orasanu, J. (1990). Shared Mental Models and Crew Decision Making. Cognitive Science Laboratory Report #46. Princeton, NJ: Princeton University.

78. Zaccaro, S. J., & Lowe, C. A. (1986). Cohesiveness and performance on an additive task: Evidence for multidimensionality. *Journal of Social Psychology, 128,* 547–58.

79. Beal, D. J., Cohen, R. R., Burke, M. J., & McLendon, C. L. (2003). Cohesion and performance in groups: A meta-analytic clarifi cation of construct relations. *Journal of Applied Psychology, 88* (6), 989–1004.

80. Ashforth, B. E., & Mael, F. (1989). Social identity theory and the organization. *Academy of Management Review, 14* (1), 20–39

81. Salas, E., Klein, C., King, H. B., Salisbury, M., Augenstein, J. S., et al. (2008). Debriefi ng medical teams: 12 evidence-based best practices. *Joint Commission Journal on Quality and Patient Safety, 34* (9), 518–27.

82. Cox, K. B. (2003). The effects of intrapersonal, intragroup, and intergroup confl ict on team performance effectiveness and work satisfaction. *Nursing Administration Quarterly, 27* (2), 153–63.

83. Fernandez, R., Vozenilek, J. A., Hegarty, C. B., Motola, I., Reznek, M., et al. (2008). Developing expert medical teams: Toward an evidence-based approach. *Academic Emergency Medicine, 15* (11), 1025–36.

84. Smith-Jentsch, K. A., Cannon-Bowers, J. A., Tannenbaum, S. I., & Salas, E. (2008). Guided team self-correction: Impacts on team mental models, processes, and effectiveness. *Small Group Research, 39* (3), 303–27.

85. Marks, M. A., DeChurch, L. A., Mathieu, J. E., & Panzer, F. J. (2005). Teamwork in multiteam systems. *Journal of Applied Psychology, 90* (5):964–71.

86. Salas, E., & Wildman, J. L. (2008). Ten critical research questions: The need for new and deeper explorations. In E. Salas, G. F. Goodwin, & C. S. Burke (Eds.), *Team effectiveness in complex organizations: Cross-disciplinary perspectives and approaches* (pp. 525–46). New York: Psychology Press.

87. Poole, M. S., & Real, K. (2003). Groups and teams in healthcare: Communication and effectiveness. In T. L. Thompson, A. M. Dorsey, K. I. Miller, & R. Parrott (Eds.), *Handbook of Healthcare Communication* (pp. 369–402). Mahwah, NJ: LEA.

88. Aldrich, H., & Herker, D. (1977). Boundary spanning roles and organizational structure. *Academy of Management Review, 2* (2), 217–30.

89. Ancona, D., & Caldwell, D. F. (1992). Bridging the boundary: External activity and performance in organizational teams. *Administrative Science Quarterly, 37* (4), 634–65.

90. Burke, C. S., Stagl, K. C., Klein, C., Goodwin, G. F., Salas, E., & Halpin, S. M. (2006). What type of leadership behaviors are functional in teams? A meta-analysis. *The Leadership Quarterly, 17,* 288–307.

91. Weick, K. E. (1995). *Sensemaking in organizations* . Thousand Oaks, CA: Sage.

92. Kelly, J. (1988). Entrainment in individual and group behavior. In J. E. McGrath (Ed.), *The social psychology of time: New perspectives* (pp. 89–110). Thousand Oaks, CA: Sage.

93. Ancona, D.G., & Chong, C. (1996). Entrainment: Pace, cycle, and rhythm in organizational behavior. In L. L. Cummings and B. M. Staw (Eds.), *Research in Organizational Behavior* (vol. 18, pp. 251–284). Greenwich, CT: JAI Press.

94. Harrison, D., Mohammed, S., McGrath, J., Florey, A., & Vanderstoep, S. (2003). Time matters in team performance: Effects of member familiarity, entrainment, and task discontinuity on speed and quality. *Personnel Psychology, 56* (3), 633–69.

95. Grol, R., & Grimshaw, J. (2003). From best evidence to best practice: Effective implementation of change in patients' care. *Lancet, 362,* 1225–30.

96. van Dijk, N., Hooft, L., Wieringa-de Waard, M. (2010). What are the barriers to residents' practicing evidence-based medicine? A systematic review. *Academic Medicine, 85* (7), 1163–70.

97. Mickan, S., Hoffman, S. J., & Nasmith, L. (2010). Collaborative practice in a global health context: Common themes from developed and developing countries. *Journal of Interprofessional Care, 24* (5), 492–502.

98. Lau, D., & Murnighan, K. (1998). Demographic diversity and fault lines: The compositional dynamics of organizational groups. *Academy of Management Review, 23,* 325–240.

99. Jehn, K., & Bezrukova, K. (2010). The fault line activation process and the effects of activated fault lines on coalition formation, confl ict, and group outcomes. *Organizational Behavior and Human Decision Processes, 112* (1), 24–42.

100. Hall, P. (2005). Interprofessional teamwork: Professional cultures as barriers. *Journal of Interprofessional Care, Suppl 1,* 188–96

101. Lingard, L., Reznick, R., DeVito, I., & Espin, S. (2002). Forming professional identities on the healthcare team: Discursive constructions

of the "other" in the operating room, *Medical Education, 36* (8), 728–34.

102. Nieva, V. F., & Sorra, J. (2003). Safety culture assessment: A tool for improving patient safety in healthcare organizations. *Quality and Safety in Healthcare, 12*, 7–23.

103. Rosenstein, A. H., & O'Daniel, M. A. (2008). A survey of the impact of disruptive behaviors and communication defects on patient safety. *Joint Commission Journal on Quality and Patient Safety, 34* (8), 64–471.

104. Saxton, R., Hines, T., & Enriquez, M. (2009). The negative impact of nurse-physician disruptive behavior on patient safety: a review of the literature. *Journal of Patient Safety, 5* (3), 180–3.

105. World Health Organization. (2009). *Patient safety curriculum guide for medical schools.* Retrieved November 9, 2010 from: http://whqlibdoc.who. int/ publications/2009/9789241598316_Eng.pdf

106. Accreditation Council for Graduate Medical Education (ACGME). (2007, February). *Common program requirements: General competencies* . Retrieved December 18, 2009 from: http:// www.acgme.org/acWebsite/dutyHours/dh_ dutyhoursCommonPR07012007.pdf

107. Grogan, E. L., Stiles, R. A., France, D. J., Speroff, T., Morris, J. A., Nixon, B., et al. (2004). The impact of aviation based teamwork training on the attitudes of health-care professionals. *Journal of the American College of Surgeons, 199* (6), 843–8. 94.

108. Weaver, S. J., Rosen, M. A., Salas, E., Baum, K. D., & King, H. B. (2010). Integrating the science of team training: Guidelines for continuing education. *Journal of Continuing Education in the Healthcare Professions, 30* (4), 1–13.

109. Helmreich, R. L., & Merritt, A. C. (1998). *Culture at work in aviation and medicine.* Aldershot, England: Ashgate.

110. Chen, H., & Hu, M. Y. (2002). An analysis of determinants of entry mode and its impact on performance. *International Business Review, 11*, 193–210.

111. Hofstede, G. (1980). Motivation, leadership,and organization: Do American theories apply abroad? *Organizational Dynamics, 9* (1), 42–63.

112. Sackmann, S. A., & Phillips, M. E. (2004). Contextual influences on cultural research: shifting assumptions for new workplace realities.*International Journal of Cross Cultural Management, 4*, 370–90.

113. De Dreu, C. K., & West, M. A. (2001). Minority dissent and team innovation: The importance

of participation in decision making. *Journal of Applied Psychology, 86* (6), 1191–201.

114. Nemeth, C. (1986). Differential contributions of majority and minority influence. *Psychological Review, 93*, 23–32.

115. Brett, J., Behfar, K., & Kern, M. C. (2007). Managing multicultural teams. *Harvard Business Review, 84* (11), 1–10.

116. Chatman, J. A., & Flynn, F. J. (2001). The influence of demographic heterogeneity on the emergence and consequences of cooperative norms in work teams. *Academy of Management Journal, 44*, 956–74.

117. McLaughlin, L. A., & Braun, K. L. (1998). Asian and Pacific Islander cultural values: Considerations for healthcare decision-making. *Health & Social Work, 23*, 116–26.

118. Meeuwesen, L., van den Brink-Muinen, A. & Hofstede, G. (2009). Can dimensions of national culture predict cross-national differences in medical communication? *Patient Education and Counseling, 75(1)*, 58–66.

119. Watson, W. E., Kumar, K., & Michaelsen, L. K. (1993). Cultural diversity's impact on interaction process and performance: Comparing homogeneous and diverse task groups. *Academy of Management Journal, 36* (3), 590–602.

120. Wendt, H., Euwema, M. C., & Hetty van Emmerik, I. J. (2009). Leadership and team cohesiveness across cultures. *The Leadership Quarterly, 20*, 358–70. 98.

121. Dovidio, J.F., Gaertner, S.L., & Kawakami, K. (2003). The contact hypothesis: The past, present,and the future. Group Processes and Intergroup Relations, 6, 5–21.

122. Lea, A. (1994). Nursing in today's multicultural society: A transcultural perspective. *Journal of Advanced Nursing, 20*, 307–13.

123. Lovering, S. (2006). Cultural attitudes and beliefs about pain. *Journal of Transcultural Nursing, 17* (4), 389–95.

124. Shavers, V. L., Bakos, A., & Sheppard, V. B. (2010). Race, ethnicity, and pain among the U. S. adult population. *Journal of Healthcare for the Poor and Underserved, 21* (1), 177–220.

125. Deschepper, R., Grigoryan, L., Lundborg, C. S., Hofstede, G., Cohen, J., Kelen, G. V., et al. (2008). Are cultural dimensions relevant for explaining cross-national differences in antibiotic use in Europe? *BMC Health Services Research, 8*, 123.

126. Harbarth, S., & Monnet, D. L. (2007). Cultural and socioeconomic determinants of antibiotic use. In I. M. Gould & J. S. Van Der Meer

(Eds.), *Antibiotic policies: Fighting resistance* (pp. 29–40). New York: Springer.

127. Betancourt, J. R., Green, A. R., Carrillo, J. E., & Ananeh-Firempong, O. (2003). Defi ning cultural competence: A practical framework for addressing racial/ethnic disparities in health and healthcare. *Public Health Reports, 118*, 293

128. Smedley, B.D., Stith, A. Y., & Nelson, A. R. (eds.). (2003). Unequal treatment: Confronting racial and ethnic disparities in health care, The Institute of Medicine. The National Academies Press, Washington, DC. http://www.nap.edu/openbook. php?record_id=12875&page=R1

129. Hope, J. M., Lugassy, D., Meyer, R., Jeanty, F., Myers, S., Jones, S., et al. (2005). Bringing interdisciplinary and multicultural team building to healthcare education: the downstate teambuilding initiative. *Academic Medicine, 80* (1), 74–83.

130. Tervalon, M., & Murray-Garcia, J. (1998). Cultural humility versus cultural competence: A critical distinction in defining physician training outcomes in multicultural education. *Journal of Healthcare for the Poor and Underserved, 9* (2), 117–25.

131. Hark, L., & DeLisser, H. M. (Eds.). (2009). *Achieving cultural competency: A case-based approach to training health professionals* .Hoboken, NJ: Wiley Blackwell.

132. Neily, J., Mills, P. D., Young-Xu, Y., Carney, B. T., West, P., et al. (2010). Association between implementation of a medical team training program and surgical mortality. *Journal of the American Medical Association, 304* (15), 1693–700.

2

WHAT FACILITATES OR HINDERS TEAM EFFECTIVENESS IN ORGANIZATIONS?

Michael W. Leonard, Allan S. Frankel, and
Andrew P. Knight

INTRODUCTION

The delivery of demonstrable clinical value and consistently good outcomes requires reliable systems of care and effective teamwork across the continuum of patient care. Effective teams are inherently necessary to achieve these goals—abundant evidence indicates that expert individuals delivering care "their way" leads to highly variable and suboptimal care.[1] One of the current cultural challenges is that the majority of healthcare practitioners were taught that individual, clinical excellence is the primary determinant of an effective healthcare delivery system.[2] The traditional and deep-seated belief that a group of expert individuals can come together without clearly agreed-upon norms or effective team behaviors and still provide flawless clinical care sustains a cultural dynamic in which it is difficult for clinicians to discuss inevitable human errors and near misses. This mindset also makes it hard to implement in healthcare high reliability principles that have been extensively applied in other high-risk industries.[3] A telling example of the current medical culture regarding error comes from Whiting's recent article describing the aftermath of a wrong site surgical procedure[4]:

> We recently had a near miss in our institution regarding wrong-side surgery when a knife hit skin on the wrong extremity. In the aftermath of this incident, the shaken surgeon was contrite and wanted to shoulder all of the blame for the episode. This surgeon did not grasp that his true failure was that he had failed to lead and establish a culture of safety and openness in his operating room (OR). He had not empowered those in his OR to speak up, he had not mastered the communication skills necessary to be a team leader, and he had not engaged in the processes and systems that might have prevented the incident. To him, surgical ownership meant "shouldering the load alone."

Achieving effective teamwork as the norm in a healthcare organization will require addressing these cultural legacies through defining effective leadership, reinforcing a culture of safety, embedding effective team behaviors, aligning reliable processes of care, and creating a culture of continual learning and improvement.[5]

Effective Leadership and Organizational Climate

Organizational climate profoundly impacts the quality of teamwork. Leadership is the essential variable in setting the tone or culture within an organization, both positively and negatively.[6,7] Creating an environment in which people both expect and support excellent teamwork is critically important. Organizational leadership that places a clear and consistent emphasis on safety is far more likely to promote effective teamwork and safe-care. An excellent example of an organization committed to safe care and continually messaging the importance thereof is the Mayo Clinic, which anchors the clinical activity in "what is in the best interest of the patient?"[8]

Transparency around the issues of safety and avoidable harm is a very powerful driver of improvement. An excellent example of this leadership surrounds the Dana-Farber's actions following the Betsy Lehman case—a terrible tragedy in which a 38-year-old woman accidentally received a lethal overdose of chemotherapy. Through full and open disclosure, and standing up for the clinicians involved when the state of Massachusetts tried to take punitive action, leadership sent a very powerful message to the organization that helped maintain a highly collaborative culture and environment of continual learning and improvement.[9]

Leadership at multiple levels of an organization is essential for effective teamwork.

Senior leaders must be able to clearly articulate organizational values, consistently model the values espoused, and create clear accountabilities regarding specific behaviors. Based on his extensive experience in multiple industries, Krause argues that the most effective leaders define very specific behaviors that create value, hold organizational members accountable for those behaviors regardless of their position or role, and continuously strive to positively improve organizational culture.[10] Knowing what behaviors are valued within the organization, and specifically what risky and negative behaviors will not be tolerated is critically important. There also needs to be "one set of rules" that applies to everyone from the chief of staff to the housekeepers. Nurses often complain bitterly that physicians are allowed to chronically exhibit disruptive behaviors without any consequences, whereas nurses would be rapidly punished and even fired for similar behavior. If nurses are held accountable and physicians are not, the recurrent message to the nurses is, "They don't care about us, so why should we really believe leadership is committed to good teamwork?" Not surprisingly, saying one thing and doing another undermines team effectiveness.

It is also important that leaders provide consistent feedback. Acknowledgment of positive behaviors is always good, but timely—within hours of an incident—face-to-face feedback concerning abusive, disrespectful behavior is absolutely necessary to demonstrate that leadership is committed to a respectful environment in which teamwork can flourish.[11] Failing to act consistently and quickly allows risky behaviors to increase; creating an environment in which it is impossible to build and sustain high performance teams.[12]

Reflecting on the Mayo Clinic experience, an organization that codified teamwork a century ago in the principles enunciated by Charles and William Mayo,[13] Swensen noted:

> Medicine cannot become highly reliable as long as autonomy, steep hierarchy, blame, independence, and opaqueness characterize an organization's culture. A basic tenet of a culture of safety is acceptance of a core of standard work based on best practice; this must be the rule and deviations from it are appropriate and expected only for patient-centered reasons, not ones that are physician-centered.[14]

One of the inherent strengths of organizations that are highly effective in creating an organizational climate that supports excellent teamwork is that there is clear and consistent messaging as to the common goal teams continually work toward. In healthcare, when it is "all about the needs of the patient," the mantra of the Mayo Clinic, teamwork flourishes.[15] When the convenience and autonomy of the physicians trumps the needs of the patient, it is very hard for effective teamwork to be an inherent part of the culture. A provider-centric culture also has much more clinical variation resulting from clinicians "doing it their way" and more clinical risk.[16,17] Highly reliable care and effective teamwork go hand in hand. Consistent execution of standardized processes requires strong cultural norms regarding how people should behave in teams. Leadership has profound influence on these factors. A valuable question within an organization that relates to autonomy and undermining teamwork comes from David Morehead, "What are the most dangerous behaviors you allow your physicians to engage in?"[18]

The strategic goals of senior leadership need to be clearly and succinctly communicated to front-line care providers, so that teams can align their efforts with those of the organization. It is critically important that senior leaders are also connected to the care process, and engaged in ongoing dialogue with both front-line providers and patients and their families. This has been found to have an effect on safety culture, which is a powerful driver of teamwork.[19] Contrary to the literature that highlights the importance of feedback,[20] Edmondson et al. found that communication alone was not enough to show front-line workers that leadership was clearly committed to a collaborative environment and supported ongoing improvement. Leaders should identify and resolve a smaller number of problems and address ongoing concerns in a manner visible to front-line staff, rather than highlighting many issues and fixing relatively few.[21]

Senior Leadership Engagement: Walk Rounds

By spending time in clinical care units, leaders have the potential to effectively reinforce teamwork norms. Leaders who spend time dialoguing with front-line staff about safety reinforce the message that safety and effective teamwork are organizational priorities. Similarly, the high reliability literature recognizes that those individuals closest to the work possess more expertise than do senior leaders.[22] Thus, leaders can gain valuable insight about problems by interacting with front-line staff.[23] Such interactions can positively influence the organizational climate for improvement as leaders gain perspective about problems faced by front-line staff and how to resolve them, and staff feel supported in their efforts.

Clinical Leadership

Effective clinical leaders are an essential factor in enhancing and embedding excellent teamwork.

Teaching clinicians to be effective clinical leaders is a fundamental need in healthcare. The current model of medical education almost exclusively focuses on the acquisition of knowledge and technical skills, with little or no emphasis on the leadership skills that allow clinicians to effectively lead teams. Effective clinical leaders are mindful that every time they walk into the room, whether a primary care office or the intensive care unit (ICU), they have a profound impact on what it feels like to be in the room for the other team members. Setting the tone in an active, positive fashion every time through sharing the plan, inviting the other team members into the conversation for both their expertise and concerns, using their names, and explicitly reinforcing that if anyone has a concern during the care process, he or she must speak up, is essential for effective teamwork.[24] Two things happen through this process: bidirectional sharing of information and inquiry and, importantly, the leader flattens hierarchy and makes himself or herself more approachable. The hallmark of an effective leader is that he or she is always approachable and continually seeks input from other team members. Part of this process or skill set is the creation of psychological safety, a team climate in which team members feel safe to speak up.

A wonderful example of effective teamwork implementation and supporting a culture of safety and learning is Paul Uhlig and his team's work in cardiac surgery. Uhlig and his team systematically implemented effective team behaviors, standardized clinical processes to enhance predictability, and multidisciplinary rounding in the ICU with the patients and their families. The result was an environment that facilitated continuous learning and improvement. Uhlig's leadership style enabled any team member to offer suggestions and voice concerns. He also broadly empowered team members to lead, because he did not want the "king of the hill cardiac surgeon" driving the process. The open dialogue and standardized processes made it much easier for team members to know what was supposed to happen, so they became effectively cross-trained and could support and provide cross-checks to insure tasks were performed, whether in the team members' domain or not. Not only did clinical outcomes improve markedly, but both patient and staff perceptions of the care process also improved substantially. This work very nicely integrated the components of leadership, safety culture, psychological safety, reliable care processes, and excellent teamwork.[25]

The positive and negative impact of clinical leaders was well illustrated by Edmondson et al. studying the implementation of minimally invasive cardiac surgery in 16 Massachusetts hospitals. Effective, collaborative teamwork with routine debriefing of cases, and a systematic process of feedback and learning that incorporated the expertise of all team members was the hallmark of the highest performing team. Interestingly, this team was led by a relatively new and junior cardiac surgeon who engaged the collective expertise of the team by debriefing every surgical case. The overall challenge was the implementation of a complex process that inherently required effective team collaboration and task coordination. Successful teams reflected what Heifetz would call adaptive leadership,[26] how to manage uncertainty and lead effectively at the same time. In contrast, another of the cardiac surgery teams was headed by a very experienced, classically hierarchical, senior physician who applied technical leadership—"We all know how to do this; if you all perform as well as I do everything will be fine"—and their learning curve lagged the high-performing teams.[27]

DeFontes' work incorporating perioperative briefings found that clear success factors for successful implementation were: (1) public commitment of physician leaders to the process; (2) active participation of all team members; (3) an ongoing process of learning as evidenced by multiple iterations of the briefing card over time; and (4) willingness of physician leaders to quickly intervene and deal with periodic resistance from individual physicians to reinforce "this is how we do it here."[28] The psychology literature indicates that when individuals publicly commit to the work, there is a greatly enhanced chance they will successfully support and reinforce the desired changes.[29] This clearly has implications for the successful implementation of enhanced teamwork. Rather than letting individuals in leadership roles sit in the room and nod their heads and shrug their shoulders, requiring public commitment is a far better strategy.

In an observational study of almost 300 surgical procedures, Mazzocco et al. found that within seconds the surgeon profoundly set the tone for teamwork on entering the operating room. Surgeons who engaged other team members, shared information, and invited them into the conversation set an active, positive tone that enhanced teamwork and made it easy for people to speak up. Conversely, surgeons who did not engage the team and pressured them to "hurry up, because I'm running late" or even criticized the team "for not being able to start a case on time" set a set a negative tone in which it was clearly harder to speak up. People tended to "keep their heads down," and poorer teamwork ensued. The study concluded that patients whose surgical teams exhibited less teamwork behaviors were at a higher risk for death or complications, even after adjusting for clinical risk.[30]

SAFETY CULTURE AND ACCOUNTABILITY

Leaders enable safety culture by focusing on the importance of safety and communicating that they believe it is a priority. A safety culture is also supported when leaders create an environment in which employees are empowered to speak up and act to resolve threats to patient safety. Psychological safety is reinforced through the behavior of senior and clinical leaders.[31,32] When leaders acknowledge and show appreciation for the contributions of other team members,[33] and make it safe for individuals to share their unintentional errors, the environment facilitates better teamwork.[34]

In a study of trauma teams, Klein et al. found the best leaders used "dynamic delegation," in which they afforded junior team members the opportunity to assume leadership roles based on the acuity of the clinical event and a combination of the leader's and junior team member's expertise and experience. Dynamic delegation provided protected "stretch opportunities" for junior leaders, in which learning was supported, but high-quality patient care remained paramount.[35,36]

Given that the majority of medical errors are derived from system flaws, and that the error chains that allow the multiple factors to progress and hurt patients are usually not obvious to the skilled clinicians (i.e., is transparent), why is there such hesitation to discuss these issues openly? Much of the resistance and fear stems from a culture that says highly trained practitioners trying hard will not make mistakes, and because the overwhelming majority of the time team members do not know what the rules are when they do make a mistake. Having a clear algorithm or definition of how unsafe individuals are differentiated from skilled practitioners working in unsafe systems is quite important. A model derived from James Reason's Unsafe Act Algorithm[37] and David Marx's Just Culture model[38] results in being able to ask a short list of questions: Was the harm intentional? Was the individual knowingly impaired? Did the individual consciously decide to engage in an unsafe act—knowingly take on unacceptable risk? Did the caregiver make a mistake that individuals of similar and training would be likely to make under the same circumstances (substitution test)? Does the individual have a history of unsafe acts? This short list of questions provides a clear model of accountability and also tells providers what the rules are, so they feel safe to speak up so we can learn and continually improve.[39] This is essential for effective teamwork.

Culture has a profound impact on behavior and the ability to consistently deliver safe care. Safety culture lives at a clinical unit level and has to be measured as such. With more than five times more variation at the clinical unit level than at the hospital level, hospital level measurement will dilute out the profound insights that can be gleaned from the perceptions of the various caregivers in that particular unit. Accurately reflecting the various perceptions of different caregivers working together is essential.[40] Often physicians, higher in the hierarchy, perceive that "we have great teamwork, nursing input is well received, and everyone is comfortable speaking up and voicing a concern about a patient." What is critically important is whether other caregivers—the nurses, technicians, and other personnel—share the same perception. When caregivers have very positive, concordant views of their care area, the culture is much healthier, being part of the team is a more positive experience, and the teams are able to consistently deliver better and safer care.[41-43] Patients and their families pay close attention to the social dynamics among the care team and themselves, and they are quick to pick up on the level of teamwork and respect among the caregivers.

One of the early pieces of literature that examined the impact of safety culture is Knaus' multicenter study of critical care outcomes. In the higher collaboration units with enhanced teamwork, patients were far more likely to survive the same risk adjusted

diagnosis than in units with poor safety culture.[44] Further evidence that highly collaborative cultures deliver better care comes from the work done to reduce central line infections across the state of Michigan. Before the Keystone project and the implementation of a central line insertion bundle and checklist, the aggregate measure of safety culture in 103 intensive care units was measured. As noted by Sexton, there was a wide range of perceptions of teamwork across these units, ranging from very poor to quite positive. Interestingly, 44% of the units in the upper one-third of teamwork scores were able to achieve the goal of no central line infections for 5 or more months, whereas only 21% of the units in the lower third of scores were able to achieve that goal. The most predictive question correlated with clinical outcomes was that caregivers felt comfortable speaking up when they were concerned about a patient.[45]

High-quality, unit level safety culture data allows the team to identify specific areas of cultural strength they can build on, and focus on specific areas of weakness or opportunities for improvement. Perceptions of leadership, comfort voicing a concern about a patient, conflict resolution, how positively nursing input is received, perceptions of teamwork, and how openly errors can be safely discussed are important aspects of safety culture. There is tremendous power in having individuals debrief their safety culture data and identify opportunities for measurable improvement.[46]

A critical care collaborative in Rhode Island found significant increases in safety culture scores and clinical outcomes after adopting a structured debriefing process, an essential behavior for high-performance teams (Table 2.1).[47-48]

A fundamental cultural norm with profoundly negative impact on teamwork is whether abusive disrespectful behavior is tolerated. If so, there is inherent risk that someone will be hesitant to speak up about a concern. Sadly, this behavior is all too common, and has been identified as a major source of avoidable harm and a primary factor in impeding good teamwork.[49] Rosenstein et al. found that significant numbers of operating room personnel had experienced overtly disrespectful behavior.[50] The American Association of Critical Care Nurses in their publication, *Silence Kills,* noted the extent of the problem and the impact on the care of critically ill patients.[51]

Table 2.1   Factors Enhancing Teamwork and Factors Inhibiting Teamwork

Effective Leadership—model the appropriate behaviors, set a positive tone, respectful	Poor Leadership—say one thing, do another, lack of respect
Clear organizational commitment to safety for patients and providers	Not clear a safe environment for patients and caregivers is the priority
Effective team behaviors—structured communication, critical language, psychological safety	Behaviors are variable, lack of consistency in how the team works together
Reliable clinical processes providing standard work and predictability	High degrees of clinical variation—"everyone does it their way"
Continual learning and improvement—items identified during debrief are captured, acted upon, and resolved	No consistent mechanism for learning and feedback—"we tell them and never hear back"

Sadly, there are all too many examples of where lack of psychological safety undermines teamwork and places patients at unacceptable risk. Blatt found that medical house staff spoke up only 14% of the time they observed an error and only 39% of the time in the presence of a known, specific opportunity to prevent patient harm.[52] The impact of poor safety culture and lack of psychological safety was explored in a pediatric cardiac surgical service line: "Many respondents felt unable to express disagreement and had difficulty raising safety concerns. Respondents admitted that errors occurred repeatedly, and that guidelines and policies were often disregarded."[53] A survey by the Institute for Safe Medication Practices examined intimidation in the workplace and its association with medication error: 49% of all respondents said intimidation had altered the way they handle order clarifications or questions about medication orders, 31% of respondents suggested or allowed a

physician to give a medication the respondent felt was inappropriate, and 49% felt pressured to accept the order, dispense a product, or administer a medication despite their concerns. The result was that 7% of respondents reported that they had been involved in a medication error during the past year in which intimidation clearly played a role.[54]

A medical example reflecting the fragility of a culture and effective teamwork that is dependent on specific leaders is Robert's study of a pediatric ICU (PICU), in which two physician leaders promoted a high reliability environment by defining specific behaviors that enhanced teamwork and led to better clinical outcomes as measured by mortality, returns to the PICU, length of stay, and numbers of patients accepted in transport. They promoted effective teamwork by engaging and educating other team members with regard to assessment of clinical risk and appropriate responses, involving them in decision making, maintaining situational awareness, and enhancing predictability through standard work. They created a safety culture in which problem solving was the focus, not blaming individuals in the aftermath of errors or adverse events. Unfortunately, after the two physician leaders left, the PICU reverted to a traditional, hierarchical model and both the quality of care and the culture of the unit degraded measurably.[55]

EFFECTIVE TEAM BEHAVIORS

In the absence of effective teamwork, it is difficult if not impossible to consistently deliver safe, high-quality care. Helmreich, in observations in the operating room, noted that the absence of structured, effective teamwork led to numerous communication failures and "surprises" among members of the surgical team.[56] Having predictability and clear agreed-on practical tools and behaviors is essential for effective teamwork.[57] Communication and teamwork failures are a central factor in the large majority of medical errors. One study in emergency medicine found an average of 8.8 teamwork failures occur per case and judged more than half of the deaths and permanent disabilities that occurred avoidable.[58] In the world of cardiac surgery, one major and six minor errors are observed per case during complex cardiac surgery.[59] It is the ability of the team to detect these threats early and mitigate them that profoundly affects clinical outcomes and team performance.

We see the ramifications of poor teamwork in medical surgical units, where lack of teamwork (i.e., the ability to articulate a common set of goals for the patient), leads to nurses trying to complete about 100 tasks lasting about 3 minutes each per 8-hour shift, with continual interruption and distraction.[60] Evanoff found on a large medical service that when asked what three things the patient needed to get better and go home; nurses, physicians, and patients could only articulate the same three goals about 30% of the time. In this study, the nurses and doctors had spoken to each other about 50% of the time each day by late afternoon.[61] Effective teamwork is not possible without a structured approach that gets all the team members on the same page as the goals of care for the patient. Briefings and standard guidelines greatly enhance teamwork and the care process. The amount of time nurses are taken away from the bedside for documentation and nonclinical work is a major factor in the quality of teamwork and care delivered. Hendrich et al. found that nurses spent more than one-third of their time on documentation, and less than one-third in direct patient care.[62] Arguably, effective teamwork can be seen as a very effective countermeasure for identifying and mitigating error during clinical care.

Effective Teamwork Tools and Behaviors

There are basic components of effective teamwork and communication: structured communication, effective assertion/critical language, psychological safety, situational awareness, and effective leadership behaviors. Structured communication relates to tools such as briefings, multidisciplinary rounds, huddles, using checklists, situational briefing models like Situation-Background-Assessment-Recommendation (SBAR) and debriefings. High-risk industries routinely use briefings to share the plan and "get everyone on the same page." Briefings are applicable in every care setting, from high-acuity interventional areas to a primary care office. In a procedural setting such as cardiology or surgery, the team can spend 1 minute briefing to both look broadly at the schedule for the day, anticipating needs, equipment, information, and specific skills. Now they have the "big picture" and

can be proactive rather than reacting to events as they unfold. Additionally, the team can quickly and efficiently brief each procedure to insure everyone knows the plan, and has the necessary equipment, skills, medication, and resources to work effectively and deliver optimal care. Studies show that briefing can reduce avoidable delays, which are both frustrating and a waste of valuable resources.[63,64]

Building structure around briefings with checklists provides additional value. Examples include daily goals in intensive care and enhancing teamwork through a comprehensive safety program.[65] Use of a checklist in the Michigan Keystone initiative to eradicate catheter-related bloodstream infections provided clear structure that enhanced team behaviors. In every ICU there was a physician–nurse leadership dyad. This was a critical factor, because nurses were instructed to stop physicians who were not following the checklist during central line insertion. Knowing the correct steps in the procedure was important, but probably more important was the nurses' knowledge that if they asked someone to stop or conform to the checklist they would be backed up by a clinical leader immediately and the correct behaviors would be reinforced.[66,67]

Recent experience with the World Health Organization Surgical Checklist has shown clear clinical benefit and fewer surgical complications.[68] Devries and his colleagues, in a Dutch multicenter study, examined the impact of the SURgical PAtient Safety System (SURPASS) that incorporated 11 checklists across the patient's continuum of surgical care. The benefit was striking, as shown by a 30% reduction in surgical complications and almost a 50% reduction in mortality across a broad population.[69]

Debriefing is an essential tool for effective teamwork and an environment of continuous learning and improvement. Get the team together for 1 to 2 minutes and ask three questions: what did we do well, what did we learn, and what would we like to do differently the next time? This can be done at the end of a procedure, the end of a shift on a medical-surgical unit, or the end of the day in a medical office practice. It is critical to create a safe place to have the conversation. Effective debriefings are never judgmental or critical. If the leaders have concerns with someone's behavior or technical performance, that is a separate, individual conversation; it is never done publicly. The process of debriefing requires building trust and psychological safety for learning. The role of the leader is to always keep the dialogue framed to the positive and geared toward learning. If the debriefing process does not feel safe, team members will very quickly become quiet, which not only leads to lost valuable opportunities to learn, but can also degrade teamwork more broadly. Two things are critical to the success of a debriefing process: (1) an environment rich with psychological safety, and (2) a systematic process to capture the information from the debriefing, take action, and provide feedback to the front-line staff who provided insights for the debrief. This is an area of fundamental need and opportunity within healthcare. Rarely are there effective mechanisms in place to capture information from frontline providers as a source of consistent learning and improvement. Building in effective debriefing can be done in any care environment. If done well, debriefing provides valuable insight into the opportunities and care failures that exist within an organization. This helps to guide leaders as to where to provide resources and engage clinicians not only to enhance the care process, but also where waste can be cut out of the system. The more that leadership understands the context in which front-line providers are providing care and the basic system failures they are working around, the greater the opportunity for improvement. High-performance healthcare organizations constantly work to learn about opportunities to not only provide better care, but also make the care process more efficient and reliable.

Effective assertion/critical language refers to a single phrase or word that when spoken everyone knows means "please stop and talk to me, and let's take a minute to insure we're doing the right thing for this patient." Often providers see things that are concerning or do not make sense but are hesitant to speak up for fear of looking dumb or offending another team member. Having one clear term that everyone has agreed to makes it much easier to speak up. A very effective term that came out of Allina Hospitals in Minnesota is, "I need a little clarity." Also in a culture in which people keep score by knowing the answers and being competent, asking for "clarity" is a very neutral request and is not perceived as questioning anyone's judgment or skills.[70]

Effective leaders always set a positive, active tone within seconds of the team coming together. They also share the plan of care and continuously invite the other team members into the conversation both for their expertise and to voice concerns. This results not only in a bidirectional sharing of information, but actively reduces the inherent power distance between the leader and the other team members. Large power distances are dangerous, making it harder for people to speak up. Effective leaders are always approachable because they have actively worked to reduce power distance.

The Role of Teamwork Training in Building and Sustaining Effective Teams

Effective teamwork training must be multidisciplinary and interactive, with physicians playing an active role. As team members must interact and use agreed upon tools and behaviors, the only way to ensure they have procedural knowledge and social agreement is to have them learn and practice together. Procedural knowledge means, "I know how to do a briefing because we have done one" and social agreement speaks to the fact that "I know how to use these tools because you and I have agreed how we're going to use them." Multidisciplinary learning and practicing together addresses both of these important elements. Because effective patient care is a team function, it is very hard to learn without structured team interaction. Kaiser Permanente, in their systematic work in perinatal safety, used three levels of training: (1) multidisciplinary effective communication and teamwork training, (2) the teaching of reliable clinical processes in an interactive, multidisciplinary environment—how to interpret, communicate, and act in response to specific fetal heart rate tracings, a systematic approach to obstetrical emergencies such as shoulder dystocia, and responding to emergencies such as fetal bradycardia; and (3) simulation training in which teams could practice scenarios on their clinical units. The learning was that the simulation experience cemented the other components together and sustained these behaviors in clinical practice.[71]

Lockwood's experience with perinatal team training and standard processes demonstrated a 60% reduction in adverse events and claims.[72] Within the Veterans Healthcare system, which has a very robust and systematic approach to team training including clear leadership designation, safety culture measurement, clinicians teaching multidisciplinary groups and metrics. Neilly et al. demonstrated an 18% reduction in mortality post surgical team training.[73] Both of these studies speak to the importance of having a formalized process and infrastructure of team training and support within organizations to be successful and sustain the gains. Paull examined the factors that predicted successful implementation of surgical team behaviors, and not surprisingly found that assigning a nurse leader to own and manage the process was a critical success factor.[74]

An Environment of Continuous Learning: Reliable Processes

Having reliable clinical processes enhances team performance by increasing predictability. Knowing what the team is seeking to achieve and being able to compare against a clear process or goal is very helpful. Having predictable processes allows the team to have earlier recognition that they are going the wrong direction or making errors. It also allows teams to improve performance, as they have metrics to benchmark against. Having predictability within the care process allows team members to proactively work to solve problems and save their mental energy for managing uncertainty in the care process. Therefore, reliability and predictability not only make the work easier and the teamwork better, but also support collaboration and process improvement.

A surgical observation study highlights the negative impact on teamwork when there is not an effective way to coordinate workflow and enhance predictability. During 10 general surgical cases, there were 19 intraoperative delays, 30 instances of uncertainty among the care team, the circulating nurses left the operating room an average of 33 times per case, and the observers felt every surgical case was affected with regard to teamwork, safety, and operational performance.[75] By contrast, Makary et al. demonstrated that the use of perioperative briefings reduced intraoperative delays in surgery 31%, and the surgeon's perception of avoidable delays 82%.[76] Greenberg et al. studied the entire spectrum of surgical care, not just intraoperative care, and identified communication breakdowns during surgeon communication with other caregivers. They recommended defined triggers that mandate communication with an attending surgeon, structured handoffs and transfer protocols, and standard use of read backs.[77]

Clear indications or triggers were recently implemented in the major Harvard hospitals in response to surgical complications. When postoperative patients experienced the significant complications of unanticipated ICU admission, hemodynamic instability, intubation with ventilatory support, unanticipated transfusion, or required an unplanned procedure, the resident physicians were required to call the attending surgeon. A forcing function that requires the communication to occur day or night drives the team to work toward the best interest of the patient, and creates the psychological safety so the call is made. Instead of possibly being perceived as an indication that the resident physician is incapable of dealing with the problem, now the conversation is, "I am required to call you. How can we best take care of this patient's problem?"[78]

In obstetrics, having clear guidelines and systematic approaches to common, high-risk problems such as postpartum hemorrhage and shoulder dystocia have been shown to significantly reduce harm.[79,80] In the units that practice intrapartum drills, when faced with an emergency they will describe "we just go into drill mode. We all know what to do and what's going to happen. We can work interchangeably because we know what's supposed to happen."[81]

SUMMARY

We have described the factors within organizations that either support and enhance effective teamwork or make it very difficult. High-quality leadership at both a senior and clinical level, a culture of safety in which individuals are comfortable speaking up and voicing concerns, an organizational climate that acts on the concerns of front-line providers, and structured, agreed-on norms of team behavior are all essential factors.

REFERENCES

1. McGlynn, E. A., Asch, S. M., Adams, J., et al. (2003). The quality of healthcare delivered to adults in the United States. *New England Journal of Medicine, 348*(26), 2635–44.
2. Bosk, C. (1979). *Forgive and Remember: Managing Medical Failure.* Chicago: University of Chicago Press.

3. Leape, L. L. (1994). Error in medicine. *Journal of the American Medical Association, 272*(23), 1851–7.

4. Whiting, J. F. (2010). Puppies and dinosaurs: Why the 80 hour work week is the best thing that ever happened in American surgery. *Archives of Surgery, 145*(4), 320–1.

5. Leonard, M. W., & Frankel, A. (2010). The path to safe and reliable healthcare. *Patient Education and Counseling,* 80:288–92.

6. Schein, E. H. (2004). *Organizational culture and leadership.* San Francisco: Jossey-Bass.

7. Kozlowski, S. W. J., & Doherty, M. L. (1989). Integration of climate and leadership: Examination of a neglected issue. *Journal of Applied Psychology, 74,* 546–53.

8. Clapesattle, H. *The Doctors Mayo.* Rochester, MN: Mayo Foundation, 1969.

9. Conway, J. B., Nathan, D. G., Benz, E. J., et al. (2006). Key learning from the Dana Farber Cancer Institute's 10-year patient safety journey. *American Society of Clinical Oncology 2006 Educational Book.* Alexandria, VA: American Society of Clinical Oncology.

10. Krause, T. R. (2005). *Leading with Safety.* Hoboken, NJ: Wiley-Interscience.

11. Hickson, G. B., Pichert, J. W., Webb, L. E., & Gabbe, S. G. (2007). A complementary approach to promoting professionalism: Identifying, measuring, and addressing unprofessional behaviors. *Academy of Medicine, 82,* 1–9.

12. Dorner, D. (1996). *The Logic of Failure: Recognizing and Avoiding Error in Complex Situations.* Cambridge, MA: Perseus Books.

13. Clapesattle, H. (1969). *The Doctors Mayo.* Rochester, MN: Mayo Foundation.

14. Swensen, S. J., James, A., Dilling, J. A., Dawn, S., Milliner, D. S., et al. (2009). Quality: The Mayo Clinic approach. *American Journal of Medical Quality, 24,* 428.

15. Berry, L. L., & Seltman, K. D. (2008). *Management Lessons from the Mayo Clinic.* New York: McGraw-Hill.

16. Dartmouth Health Atlas. Retrieved March 1, 2011 from: http://www.dartmouthatlas.org/

17. Knox, E., Simpson, K. R. High reliability perinatal unit: An approach to the prevention of patient injury and medical malpractice claims. *Journal of Healthcare Risk Management, 19*(2), 24–32.

18. Morehead, D. Personal communication.

19. Thomas, E. J., Sexton, J. B., Neilands, T. B., et al. (2005). Correction: The effect of executive walk rounds on nurse safety climate attitudes: A randomized trial of clinical units. *BMC Health Services Research, 5,* 46.

20. Frankel, A., Grillo, S. P., Baker, E. G., et al. (2005). Patient safety leadership WalkRounds at partners healthcare: Learning from implementation. *Joint Commission Journal on Quality and Patient Safety, 31,* 423–37.

21. Tucker, A. L., & Singer, S. J. *Going Through the Motions: An Empirical Test of Management Involvement in Process Improvement.* Harvard Business School Working Paper 10-047. Retrieved March 1, 2010 from: http://www.hbs.edu/research/pdf/10-047.pdf

22. Roberts, K. (1990). Some characteristics of one type of high reliability organization. *Organization Science, 1*(2), 160–76.

23. Frankel, A., Graydon-Baker, E., Neppl, C., et al. (2003). Patient safety leadership WalkRounds. *Joint Commission Journal on Quality and Patient Safety, 29,* 16–26.

24. Mazzocco, K., Petiti, D. B., Fong, K. T., et al. (2009). Surgical team behaviors and patient outcomes. *American Journal of Safety, 197*(5), 678–85.

25. Uhlig, P. N., Brown, J., Nason, A. K., et al. (2002). System innovation: Concord Hospital. *Joint Commission Journal on Quality and Patient Safety, 28*(12), 667–72.

26. Heifetz, R. A. M., Grashow, A., & Linsky, M. (2009). *Practice of Adaptive Leadership: Tools and Tactics for Changing Your Organization and the World.* Cambridge, MA: Harvard Business School Press.

27. Edmondson, A., Bohmer, R., & Pisano, G. (2001). Speeding up team learning. *Harvard Business Review, November,* 5–11.

28. Defontes, J., & Surbida, S. (2004). Perioperative safety briefing project. *The Permanente Journal, 8*(2), 21–7.

29. Cialdini, R. (2001). *Influence: Science and Practice.* 4th ed. Needham Heights, MA: Allyn & Bacon.

30. Mazzocco, K., Petiti, D. B., Fong, K. T., et al. (2009). Surgical team behaviors and patient outcomes. *American Journal of Surgery, 197*(5), 678–85.

31. Edmondson, A. (1999). Psychological safety and learning behavior in work teams. *Administrative Science Quarterly, 44*(4), 350–83.

32. Edmondson, A. C. (2003). Managing the risk of learning: Psychological safety in work teams. In: West, M, ed. *International Handbook of Organizational Teamwork.* London: Blackwell.

33. Nembhard, I. M., & Edmondson, A. (2006). Making it safe: The effects of leader inclusiveness

and professional status on psychological safety and improvement efforts in healthcare teams. *Journal of Organizational Behavior, 27*(7), 941–66.

34. Edmondson, A. (2003). Speaking up in the operating room: How team leaders promote learning in interdisciplinary action teams. *Journal of Management Studies, 40*(6), 1419–52.

35. Klein, K. J., Ziegert, J. C., Knight, A. P., & Xiao, Y. (2006). Dynamic delegation: Shared, hierarchical, and deindividualized leadership in extreme action teams. *Administrative Science Quarterly, 51*(4), 590–621.

36. Vogus, T. J., Sutcliffe, K. M., & Weick, K. (2010). Doing no harm: Enabling, enacting and elaborating a culture of safety in healthcare. *Academy of Management Perspectives,* November, 60–77.

37. Reason, J. (1997). *Managing the Risk of Organizational Accidents*. Brookfield, VT: Ashgate.

38. Marx, D. *Just Culture*. Retrieved March 1, 2011 from: http://www.webmm.ahrq.gov/perspective. aspx?perspectiveID=49

39. Leonard, M. W., & Frankel, A. (2010). The path to safe and reliable healthcare. *Patient Education and Counseling,* 80, 288–92.

40. Hudson, D. W., Sexton, J. B., Thomas, E. J., et al. (2009). A safety culture primer for the critical care clinician: The role of culture in patient safety and quality improvement. *Contemporary Critical Care, 7*(5), 1–13.

41. Defontes J., & Surbida, S. (2004). Perioperative safety briefing project. *The Permanente Journal, 8*(2), 21–7.

42. Hudson, D. W., Sexton, J. B., Thomas, E. J., et al. (2009). A safety culture primer for the critical care clinician: The role of culture in patient safety and quality improvement. *Contemporary Critical Care, 7*(5), 1–13.

43. Neily, J., Mills, P. D., Young-Xu, Y., et al. (2010). Association between implementation of a medical team training program and surgical mortality. *Journal of the American Medical Association, 304*(15), 1693–700.

44. Knaus, W. A. (1986). An evaluation of outcome from intensive care in major medical centers. *Annals of Internal Medicine,* 104, 410–8.

45. Hudson, D. W., Sexton, J. B., Thomas, E. J., et al. (2009). A safety culture primer for the critical care clinician: The role of culture in patient safety and quality improvement. *Contemporary Critical Care, 7*(5), 1–13.

46. Sexton, J. B., Paine, L. A., Manfuso, J., et al. (2007). A check-up for safety culture in "my patient care area." *Joint Commission Journal on Quality and Patient Safety, 33*(11), 699–703.

47. Depalo, V. A., McNicoll, L., Cornell, M., et al. (2010). The Rhode Island ICU collaborative: A model for reducing central line-associated bloodstream infection and ventilator-associated pneumonia statewide. *Quality and Safety in Health Care, 19*(6), 555–61.

48. Rhode Island Quality Institute. *A Statewide Partnership to Improve Healthcare Quality.* Retrieved March 01, 2011 from: http://www. commonwealthfund.org/~/media/Files/ Publications/Case%20Study/2010/Dec/1465_ Chase_Rhode_Island_quality_inst_case_study.pdf

49. JCAHO Sentinel Event Alert #40, July 2008. Retrieved March 1, 2011 from: http://www. jointcommission.org/sentinel_event_alert_ issue_40_behaviors_that_undermine_a_culture_ of_safety/

50. Rosenstein, A. H., & O'Daniel, M. O. (2006). Impact and implications of disruptive behavior in the perioperative arena. *American College of Surgeons, 203*(1), 96–105.

51. Silence Kills. http://www.silencekills.com/ UPDL/PressRelease.pdf

52. Blatt, R., Christianson, M. K., Sutcliffe, K. M., Rosenthal, M. M., Blatt, R., & Christianson, M. (2006). A sensemaking lens on reliability. *Journal of Organizational Behavior, 27*(7), 897–917.

53. Bognár, A., Barach, P., Johnson, J. K., et al. Errors and the burden of errors: Attitudes, perceptions, and the culture of safety in pediatric cardiac surgical teams. *Ann Thorac Surg.* 2008;85(4):1374–81.

54. Institute for Safe Medication Practices Medication Safety Alert, Intimidation. Practitioners speak up about this unresolved problem (Part I), March 11, 2004. Retrieved March 1, 2011 from: http://www.ismp.org/ Newsletters/acutecare/articles/20040311_2.asp

55. Roberts, K. H., Madsen, P., Desai, V., & Van Stralen, D. (2005). A case of the birth and death of a high reliability healthcare organization. *Quality and Safety in Health Care, 14,* 216–20.

56. Sexton, B., Marsch, S., Helmreich, R. L., et al. (1997). Jumpseating in the operating room. *Proceedings of the Second Conference on Simulators in Anesthesiology Education.* New York: Plenum, 107–8.

57. Leonard, M., Graham, S., & Bonacum, D. (2004). The human factor: The critical importance of effective teamwork and communication in providing safe care. *Quality and Safety in Health Care, 13*(Suppl), i85–90.

58. Risser, D. T., Rice, M. M., & Salisbury, M. L. (1999). The potential for improved teamwork to reduce medical errors in the emergency department. *Annals of Emergency Medicine, 34*(3), 373–83.

59. Carthey, J., de Leval, M. R., & Reason, J. T. (2001). The human factor in cardiac surgery: Errors and near misses in a high technology medical domain. *Annals of Thoracic Surgery, 72*(1), 300–5.

60. Tucker, A. L., & Spear, S. J. (2006). Operational failures and interruptions in hospital nursing. *Health Services Research, 41*(3 Pt 1), 643–62.

61. Evanoff, B., Potter, P., Wolf, L., et al. Can we talk? Priorities for patient care differed among healthcare providers. In: Henriksen K, Battles JB, Marks ES, Lewin DI, eds. *Advances in Patient Safety: From Research to Implementation (Volume 1: Research Findings).* Rockville, MD: Agency for Healthcare Research and Quality (US), 2005.

62. Hendrich, A., Chow, M. P., Bafna, S., et al. (2009). Unit-related factors that affect nursing time with patients: Spatial analysis of the time and motion study. *HERD, 2*(2), 5–20.

63. Nundy, S., Arnab, M., Sexton, J. B., et al. (2008). Impact of preoperative briefings on operating room delays. *Archives of Surgery, 143*(11), 1068–72.

64. Neily, J., Mills, P. D., Young-Xu, Y., et al. (2010). Association between implementation of a medical team training program and surgical mortality. *Journal of the American Medical Association, 304*(15), 1693–00.

65. Pronovost, P., Weast, B., Rosenstein, B., et al. (2005). Implementing and validating a comprehensive unit-based safety program. *Journal of Patient Safety, 1*(1), 33–40.

66. Pronovost, P., Needham, D., Berenholtz, S., et al. (2006). An intervention to decrease catheter-related bloodstream infections in the ICU. *New England Journal of Medicine, 355,* 2725–32.

67. Sexton, B. Personal communication.

68. Haynes, A. B., Weiser, T. G., Berry, W. R., et al. (2009). A surgical safety checklist to reduce morbidity and mortality in a global population. *New England Journal of Medicine, 360,* 491–9.

69. de Vries, E. N., Prins, H. A., Crolla, R., et al. (2010). Effect of a comprehensive surgical safety system on patient outcomes. *New England Journal of Medicine, 363,* 1928–37.

70. Frankel, A., Leonard, M., Simmonds, T., & Haraden, C. (2009). *The Essential Guide for Patient Safety Officers.* Oakbrook Terrace, IL: Joint Commission Resources.

71. McFerran, S., Nunes, J., Pucci, D., et al. (2005). Perinatal patient safety project: A multicenter approach to improve performance reliability at Kaiser Permanente. *Journal of Perinatal & Neonatal Nursing, 19*(1), 37–45.

72. Pettker, C. M., Thung, S. F., Norwitz, E. R., et al. (2009). Impact of a comprehensive patient safety strategy on obstetric adverse events. *Am J Obstet Gynecol. 200*(5), 492.

73. Neily, J., Mills, P. D., Young-Xu, Y., et al. (2010). Association between implementation of a medical team training program and surgical mortality. *Journal of the American Medical Association, 304*(15), 1693–700.

74. Paull, D. E., Mazzia, L. M., Izu, B. S., et al. (2009). Predictors of successful implementation of preoperative briefings and postoperative debriefings after medical team training. *American Journal of Surgery, 198,* 675–8.

75. Christian, C. K., Gustafson, M. L., Roth, E. M., et al. (2006). A prospective study of patient safety in the operating room. *Surgery. 139*(2), 159–73.

76. Nundy, S., Arnab, M., Sexton, J. B., et al. (2008). Impact of preoperative briefings on operating room delays. *Archives of Surgery, 143*(11), 1068–72.

77. Greenberg, C. C., Regenbogen, S. E., Studdert, D. M., et al. (2007). Patterns of communication breakdowns resulting in injury to surgical patients. *J American College of Surgeons, 204,* 533–40.

78. El Bardissi, A. W., Regenbogen, S. E., Greenberg, C. C., et al. (2009). Communication practices on 4 Harvard surgical services: A surgical safety collaborative. *Annals of Surgery, 250,* 861–5.

79. Draycott, T., Crofts, J., Ash, J. P., et al. (2008). Improving neonatal outcome through practical shoulder dystocia training. *American Journal of Obstetrics and Gynecology, 112*(1), 14–20.

80. Draycott, T., Sibanda, T., Owen, L., et al. (2006). Does training in obstetric emergencies improve neonatal outcome? *British Journal of Obstetrics and Gynecology, 113,* 177–82

81. Michael Leonard interview with staff at the Bristol Southmead maternity unit. Personal communication.

PART TWO

THE SCIENCE OF TEAM TRAINING:
WHAT WORKS IN HEALTHCARE

3

BUILDING TEAMWORK SKILLS IN HEALTHCARE: THE CASE FOR COMMUNICATION AND COORDINATION COMPETENCIES

Alexander Alonso and Dana M. Dunleavy

SARA, A 19-YEAR-OLD college student, has been brought into the emergency room by her roommate. The patient reports that her mom is 3 hours away by plane. The patient has been diagnosed with pyelonephritis and is admitted for intravenous (IV) antibiotics and hydration. The roommate reports that Sara has not been getting much sleep and has looked tired and run down over the past few days. The nurse tells her that Sara should be feeling much better after 24 hours of IV fluids and antibiotics. The following morning, the nurse is surprised to see that Sara's temperature is higher despite antipyretics and her heart rate has increased. Following the report, she is concerned about potential sepsis. During her morning assessment, she recognizes that Sara is showing signs of acute deterioration and needs help. The nurse activates the rapid response team, whose responders arrive shortly to stabilize the patient. While initiating treatment, the team seeks information from the nurse, but reacts harshly because there is no clear indication for their activation. Later during treatment, the three members of the responder team are struggling to coordinate actions and resolve information conflicts. Because the team is struggling to stabilize Sara, the hospitalist calls for an immediate transfer to the intensive care unit.

The situation described in the preceding is all too common in healthcare. It describes an encounter in which a patient's life depends on the skills of a network of healthcare professionals. Their clinical skills are called on to detect, analyze, and respond to a problem. This situation, however, could not have been addressed by clinical skills alone. Too often the breakdowns in healthcare result not from failure in clinical skills, but rather those in nonclinical skills. For example, in this case Sara's care providers were able to detect the potential problem—sepsis. They did not, however, communicate clearly or coordinate their actions resulting in her unnecessary deterioration. Their ability to respond to the problem was crippled by their inability to act as a team. It is these types of failures that make teamwork training critical in healthcare.

Teamwork training is pervasive in healthcare. It is manifested in a myriad of ways covering a variety of different skills. A recent Google search of "team training in healthcare" resulted in approximately 4 million hits all focusing on at least communication. Communication alone does not constitute teamwork. Teamwork in healthcare requires a host of teamwork skills ranging from resource management to conflict management. Healthcare professionals must be able to monitor potential medication errors and back each other up when a potential error is imminent. They must be able to understand their roles and responsibilities in stressful situations that do not always allow for clear direction. This chapter addresses this need.

This chapter focuses primarily on describing the core teamwork skills needed by all healthcare professionals. First, it provides a brief history of the patient safety movement and how teamwork became a lever for reducing medical error. Second, it describes the team training and its evolution in healthcare. Third, it reviews the core teamwork skills needed by healthcare professionals and the outcomes one can anticipate from building teamwork proficiency. Finally, it provides guidelines for ensuring that team training effectively builds proficiency in the skills.

History of Team Training in Healthcare

In 1999 the Institute of Medicine (IOM) published, *To Err Is Human: Building a Safer Health System*, a frightening indictment of the inadequate safety that the United States medical establishment too often provides its patients.[1] Extrapolating from data gathered through the Harvard Medical Practice Study and the Utah-Colorado Medical Practice Study, the IOM report concluded that medical errors cause between 44,000 and 98,000 deaths annually—more than result from automobile accidents (43,458), breast cancer (42,297), or AIDS (16,516).

The report also noted that in addition to causing human suffering and death, medical errors are financially costly. With regard to direct costs, the IOM estimated that, among US hospital inpatients, *medication* errors alone cost approximately 2 billion dollars annually. With regard to indirect costs, errors result in opportunities lost, given that funds spent in correcting mistakes cannot be used for other

purposes, as well as in higher insurance premiums and copayments. In addition, because of their effect on diminished employee productivity, decreased school attendance, and a lower state of public health, such errors exact a price from the society-at-large. Specifically, the IOM estimated that the total indirect cost of medical errors that result in patient harm lies between 17 and 29 billion dollars annually. Finally, and equally perilous in the long run, medical errors undermine patients' and health professionals' confidence in the healthcare system itself.

To alleviate this unacceptable prevalence of medical errors, the IOM recommended a four-tiered approach:

1. "Establishing a national focus to create leadership, research, tools and protocols to enhance the knowledge base about safety;
2. Identifying and learning from errors through [establishing] immediate and strong mandatory reporting efforts … [and encouraging] … voluntary efforts, both with the aim of making sure the system continues to be made safer for patients;
3. Raising standards and expectations for improvements in safety through the actions of oversight organizations, group purchasers, and professional groups; and
4. Creating safety systems inside [healthcare] organizations through the implementation of safe practices at the delivery level. This level is the ultimate target of all the recommendations" (Kohn et al., 1999, p. 5).[1]

The overwhelming message was medical errors are preventable using a variety of potential interventions designed to enhance patient safety nationally. Since *To Err is Human*, the continued emphasis on safety and the strategies to improve it have not lost any momentum. Then-President Clinton established the Quality Interagency Coordination (QuIC) Task Force to develop a coordinated federal plan for reducing the number and severity of medical errors. The QuIC was comprised of participants from the Department(s) of Health and Human Services, Labor, Defense, and Veterans Affairs (VA), among other agencies. The QuIC's charge was to respond to the IOM's advice and propose specific actions for improving patient safety and reducing medical errors.

The Agency for Healthcare Research and Quality (AHRQ) is the primary federal agency responsible for conducting and supporting research to promote patient safety. The AHRQ's responsibility is drawn from the IOM's recommendations and the QuIC's action items and encompasses three broad areas: (1) identifying the causes of errors and injuries in the delivery of healthcare; (2) developing, demonstrating, and evaluating error-reduction and patient-protection strategies; and (3) distributing effective strategies throughout the US healthcare community. However, other agencies, such as the Department of Defense's TRICARE Management Activity have also been responsible for promoting the goal of national patient safety. A major focus of these agencies has been supporting research and development activities centered on improving team performance in the delivery of care. Many organizations, such as The Joint Commission, Institute for Healthcare Improvement (IHI), the National Patient Safety Foundation (NPSF), the National Quality Forum (NQF), the Association of Registered Nurses (AoRN), the Association of American Medical Colleges (AAMC), and the Accreditation Council for Graduate Medical Education (ACGME), to name a few, have cited the importance of teamwork in patient safety.

Numerous reports, professional meetings, and publications have continued to champion the need to improve safety, and many have identified team training as a significant strategy in achieving that goal.[2-6] For example, the October 2004 issue of *Quality and Safety in Healthcare* was dedicated to improving team performance through the use of simulation and training. Moreover, Salas and colleagues published numerous articles outlining critical teamwork processes in healthcare and they align with team skills training.[7,8] Some publications, such as Baker et al.'s, highlight how team competencies, training, and the assessment of these skills might be incorporated into the professional education of physicians. Others such as Alonso et al.'s, highlight specific examples of team skills needed for training healthcare professionals in a variety of contexts.[9] The preponderance of evidence available makes one thing abundantly clear—there are many ways to skin the team training cat in healthcare. The following section provides a review of the most commonly used team skills models in healthcare.

Common Models of Teamwork Skills for Healthcare

Teamwork has been studied extensively over the past 20 years. Teamwork is defined by a set of inter-related knowledge, skills, and attitudes (KSAs) that facilitate coordinated, adaptive performance in support of one's teammates, objectives, and mission.[4-7] Teamwork is distinct from taskwork (i.e., operational skills), but both are required for teams to be effective in complex environments.[8] For many teams task-related knowledge and skills are not enough for effective functioning. Effective teamwork is dependent on each team member being able to:

- Anticipate the needs of others;
- Adjust to each other's actions and to the changing environment; and
- Have a shared understanding of how a procedure should happen to identify when errors occur and how to correct for these errors.

Given the interdisciplinary nature of healthcare and the necessity of cooperation among the workers who treat patients, teamwork is critical to ensure safety as well as error recovery and mitigation. Teams make fewer mistakes than do individuals, especially when each team member knows his or her responsibilities and those of other team members.[10-12] However, simply installing a team structure does not automatically ensure that a team will operate effectively. Teamwork is not an automatic consequence of co-locating people together, and it depends on a willingness to cooperate toward a shared goal. Although teamwork does not require team members work together on a permanent basis, neither does teamwork result from simply having permanent assignments that carry over from day to day.[13] Teamwork is sustained by a commitment to a shared set of team KSAs that foster a series of teamwork processes.[14] Team performance remains a function of the inputs brought to a team by each individual and the processes they engage in to produce a common result. An example is the interaction between one's skill in providing clear and concise patient histories and the need for efficient and complete information exchange to prevent medical errors. If a healthcare professional lacks proficiency, a critical team process (i.e., communication) will be crippled and team performance will be limited.

All common models of team training in healthcare focus primarily on enhancing the relationship between skills and processes. The primary emphasis is to identify individual skills where professionals can improve proficiency supporting a specific process. Next, we review the generational evolution of team training models. First, we review crew resource management-based models for healthcare professional teamwork. Second, we review the work of the ACGME and the American Association of Medical Colleges (AAMC) to enhance physician teamwork through curriculum enhancements. Third, we review AHRQ and DoD's Team Strategies and Tools to Enhance Performance and Patient Safety (aka TeamSTEPPS®) model. All three are pervasive in healthcare and represent a general model for team training.

The study of teams in healthcare and how best to train them has evolved rapidly since the publication of the IOM report, *To Err is Human*. This section provides a brief review of the significant developments in the study of healthcare teams and team training that have occurred since 1999. Similar to Helmreich, we argue that team training in healthcare is evolving through a series of generations.[15] The first generation of these programs was primarily derived from aviation and crew resource management (CRM) and focused on building situational awareness. The second generation (which we are now in) has produced healthcare-specific team training that is evidenced-based and allows for more opportunities for skills practice. The following briefly reviews both generations of healthcare team training. After which, it is argued that future generations of healthcare team training should strive to expand lessons learned beyond the team and concentrate on enhancing the performance of the larger the multi-team system (MTS).[16]

First Generation

The first generation of team training in healthcare concentrated on adapting team training and error reduction programs from aviation, specifically CRM, to the healthcare community.[17] Crew resource management training is perhaps the most widely recognized team training program designed to improve

the margin of safety in aviation. It was designed to counter the high-risk aviation environment in which there is the potential for great loss of life and property. Crew resource management is a family of instructional strategies that seeks to improve teamwork in the cockpit by applying well-tested training tools (e.g., simulators, lecture, videos) targeted at specific teamwork behaviors.[17-19] The behavioral skills typically addressed by CRM training include: adaptability/flexibility, assertiveness, communication, decision making, leadership, mission analysis, and situational awareness.

Proponents of adapting CRM training to healthcare point to the fact that CRM has been successful in reducing errors in aviation, which is a high-risk industry just like the healthcare industry.[20-22] A meta-analysis of 58 studies conducted on CRM training programs by Salas et al. found that trainees of CRM training programs in the aviation industry had positive reactions, enhanced learning, and behavioral change in terms of awareness and communication patterns.[23]

Crew resource management training in healthcare was used by the MedTeams™ and Medical Team Management programs to train key teamwork skills.[7,24] Originally designed for teams in emergency medicine, the primary goal of MedTeams™ was to reduce medical errors through interdisciplinary teamwork. MedTeams™ training was developed as an evaluation-driven CRM-based course. MedTeams™ designers defined a core team as a group of 3 to 10 medical employees who are trained to use specific teamwork behaviors to coordinate their clinical interactions and who work interdependently during a shift. To ensure that team members easily recognize one another, they wear visible armbands, badges, or colored scrubs that identify them as members of a particular core team.[25] MedTeams™ was taught using a train-the-trainer approach in which the course itself consisted of an 8-hour block of classroom instruction containing an introduction module, five learning modules, and an integration unit.

Medical Team Management was developed by the United States Air Force in response to an incident at an air force facility in which poor teamwork caused a newborn to develop neurological problems.[26] Similar to MedTeams™, the primary purpose of Medical Team Management was to reduce medical errors, in this case by teaching human-factors concepts to interdisciplinary teams of medical professionals.[27,28] A secondary purpose was to change the military's traditional medical culture to one that emphasizes open communication as opposed to individual performance. Medical Team Management specifically fostered a culture that values team performance and encourages effective communication.[29] The Medical Team Management curriculum included an introduction to the program, overviews of key patient safety and CRM issues, and specific modules for each of CRM's seven foundational elements. Finally, Medical Team Management uses a number of tactics for continued use by practitioners to sustain and reinforce the human-factors concepts that are learned as trainees.

Three evaluations were conducted of these early courses. The first by Baker et al. involved a detailed case study analysis of MedTeams™ and Medical Team Management.[24] For each course, Baker et al. reviewed actual team training materials such as student and instructor guides, slides, and other audiovisual materials; attended at least one training session, and collected independent data on training effectiveness from class participants. Based on their findings, the researchers reported that each program possessed several desirable characteristics, such as using active learning techniques to develop teamwork-related competencies and offering interdisciplinary training to teams of physicians, nurses, technicians, and other healthcare professionals. Nevertheless, each program also had a number of limitations. For example, none of the programs was based on a comprehensive pretraining needs analysis, limited opportunities existed for participants to receive structured practice and feedback on critical teamwork skills, and few strategies were available for sustaining and reinforcing teamwork principles in the post-training environment.

The second evaluation of early CRM-derived medical team training programs involved a random clinical trial of MedTeams™ conducted in 24 labor and delivery (L&D) units. Sachs et al. randomly assigned 24 hospital L&D units to participate in either the experimental or control conditions.[30] This study involved multiple performance measures that focused on patient outcomes, team process, and staff and patient satisfaction. Outcome measures such as the time it took for new patients to be processed through hospital admissions and the time interval

between deciding to do a C-section and initial incision, were recorded for training evaluation purposes. Although CRM-based team training was shown to have a positive impact on behaviors, no effect of CRM-based team training was found with important L&D patient safety outcomes. These results reinforce the notion that CRM-based training is a good basis for developing medical team training, but in itself, it is not a universal solution.

The final evaluation of early CRM-derived medical team training programs was conducted by Salas et al., who performed a systematic review of CRM in the healthcare industry.[31] This review yielded results similar to those in the previous metaanalysis. Twenty-eight accounts (11 within the medical community) of the implementation of CRM training were systematically reviewed. As in previous work, links between CRM training and reactions, declarative and procedural knowledge of awareness, and communication techniques were established. However, as in the aviation industry, a limited number of organizational safety outcomes could be established, thus preventing researchers from identifying an impact of CRM on safety. Despite this, Salas et al. noted that CRM is not an exhaustive solution when attempting to extend teamwork training to the healthcare domain.

Second Generation: Accreditation Council for Graduate Medical Education and American Association of Medical Colleges Competencies for Training

Following the initial rush of CRM-based team skills models, practitioners turned to models developed by accrediting bodies such as ACGME and AAMC. These models were more heuristic, calling for a gestalt focus on competencies such as interprofessional collaboration, professional communication, organizational citizenship, and systems-based practice.[1,32,33] Table 3.1 provides a summary of teamwork competencies identified by ACGME as critical for effective practitioner performance.

The ACGME added these competencies to core curriculum ones in the mid-2000s. They were designed to be incorporated and assessed as part of medical education across all components of learning. For example, for any learning activity (e.g., a practicum or class) medical students would be

Table 3.1   Accreditation Council for Graduate Medical Education Teamwork Competencies

Teamwork Knowledge, Skills, and Attitudes Competencies	Definition
Interpersonal and Communication Skills	Competency in interpersonal and communication skills will be assessed using direct observation of the resident during communications with other residents, with otolaryngology attending physicians, with physicians from other services, with nonphysician clinical staff, with nonphysician nonclinical staff, and with patients and their families. These competencies in communication with physicians and nonphysicians are already addressed on the existing quarterly evaluation form. Reporting back through the resident's mentor will serve as another mechanism for assessing competency in interpersonal and communication skills.
Professionalism	Competency in professionalism will be assessed by direct observation of the resident's responsibility in carrying out their professional duties—including continuity of care, responsiveness to changes in clinical situations, overall responsiveness and availability, and self-sacrifice, and their following of ethical principles in their dealings with patients, their families, and other physicians and healthcare workers. The resident's sensitivity to different patient populations will be evaluated by direct observation and comparison of the professionalism and responsibility demonstrated when caring for patients of different ethnic and economic backgrounds that are treated in the different hospitals.
Systems-Based Practice	Competency in systems-based practice will be assessed by direct observation of the resident's use of the entire healthcare system in caring for their patients, as well as their teamwork within the system. This will be addressed using both the regular quarterly evaluations, as well as direct observation at the briefings and meetings, and during clinical care, as well as during discussions at clinical care conferences.

Adapted from ACGME Core Competencies. ©2001 by Michael G. Stewart, MD, MPH. Reprinted with permission.

evaluated on their proficiency in all these competencies. Currently, all ACGME-accredited medical education programs must report how each learning activity encompasses competencies in interpersonal and communication skills, professionalism, and systems-based practice.

During the same period, AAMC began focusing efforts to assess medical school students' proficiencies in teamwork-oriented competencies such as organizational citizenship and interpersonal skills. In 2007, The Office of Faculty Affairs began sponsoring the adoption and implementation of teamwork skills in educational programs for medicine.[33] Specifically, they instituted the Team*Works!* Program, a professional development program designed to put the knowledge, skills, and attitudes of high-performing teams to work in medical schools and teaching hospitals. The program currently provides coaching for team skills over the course of 6 months, using online support of active learning, workshops, and peer analysis of team function. Team skills addressed over the professional development opportunity included team goal-setting, conflict management, and integration of different experiences and work styles into daily work.

The Current Generation—TeamSTEPPS®

Several researchers argued that the first generation of teamwork skills models in healthcare were too narrowly focused on CRM (a subdomain of team training) and did not take advantage of the 20+ years of research that has been conducted on teams and team performance in such fields as industrial, social, military, and human factors psychology. Still, these same researchers argued that the ACGME and AAMC efforts did not fully operationalize competencies related to teamwork skill in the current form.[1,33] The conventional thinking on teamwork skills left a void where the appropriate teamwork skills identified were not specified for healthcare, and tools and strategies for building proficiency in these skill domains were not readily available. Then came the work of Salas, Baker, and colleagues who worked to identify teamwork skills that were clearly operationalized and linked to teamwork tools and strategies for enhancing processes like communication, backup behavior, cross-monitoring, and leadership.[1,8,34,35]

Salas et al. conducted a review of existing teamwork processes and identified a framework of critical components to teamwork (i.e., The Big Five of Teamwork). Then, Baker et al. along with Salas developed a comprehensive model for enhancing performance by building teamwork skills competency in easily trainable individual skill domains. This model was first published as the foundation for the TeamSTEPPS program, which is now the federal standard for medical professional team training. Its components were first published in 2006 by Alonso et al., who delineated the implementation of this program in the Department of Defense Military Health System.

The critical aspects, or core competencies, of teamwork include: team leadership, mutual performance monitoring (i.e., situation monitoring), backup behavior (i.e., mutual support), and communication. These core competencies lead to such important team outcomes as enabling teams to be adaptable to changing situations, having team members with compatible shared mental models, and yielding team members with stronger orientations toward teamwork. Table 3.2 presents these competencies along with their definitions, behavioral examples, and selected references.

Because the current generation of research produced more healthcare specific skills that were derived from the emerging evidence base, there was a need to develop a new approach for teaching teamwork skills to healthcare professionals. Building on the earlier reviews, Baker et al. and Alonso et al. developed a framework integrating core teamwork skills according to key teamwork outcomes for team training.[7,9,31] In this framework, core teamwork KSAs were linked to specific teamwork outcomes that could be attained via team training. The overarching goal of this framework was to address two key deficiencies. The first deficiency stemmed from a focus on CRM, which serves as a good first step in conducting team training but does not completely generalize to all types of teams and teamwork. The second deficiency focused on the goal to make team training more effective than basic CRM training, which aimed to provide information about teamwork but lacked the training and development of key skills that would build proficiency in teamwork. This distinction is critical when considering the difference between training a skill versus training toward an outcome. For example, theories of teamwork point to the importance of adaptability/flexibility as a central skill.[8] However, it is hard to directly train adaptability/ flexibility, because it is required when responding to an unpredictable situation that the team encounters. Therefore, Alonso et al. concluded based on the available evidence that it is more appropriate to teach team members to monitor the performance of others and provide assistance, plan and organize team roles, and communicate with one another efficiently. Combined, these skills yield a highly adaptable and flexible team.

The current generation of medical team training then only focused on the core skills of teamwork that could be directly trained. These skills were linked to performance, knowledge, or attitude-based outcomes that earlier CRM-derived courses had often targeted during training. For example, shared mental models (a topic covered in many CRM courses) were viewed as a result of using monitoring and backup behaviors. Table 3.3 presents teamwork outcomes along with their definitions, behavioral examples, and selected references.

The framework that drives the second generation of healthcare team training is presented in Figure 3.1, in which the circle in the middle includes the trainable skills of leadership, situation monitoring (mutual performance monitoring), mutual

Table 3.2   Team Knowledge, Skills, and Attitudes Competencies

Teamwork Knowledge, Skills, and Attitudes Competencies	Definition	Behavioral Examples	Medical Relevance
Team Leadership	Ability to direct and coordinate the activities of other team members, assess team performance, assign tasks, develop team knowledge, skills, and attitudes, motivate team members, plan and organize, and establish a positive atmosphere.	➤ Facilitate team problem solving. ➤ Provide performance expectations and acceptable interaction patterns. ➤ Synchronize and combine individual team member contributions. ➤ Seek and evaluate information that affects team functioning. ➤ Clarify team member roles. ➤ Engage in preparatory meetings and feedback sessions with the team.	Emergency medicine, surgical, and labor and delivery teams must conduct assessments on patient intake. Leaders must facilitate briefings and huddles to ensure shared visions for treatment plans. They must also conducts debriefs such as M&M meetings following treatment to allow for process improvement.
Mutual Performance Monitoring (aka., Situation Monitoring)	The ability to develop common understandings of the team environment and apply appropriate task strategies to accurately monitor teammate performance.	➤ Identify mistakes and lapses in other team members' actions. ➤ Provide feedback regarding team members' actions to facilitate self-correction.	All healthcare teams conduct patient diagnosis and assessments. For that reason, providers must use situation monitoring to gather information about patients and their condition. However, patients are not the only part of the equation that must be monitored. Healthcare professionals can use cross-monitoring to each other's ability to work effectively. They can also prevent potential lapses in quality of care by ensuring that staff suffering from fatigue or other factors are backed up.

Backup Behavior (aka., Mutual Support)	Ability to anticipate other team members' needs through accurate knowledge about their responsibilities. The ability to shift workload among members to achieve balance during high periods of workload or pressure.	➢ Recognition by potential backup providers that there is a workload distribution problem in their team ➢ Shift work responsibilities to underused team members. ➢ Complete the whole task or parts of tasks by other team members.	Healthcare providers in a variety of settings use backup behavior or mutual support to assist others. Providers in the emergency room back each other up during trauma events and other critical care situations. Providers in the labor and delivery unit support one another by completing tasks when others are interrupted. Primary care healthcare providers often back each other up by filling in for one another during patient testing and diagnoses.
Communication	The exchange of information between a sender and a receiver irrespective of the medium.	➢ Follow up with team members to ensure the message was received. ➢ Acknowledge that a message was received. ➢ Clarify with the sender of the message that it was received is the same as the intention.	Communication is the cornerstone support mechanism of teamwork. Without it, trauma teams would not confirm orders as they barked out by team leaders. Without communication, labor and delivery team members would not have a means for advocating and asserting patient needs or resolving critical differences in professional opinion. Without communication, primary care physicians would not be able to gather information from specialists and laboratories. Each of these represents a potential breakdown in communication during care or transitions in care. Handoff protocols and structured communication formats allow teams to transfer information without restrictions from extraneous or missing information.

Table 3.3	Team Outcomes	
Teamwork Outcomes	**Definition**	**Behavioral Examples**
Mutual Trust	The sense of trust experienced by team members after continued successful performance	➤ Express a sense of trust in other team members during task. ➤ Accept the judgment of team members without question.
Adaptability	Ability to adjust strategies based on information gathered from the environment through the use of compensatory behavior and reallocation of intra-team resources. Altering a course of action or team repertoire in response to changing conditions (internal or external)	➤ Identify cues that a change has occurred, assign meaning to that change, and develop a new plan to deal with the changes. ➤ Identify opportunities for improvement and innovation for habitual or routine practices. ➤ Remain vigilant to changes in the internal and external environment of the team.
Shared Mental Models	An organizing knowledge structure of the relationships between the task the team is engaged in and how the team members will interact	➤ Anticipate and predict each other's needs. ➤ Identify changes in the team, task, or teammates and implicitly adjust strategies as needed.
Team Orientation	The expression of one's motivation to be part of a team	➤ Express a desire to want to perform tasks as a team. ➤ Actively seek team tasks to be performed in group settings.

support (backup behavior), and communication. Performance outcomes, knowledge outcomes, and attitudinal outcomes are then depicted in the corners as resulting from proficiency on the central skills. This framework is referred to as the TeamSkills Triangle.

The TeamSkills Triangle framework treats the common teamwork competencies as specific, learnable skills (i.e., leadership, situation monitoring, mutual support, and communication)[9,36] and teamwork outcomes as specific, key learning outcomes that can be attained after developing proficiency in the core teamwork skills (i.e., competencies). TeamSTEPPS® training teaches specific tools and strategies that can be used to improve teamwork performance in the medical environment. The core teamwork skills or competencies are described in detail next.

Leadership

Leadership is a critical component of effective team performance. Regardless of team type, whether healthcare or not, leaders influence team effectiveness by facilitating team actions and making sure that teams have all the necessary resources for optimal performance. Facilitation of team actions often involves such activities as ensuring that team actions are understood by all and that changes in information are shared by team members. In addition, leaders must also provide team members with the appropriate material and human resources (e.g., team members with proper skills) to perform. Facilitating team actions results in the development of a shared mental model (or a shared understanding of the current situation) among team members, and managing resources ensures that teams can be adaptable.

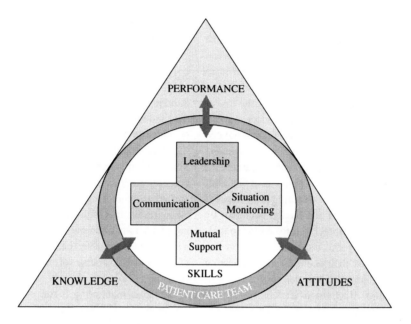

Figure 3.1
The TeamSkills Triangle

Leadership and Team Effectiveness

Leadership is defined by McGrath (p. 365) as a responsibility "to do, or get done, whatever is not adequately handled for the group needs."[37] Others have defined it as the means by which designated leaders or leaders in action affect team effectiveness before, during, and after a task. This is done by ensuring that team members are seeking information, planning team duties, coordinating team actions, resolving conflict among themselves, and providing coaching and feedback. More specifically, it is the duty of those entrusted with leadership responsibilities to ensure team actions like monitoring and information sharing take place. Leaders do this by performing two key behaviors: managing resources and facilitating team actions.

How important is leadership in promoting team effectiveness? Leadership has been identified by team researchers as an important piece in the teamwork skills puzzle. Salas et al. point out that leaders impact team effectiveness not by handing down solutions to teams, but rather by facilitating team problem-solving through cognitive processes (e.g., shared mental models), coordination processes (e.g., environmental monitoring; resource management),

and the team's collective motivation and behaviors (e.g., performance expectations).[8]

Leadership and Teams

Organizational researchers have long focused on the value of teams as a unit of task work, with leadership serving as a means for improving employee performance and attitudes. Some researchers have taken on the added burden of assessing the role of leaders and leadership strategies so as to best facilitate not only individual, but also team outcomes. Fleishman et al. provided a taxonomy of task-based leader skills that can be used to demonstrate the role of leaders when facilitating team actions. Researchers identified skills such as planning, organizing, problem-solving, facilitating, and supporting the team action process. These skills were identified as the essential behaviors that leaders need to take to ensure teams perform effectively and attain their desired outcomes.

Later, Morgeson expanded on Fleishman's taxonomy by grouping the key leadership skills into one of three categories: monitoring, diagnosis, and intervention.[38] In this model, monitoring refers to the continual monitoring of the team and environmental cues. Diagnosis refers to using information to make decisions and draw up action plans. Intervention can include team establishment, motivation, and team member development. DeChurch and Marks combined taxonomies to develop a theory of the role of leadership in action teams.[39] Two key leader behaviors were identified as having a vital impact on simulated fighter pilot performance: information management (i.e., resource management) and communication (i.e., facilitation). These researchers pointed out that leaders have the greatest impact on team performance if they manage information and human resources by delegating tasks and supplying information to their team members. They also illustrated the point that leaders must support their teams by communicating with them and holding information sessions to reinforce the coordinated actions to be taken. Teams with leaders who performed these behaviors reported significantly greater sharedness in mental models, committed fewer errors in flight, and performed better than teams with leaders who did not perform these behaviors. This is just one example of several leadership skills affecting team effectiveness.

Leaders have an impact on team effectiveness through ensuring that team actions are understood by all, changes in information are shared by team members, and teams and team members have the resources necessary to perform the task required. Leaders must ensure that information sharing, monitoring, helping, and other team actions are taking place by reinforcing shared mental models and modeling team actions for team members. Leaders must provide team members with the appropriate human and material resources (e.g., team members with proper skills) to perform. Facilitating team actions aids in the development of shared mental models, whereas managing resources ensures that teams can be adaptable when necessary. In summary, the evidence suggests that effective team leaders:

- Are responsible for ensuring that team members are sharing information, monitoring situational cues, resolving conflicts, and helping each other when needed;
- Manage resources to ensure teams performance;
- Facilitate team actions by communicating through informal information exchange sessions;
- Develop norms for information sharing; and

- Ensure team members are aware of situational changes to plans.

Situation Monitoring

Situation monitoring is the process of actively scanning and assessing elements of the "situation" to gain or maintain an accurate awareness or understanding of the situation in which the team is functioning. Situation monitoring was adapted from theoretical concepts such as mutual performance monitoring and cross-monitoring.[34] Successful situation monitoring results in a high degree of situational awareness, which when communicated to others, cultivates a mutual understanding (i.e., a shared mental model) of the current course of action when treating patients.[40–43]

Situation monitoring is the process of actively scanning and assessing elements of the situation to gain or maintain an accurate awareness or understanding of the situation in which the team is functioning. In this module, we have extracted elements from the literature on effective team processes to develop the status, team, environment, and progress (STEP) tool as a model for those new to monitoring situations in the delivery of healthcare. Status, team, environment, and progress includes the following elements that should be monitored and assessed: the status of the patient, team members, the environment, and progress toward the goal.

Marks et al. identified three essential elements that effective teams must monitor during action phases, defined as "periods of time when teams are engaged in acts that contribute directly to goal accomplishment" (p. 360).[34] These elements include systems (both internal and environmental), the team itself, and progress toward the goal.

Systems monitoring includes tracking internal systems components (e.g., human resources and equipment), environmental conditions (e.g., number of OR rooms available or status of other patients on the unit). Teams working in dynamic environments need to monitor and assess internal and external systems, allowing identification of changes that can affect tasks and/or the final goal. Recently, the Institute for Healthcare Improvement highlighted rapid response teams, in conjunction with the 100k Lives Campaign, to emphasize the need to respond more quickly to critical changes in the status of the patient (e.g., acute change in vital signs, acute drop in blood oxygen level, decreased urine output, altered mental function). By monitoring the patient's condition and using rapid response teams when appropriate, medical teams can help to prevent cardiac arrest or other adverse events. *Team monitoring* refers to the process of observing, or cross-monitoring, the actions of fellow team members in an effort to identify errors, performance discrepancies, and areas in which another member can provide support. Support encompasses feedback, coaching, performing backup behaviors, and assuming or completing taskwork for another member.

Monitoring progress toward the goal refers to assessing the status of the team's taskwork in relation to achieving the goal. This type of information allows the team to continually assess the plan of care, the need for additional resources, and whether the established goals are being met by the team.

Shared Mental Models

The act of sharing and discussing information gained from situation monitoring provides the opportunity to gather more information about the situation and helps cultivate a mutual understanding. This mutual understanding is commonly referred to as a *shared mental model*. Shared mental models are defined as organized knowledge structures of relevant facts and relationships about a task or situation that are commonly held by members of a team. Teams develop the plan, share the plan, and monitor the plan. In their review of the literature, Mohammed and Dumville identified several constructs studied by various disciplines that are similar to the concept of shared mental models.[44] Terms used by other disciplines include information sharing, transactive memory, and cognitive consensus.

The information sharing literature, as summarized by Mesmer-Magnus and DeChurch, examined information pooling behaviors in groups, and distinguished shared information (information held by all members) from unshared information (information held by only one member).[35] Given that teams are typically composed of members with distinct roles who tend to have unique information, it is important to pay attention to the factors that promote and undermine the opportunity for team members to present and discuss their diverse information and observations.

The transactive memory literature advanced the concept of individual team member's memory systems regarding knowledge and expertise possessed by other team members. The important point of this literature is that each team member needs to be aware that he or she may have unique information that would benefit the team as a whole. As a result, opportunities for "sharing" information will be less about rehashing information that all members already possess and focus more on discussing and pooling unique and unshared information.

The literature on cognitive consensus defined this construct as the "similarity among [team] members regarding how key issues are defined and conceptualized" (p. 274).[43] In other words, team members who have cognitive consensus are more likely to interpret situational cues and other issues similarly. This literature adds to the shared mental model concept that team members share adequate knowledge of taskwork and teamwork, in addition to having a common understanding of the assumptions underlying significant issues. However, it should be noted that extreme levels of consensus can be dysfunctional in many situations; therefore, there must be a balance between diversity and consensus for optimal team effectiveness.

The basic premise regarding the relationship of shared mental models and teamwork is that team effectiveness will improve if team members have a shared understanding of the situation. Currently, there are many papers postulating the theoretical impact of shared mental models on team effectiveness; however, there is little empirical evidence substantiating this relationship because of the difficulty of measuring this cognitive construct at the group level. Nonetheless, the theoretical, empirical, and anecdotal evidence suggest that team members who possess shared mental models resulted in teams that:

- Can anticipate;
- Backup and fill-in for one another;
- Communicate to ensure team members have the necessary information for task performance; and
- Team members understand each others' roles, and how they interplay.

In healthcare if the wrong plan is developed, potentially all actions that follow are wrong; and the patient and provider are at risk. A shared mental model serves as an error reduction strategy; providers understanding the plan monitor all actions relative to that plan.

Mutual Support

Mutual support is critical to the social and task performance of teams. It can include simple task assistance (i.e., backup behavior) and other, more complex forms of support, like helping to resolve conflicts. Some of the skills involved with successful mutual support include conflict resolution, task assistance, and verbal feedback, all of which trainable. Teams that engage in mutual support are better equipped to be adaptable in changing situations and environments.

Mutual support is commonly referred to as backup behavior in the teamwork literature. Backup behavior is considered critical to the social and task performance aspects of teams and essentially involves helping other team members to perform their tasks. The construct suggests some degree of task interchangeability among members because they must fully understand what each other does and be willing to provide and seek assistance when needed. Porter et al. define backup as "the discretionary provision of resources and task-related effort to another member of one's team that is intended to help that team member obtain the goals as defined by his or her role when it is apparent that the team member is failing to reach those goals" (p. 392).[45] Backup behavior differs from feedback in that it is usually more proactive.

A team backup behavior can be provided by offering or requesting assistance. Backup often includes filling in for a team member who is unable to perform a task and helping others correct their mistakes. A member may be unable to perform his or her tasks because the individual is inexperienced, incapable, overburdened, or has made an error. Backup behavior is also provided when a member is unable to perform all of his or her tasks, or a fellow team member is presently underused. Porter et al. note that when such underused individuals backup the individual whose capacity is being surpassed, the team is allowed to dynamically adjust. This level of performance could not have been accomplished had the members been working solely as individuals. Situation monitoring allows team members to effectively assess whether

fellow members are overloaded. Backup behavior allows reallocation of work tasks to underused team members, resulting in teams being more adaptive. In summary, mutual support is a core skill that enables teams to function effectively. Supporting teams typically:

- Backup and fill in for each other;
- Are self-correcting;
- Compensate for each other;
- Reallocate functions;
- Distribute and assign work thoughtfully; and
- Regularly provide feedback to each other (both individually and as a team).

Communication

Teamwork will only be effective if there is good communication among team members Researchers have noted that good communication is a function of two critical subskills: exchanging information and consulting with others.[42] The exchange of information involves such behaviors as closed-loop communication, information sharing, procedural talk, and volunteering and requesting information. The skill of consulting with others involves the open exchange of relevant interpretations, effectively influencing others, and evaluative interchange. Outcomes of good communication include the development of mutual trust and shared mental models, thus enabling teams to adapt quickly to changing situations. The most critical skill for healthcare professionals is communication because of constant transitions in care; one team needs to impart information to the other team when transitioning a patient or when presenting patient information.

A tremendous amount of evidence exists to support the efficacy of good communication skills for effective teamwork. For example, Cannon-Bowers et al. found that communication is comprised of two critical subskills: exchanging information and consulting with others. Information exchange was defined by such behaviors as closed-loop communication, information sharing, procedural talk, and volunteering and requesting information. Consulting with others consisted of effective influence, open exchange of relevant interpretations, and evaluative interchange. Likewise, Dickinson and McIntyre found that effective communication required that information be exchanged in a set manner using proper terminology and acknowledgment of the information received.

Communication is an important component of team process, by serving as a coordinating mechanism, or supporting structure, for teamwork. Communication skills interplay directly with leadership, situation monitoring, and mutual support. Team leaders provide guidance through verbal feedback. Leaders also promote interaction among team members by clarifying team roles and defining team norms for conflict resolution. Effective communication skills are needed to clearly convey information, provide awareness of roles and responsibilities, or how performance impacted outcomes.

Good communication facilitates development of mutual trust and shared mental models, enabling teams to quickly adapt to changing situations. Salas et al. note, "communication is especially important as the environment increases in complexity (e.g., emergency situations) as it not only distributes needed information to other team members but also facilitates the continuous updating of the team's shared mental model and their engagement in [other team activities]."[8]

Communication is a critical skill possessed by team members, for effective teamwork to occur. Team members that possess good communication skills are able to:

- Communicate accurate and complete information in a clear and concise manner;
- Seek information from all available sources;
- Readily anticipate and share the information needs of other team members;
- Provide status updates; and
- Verify information received.

Leadership, situation monitoring, mutual support, and communication are the keys to attaining team orientation, mutual trust (especially in time-constrained events), and other important outcomes. They serve as the modern-day foundation for all team skills training programs in healthcare. Despite this undeniable fact, one major question remains about team training in healthcare—why do teamwork competencies matter in healthcare?

Why Teamwork Skills Matter for Healthcare

Determining why teamwork matters in healthcare is quite simple. One needs only examine how teamwork is triggered throughout healthcare clinical work to identify potential pitfalls of failed teamwork. These potential pitfalls make it possible to quantify the importance of teamwork competencies among healthcare professionals. Consider, for example, the emergency department in a teaching hospital in which the intake process for a patient calls for multiple assessments by a triage nurse, a clinical nurse, a physician's assistant or resident, and, ultimately, an attending physician. The purpose of conducting multiple assessments is to capture critical patient information about medical history, condition, and pain suffered through various iterations of reliable interviewing. Healthcare professionals can then cull together information from the patient and families to apply their collective expertise toward the effective diagnosis and treatment of ailments. This process requires significant amounts of teamwork beyond clinical tasks such as diagnosis and treatment. For instance, healthcare professionals must share the information gathered and develop a shared mental model for what treatment will resemble. To do so, they must leverage their situation monitoring competencies to assess the patient's complete condition, their communication skills to ensure effective information exchange, and their mutual support competencies to resolve any conflicting information. Further, they must rely on a leader to bring them together with information in hand to delineate a clear, shared course of treatment.

Leadership competencies play a vital role in healthcare. For example, in the stabilization of patients in acute deterioration, intensivists or hospitalists must play the role of designated leader in the rapid response system. These leaders serve to identify a treatment plan for patients and relay this information to their fellow intensive care nurses and respiratory therapists. This treatment team must then coordinate with floor staff like the clinical nurse and the intensive care unit that may potentially care for the patient. This is just one specific example of the importance of leadership. Clinically speaking, effective team leadership leads to the proper exchange of information and the equitable distribution of resources. These, in turn, reduce the risk of outcomes such as medication errors and failure to treat the true causes of illness. Leaders also set the norms for process improvement by facilitating debriefs.

In the context of healthcare, situation monitoring is critical at two points in delivery of care: (1) the assessment and diagnosis of patient conditions, and (2) the assessment of changes in patient conditions. All healthcare providers must assess the patient's situation before and while engaging in patient care. Nevertheless, situation monitoring serves a greater purpose in healthcare. If a fellow team or team member demonstrates proficiency in situation monitoring, that team or person can assess situations for teams further along the chain of care (e.g., a primary care physician can monitor patients along the chain of care as they engage specialists). Moreover, providers can engage in monitoring of each other to ensure that medical error does not jeopardize patient safety.

Healthcare teams must demonstrate proficiency in mutual support to ensure that task assistance and conflict management occur when needed. For example, mutual support at the team level occurs when a provider simply performs a task for another team member. Similarly, the team leaders can aid in the resolution of conflict between two team members. An example of mutual support at the system level is healthcare providers monitor the actions of a care unit during a transition in care, anticipate potential tasks that need to be performed, and act to complete those tasks. Another example of mutual support at the system level is a provider performing key tasks for another team member pulled away from treatment tasks. In the emergency department, this is an all-too-common occurrence. Providers often encounter the threat of interruptions in treatment and rely on others to assist them by substituting in their role. Teams that can actively manage their conflicts and provide task assistance ensure the effective treatment of patients. Imagine the labor and delivery team that requires an assertive nurse to stand up to the remaining team members when there is a failure to acknowledge signs of fetal deterioration. The most effective team will be able to actively manage the task conflict encountered when someone advocates for the patient, as well as have someone fill in when team members encounter interruptions during treatment. Teams that demonstrate proficiency in

this competency can avoid potential dangers such as incomplete treatment or inappropriate treatment actions such as wrong-site surgery.

The most critical teamwork competency for healthcare providers is communication. Information exchange during transitions in care presents the most fertile opportunity for medical error. Take for example the transition in care from emergency department to intensive care unit. One team needs to impart information to the other team when transitioning a patient or when presenting patient information. Imagine a situation where the intensive care unit receives only certain information about the medications a patient has been given during treatment. This can result in situations in which the intensive care unit staff inappropriately medicate the patient or lose valuable treatment time seeking further information about the patient's history. Moments lost in treatment can lead to failed stabilization and, ultimately, fatalities. But the importance of communication is not limited to transitions between teams; effective communication is important for all phases of healthcare team execution, and for all teams within the healthcare system. Effective communication is cornerstone of teamwork in that appropriate callouts and checkbacks prevent medications errors or following the wrong orders. Teams cannot build a shared mental model for patient care without effectively communicating what needs to be done. The importance of communication was made most apparent by the Joint Commission's Root Cause Analyses of medical errors completed in 2002.[46] This report stipulated that 70% of medical errors resulted from breakdowns in communication more than any other factor.

The examples presented here highlight potential costs of failing to communicate and coordinate as a team. Teams who engage in effective leadership, situation monitoring, mutual support, and communication have better team outcomes such as shared mental models, mutual trust, team orientation, and adaptability. These improved KSAs result in fewer unclear communications, less ambiguity in the patient treatment process, and reduced risk for the patient. The ability to achieve these outcomes relies on the ability to build team training for healthcare professionals that reflects these competencies. Without a focus on these competencies, healthcare professionals can only attempt to realize safer care in an incomplete fashion.

REFERENCES

1. Kohn, L. T., Corrigan, J. M., & Donaldson, M. S. (1999). *To err is human.* Washington, DC: National Academy Press.

2. Leonard, M., & Tarrant, C. A. (2001). Culture, systems, and human factors—Two tales of patient safety: The KP Colorado region's experience. *The Permanente Journal 5*(3), 46–9.

3. Leonard, M., Graham, S., & Bonacum, D. (2004). The human factor: The critical importance of effective teamwork and communication in providing safe care. *Quality & Safety in Healthcare, 13*(Suppl 1), i85–90.

4. Hammon, W. R. (2004). The complexity of team training: what we have learned from aviation and its applications to medicine. *Quality & Safety in Healthcare, 13*(Suppl 1), i72–79.

5. Barach, P., & Small, S. D. (2000). Reporting and preventing medical mishaps: Lessons from non-medical near miss reporting systems. *British Medical Journal, 320*(1), 759–63.

6. Barach P., & Weingart, M. (2004). Trauma team performance. In W. Wilson, C. Grande, & D. Hoyt (Eds.), *Trauma: resuscitation, anesthesia, surgery, & critical care.* New York: Dekker; pp. 101–14.

7. Baker, D. P., Gustafson, S., Beaubien, J. M., Salas, E., & Barach, P. (2003). *Medical teamwork and patient safety: The evidence-based relation.* Washington, DC: American Institutes for Research.

8. Salas, E., Sims, D. E., & Burke, C. S. (2005). Is there a "big five" in teamwork? *Small Group Research, 36*(5), 555–99.

9. Alonso, A., Baker, D., Day, R., Holtzman, A., King, H., & Toomey, L. S. E. (2006). Reducing medical error in the military health system: How can team training help? *Human Resources Management Review, 16,* 396–415.

10. Volpe, C. E., Cannon-Bowers, J. A., Salas, E., & Spector, P. E. (1996). The impact of cross training on team functioning: An empirical investigation. *Human Factors, 38*(1), 87–100.

11. Smith-Jentsch, K. A., Salas, E., & Baker, D. P. (1996). Training team performance-related assertiveness. *Personnel Psychology, 49*(4), 909–36.

12. Sims, D. E., Salas, E., & Burke, S. C. (2004, April). Is there a "big five" in teamwork? 19th Annual Meeting of the Society for Industrial and Organizational Psychology. Chicago.

13. Morey, J. C., Simon, R., Jay, G. D., et al. (2002). Error reduction and performance improvement in the emergency department through formal teamwork training: Evaluation results of the MedTeams project. *Health Services Research, 37*(6), 1553–81.

14. Klein, C. A., Salas, E., Burke, C. S., et al. (2009). Does team training enhance team processes, performance, and team member affective outcomes? A meta-analysis. *Journal of Applied Psychology, 93,* 57–79.

15. Helmreich, R. L., Merritt, A. C., & Wilhelm, J. A. (2000). The evolution of crew resource management training in commercial aviation. *International Journal of Aviation Psychology, 9*(1), 19–32.

16. Mathieu, J. E., Marks, M. A., & Zaccaro, S. J. (2001). Multi-team systems. In N. R. Anderson, D. Ones, H. K. Sinangil, & C. Viswesvaran (Eds.), *International handbook of work and organizational psychology.* (pp. 289–313). London: Sage.

17. Helmreich, R. L., Wilhelm, J. A., Klinect, J. R., & Merritt, A. C. (2001). Culture, error, and crew resource management. In: E. Salas, C. A. Bowers, E. Edens (Eds.), *Improving teamwork in organizations: Applications of resource management training.* (pp. 305–31). Mahwah, NJ: LEA.

18. Helmreich, R. L. (1998). Turning silk purses into sows' ears: Human factors in medicine. In L. C. Henson, & A. H. Lee (Eds.), *Simulators in anesthesiology education.* (pp. 1–8). New York: Plenum, 1998.

19. Helmreich, R. L., & Foushee, H. C. (1993). Why crew resource management? Empirical and theoretical bases of human factors training in aviation. In E. L. Weiner, B. G. Kanki, & R. L. Helmreich (Eds.), *Cockpit resource management.* (pp. 3–45). San Diego: Academic Press; 1993.

20. Helmreich, R. L., & Merritt, A. C. (1998). *Culture at work in aviation and medicine: National, organizational, and professional influences.* Brookfield, VT: Ashgate.

21. Helmreich, R. L., & Schaefer, H. G. (1994). Team performance in the operating room. In M. S. Bogner MS (Ed.), *Human error in medicine.* (pp. 225–53). Mahwah, NJ: LEA.

22. Baker, D., Day, R., & Salas, E. (2006). *Teamwork as an Essential Component of High Reliability Organizations. Health Services Research, 41*(4), 1576–98.

23. Salas, E., Burke, S. C., Bowers, C. A., & Wilson, K. A. (2001). Team training in the skies: Does crew resource management (CRM) training work? *Human Factors, 43*(4), 641–74.

24. Baker, D. P., Beaubien, J. M., & Holtzman, A. K. (2003). *DoD medical team training programs: An independent case study analysis.* Washington, DC: American Institutes for Research.

25. Simon, R., Salisbury, M., & Wagner, G. (2000). MedTeams: Teamwork advances emergency department effectiveness and reduces medical errors. *Ambulatory Outreach, Spring,* 21–4.

26. Searles, R. B. (2002). Patient safety program educating medical community. Retrieved July 2002 from: http://www.air.org/files/adv_pub_safety.pdf

27. Kohsin, B. Y., Landrum-Tsu, C., & Merchant, P. G. (2002). Implementation guidance for Medical Team Management in the MTF (Medical Treatment Facility). Bolling Air Force Base, Washington, DC: Air Force Medical Operations Agency: unpublished manuscript.

28. Stone FP. (2000). Medical team management: Improving patient safety through human factors training. Washington, DC: Military Health System Healthcare Reengineering.

29. Kohsin, B. Y. (2002). Talking paper on the status of AF [Air Force] Medical Team Management. Unpublished manuscript.

30. Mann, S., Marcus, R., & Sachs, B. P. (2006). Lessons from the cockpit: How team training can reduce errors on L&D. *Contemporary OB/GYN, January,* 1–7.

31. Salas, E., Wilson-Donnelly, K., Sims, D. E., Burke, C. S., & Priest, H. A. (2005). Teamwork training for patient safety: Best practices and guiding principles. *Joint Commission Journal on Quality and Patient Safety, 31,* 363–71.

32. ACGME. (2010). ACGME Teamwork Competencies. Chicago: Accreditation Council for Graduate Medical Education.

33. Leadley, J. (2012). TeamWorks: A Physician Team Training Initiative. Retrieved April 17, 2012 from https://www.aamc.org/members/gfa/faculty_vitae/269828/06-06-00fvspotlightteamcatalyst.html.

34. Marks, M. A., Mathieu, J. E., & Zaccaro, S. J. (2001). A temporally based framework and taxonomy of team processes. *Academy of Management Review, 26,* 356–76.

35. Mesmer-Magnus, J. R., & DeChurch, L. A. (2009). Information sharing and team performance: A meta-analysis. *Journal of Applied Psychology, 94*(2), 535–46.

36. Baker, D. P., Beaubien, J. M., & Harvey, A. K. (2003). *Program evaluation of medical team training in the Department of Defense: Team performance measures.* Washington, DC, American Institutes for Research.

37. McGrath, J. E. (1984). *Groups: Interaction and performance.* Englewood Cliffs, NJ: Prentice-Hall.

38. Morgeson, F. P. (1997). *Leading as event management: Toward a new conception of team leadership.* Poster session presented at meeting of the Society of Industrial and Organizational Psychology, St. Louis.

39. DeChurch, L. A., & Marks, M. A. (2006). Teams leading teams: Examining the role of leadership in multi-team systems. *Journal of Applied Psychology, 91,* 311–26.

40. Stout, R. J., Prince, C., Salas, E., & Brannick, M. T. (1999). Beyond reliability: Using crew resource management (CRM) measurements for training. In R. S. Jensen (Ed.), *Proceedings of the 10th International Symposium on Aviation Psychology.* Columbus, OH: The Ohio State University Press; pp. 61–71.

41. Klimoski, R., & Mohammed, S. (1994). Team mental model: Construct or metaphor? *Journal of Management, 20*(2), 403–47.

42. Cannon-Bowers, J. A., Tannenbaum, S. I., Salas, E., & Volpe, C. E. (1995). Defining competencies and establishing team training requirements. In R. A. Guzzo, & E. Salas (Eds.), *Team effectiveness and decision-making in organizations.* (pp. 333–80). San Francisco: Jossey-Bass 1995.

43. Mathieu, J. E., Heffner, T. S., Goodwin, G. F., & Salas, E. (2000). The influence of shared mental models on team process and performance. *Journal of Applied Psychology, 85,* 273–83.

44. Mohammed, S., & Dumville, B. C. (2001). Team mental models in a team knowledge framework: Expanding theory and measurement across disciplinary boundaries. *Journal of Organizational Behavior, 22,* 89–106.

45. Porter, C. O. L. H., Hollenbeck, J. R., Ilgen, D. R., Ellis, A. P. J., West, B. J., & Moon, H. (2003). Backup behavior in teams: The role of personality and legitimacy of need. *Journal of Applied Psychology 88,* 391–403.

46. JCAHO. (2002). Root Causes—A failure to communicate: Identifying and overcoming communication barriers. *Joint Commission Perspectives on Patient Safety, 2*(9), 4–5.

4

HOW CAN TEAM PERFORMANCE BE MEASURED, ASSESSED, AND DIAGNOSED?

Michael A. Rosen, Nicola Schiebel, Eduardo Salas, Teresa S. Wu, Salvatore Silvestri, and Heidi B. King

INTRODUCTION

In team training, the overarching reason for measuring and assessing team performance is to improve it. Here, measurement can drive increases in quality and quantity of teamwork behaviors via feedback to learners as well as providing the basis for systematic decisions about how to refine the teamwork implementation itself (i.e., what aspects of the training are or are not effective and how can they be improved?). Of course, there are other reasons to measure team performance (e.g., certifications, research); however, these applications are not the present focus. Consequently, this chapter is not a comprehensive review of team performance measurement and assessment, but a focused look at how team performance measurement can be used to drive effective implementations of teamwork training initiatives in healthcare. Interested readers are referred to more general sources for comprehensive reviews.[1,2]

This chapter is intended to provide a practical guide to navigating the complexities of designing and implementing a team performance measurement system within the context of a healthcare safety and quality improvement initiative. To this end, the present chapter is organized in three main sections.

First, key concepts in team performance measurement are defined. Second, a series of decision points in the design and implementation process, potential options, and considerations for making each decision are provided. These questions represent the fundamental decisions made when developing and implementing a team performance measurement system. Third, a set of overarching strategies for meeting some of the prominent goals of most team training implementations is provided: (1) acquisition of teamwork competencies during initial training, (2) transfer of learned behaviors to the job, and (3) sustainment and continuous improvement of gains in performance over time.

KEY DEFINITIONS

This section seeks to establish a common language by defining concepts central to any discussion of team performance measurement systems. First, concepts related to teams are defined. Second, definitions related to the process of measuring and understanding performance are provided. The terminology adopted here stems from the science of teams and human performance.

Teams, Teamwork, Team Performance, and Team Effectiveness

There is a large research base dedicated to understanding the nature of teams,[3,4] as well as how to train,[5] develop,[6] and manage[7] them. This section provides definitions rooted in this research as well as a discussion of these concepts in the context of healthcare.

First, a *team* is a collection of two or more individuals working interdependently towards a shared and valued goal(s).[8,9] This definition emphasizes: (1) meaningful interdependence (i.e., team members rely on one another to accomplish their work), and (2) some type of common purpose and specific aims valued by all members. Team members do not necessarily share all goals in common (i.e., team members can have unique individual goals), but team members are striving to achieve something in common (e.g., providing safe and high-quality care).

When developing a team performance measurement system, it is critical to identify the roles and boundaries of a team. Although the conceptual definition of a team presented in the preceding is relatively simple, defining a team within a healthcare organization is not always so straightforward. Team membership can be transient and frequently changing (e.g., a trauma team with members joining and leaving the team during a case). Additionally, some team members may be more central to that team's performance than others.[10] For example, an operating room (OR) team has several core members (e.g., surgeon, physician's assistant, circulating nurse, technicians). However, the administrator overseeing that room has an impact on how the team performs (e.g., scheduling), as do the allied health professionals (e.g., staff working in supply or room turnover). These staff can be viewed as a part of the OR team because their work is interdependent to some extent and they share a similar goal of safe, high-quality patient care. Defining the boundaries of who will and will not be considered a part of the target team of interest is critical for measurement to be effective.

Second, *teamwork* is the "dynamic, simultaneous and recursive enactment of process mechanisms which inhibit or contribute to team performance and performance outcomes" (p. 190).[11] Essentially, this involves the *actions* taken by team members for the purpose of working together—of coordinating, cooperating, and collaborating.[12] It is a process (i.e., actions taken), and not an outcome (i.e., the result or effect of what someone does). Additionally, the distinction between teamwork and taskwork is useful. *Taskwork* is associated with an individual. In healthcare, this can be equated roughly to some aspects of clinical competence. However, *teamwork competencies* are the knowledge, skills, and attitudes (KSAs) underlying effective teamwork.[13] For example, the TeamSTEPPS® (Strategies and Tools to Enhance Performance and Patient Safety) program (teamstepps.ahrq.gov) is a teamwork curriculum rooted in the science of teams[14] that includes the general teamwork competency areas of leadership, communication, situation monitoring, mutual support, and team structure. Team competencies are discussed in more detail in following sections.

Third, *team performance* is a dynamic process involving both teamwork and taskwork behaviors.[11] It is the sum of *both teamwork and taskwork behaviors*. The major challenges associated with measuring team performance are rooted in its *multilevel* (i.e., it is comprised of both teamwork and taskwork processes) and *dynamic* (i.e., it unfolds and varies over time) nature. Much of the remainder of the chapter deals with methods and strategies for capturing and understanding dynamic multilevel team performance.

Fourth, *team effectiveness* is a judgment of the quality of a team's performance outcomes or an assessment of the team's outcomes relative to set criteria.[11] This can include the quantity and quality of specific outcomes (e.g., efficiency, error counts, resource use, patient outcomes), team member satisfaction, and viability (i.e., the team's ability to continue to work together in the future).[15]

Measurement, Evaluation, Assessment, and Performance Diagnosis

This section provides a review of measurement concepts related to team performance measurement systems.

Most fundamentally, *measurement* involves a systematic process of: (1) assigning numbers to events, objects, occurrences, or other phenomena; or (2) classifying those phenomena into groups.[16] At a high level, the quality of a measurement system is determined by conceptual characteristics of the rules for assigning numbers or classifying phenomena (i.e., construct validity) as well as the consistency by which the rules can be applied (i.e., reliability). Consequently, *team performance measurement* is a systematic process for quantifying different aspects of a team's functioning, specifically capturing teamwork and taskwork processes. *Evaluation* and *assessment* refer to what is done with the measurement data. Both involve comparing the measurement data with some type of prespecified criterion or expectations for good or poor team performance. Although usage of these terms can vary widely, assessment generally refers to a summative judgment of competence (or lack thereof) and evaluation refers to a more formative process of identifying strengths and weaknesses that can be used for developmental purposes. *Performance diagnosis* involves

determining the underlying causes of an effective or ineffective performance.[17] Here measurements of performance are used to make inferences about the reasons behind the observed levels of performance. Performance diagnosis is most commonly discussed in the context of training programs in which the goal is to understand why a team performed the way it did so that: (1) deficiencies in teamwork competencies can be identified and corrected, (2) good teamwork can be reinforced, and (3) decisions about what types of learning activities are needed in the future can be made. Table 4.1 describes several characteristics of a team performance profile—a collection of measures used to generate a robust picture of and subsequently diagnose a team's performance. These characteristics are discussed throughout this chapter as they define many useful features of a team performance measurement system.

Table 4.1 Characteristics of a Team Performance Profile

Characteristic: A Team Performance Measurement System Should …	Description/Rationale
Capture and discriminate between multiple levels of performance	By distinguishing between teamwork and taskwork—between individual and team level processes—a better understanding of the reasons or causes of performance outcomes can be understood. This enables feedback to be provided appropriately (e.g., to correct or reinforce individual or team-level performance).
Be contextualized and task-relevant	Measures should take into account the specific context (e.g., clinical domain) of the team and do not apply overly generic descriptions of teamwork. If teamwork measures are overly abstract or generic, it complicates the process of training raters and maintaining interrater reliability.
Be competency based or theory driven	Measures should focus on the specified *teamwork* KSAs being trained or more generally measures should capture what is targeted for change or improvement.
Be descriptive of team performance	Measures should provide information about what actually happened instead of a high-level summary score. More fine-grained measurements can be more useful for identifying specific problems and providing corrective and process-oriented feedback.
Collect from multiple sources	Multiple sources (e.g., team members, observers) are a way of *triangulating* with measurement—capturing different aspects of teamwork from different vantage points. Incorporating multiple perspectives and methods can provide a more complete picture of a team's performance.

(Continued)

Table 4.1   (Continued)

Characteristic: A Team Performance Measurement System Should ...	Description/Rationale
Capture the dynamic and longitudinal nature of team performance	Measures should capture variations in teamwork: (1) during a performance episode, as well as (2) a historical record of team performance across performance episodes for comparisons and to assess improvement and sustainment.

Source: Salas, E., Rosen, M. A., Burke, C. S., Nicholson, D., & Howse, W. R. (2007). Markers for enhancing team cognition in complex environments: The power of team performance diagnosis. *Aviation, Space, and Environmental Medicine Special Supplement on Operational Applications of Cognitive Performance Enhancement Technologies, 78*(5), B77–85.

CORE QUESTIONS IN THE DESIGN AND IMPLEMENTATION OF A TEAM PERFORMANCE MEASUREMENT SYSTEM

Unfortunately, there is no perfect, one-size-fits-all, or off-the-shelf solution to team performance measurement, evaluation, assessment, or diagnosis. In many cases, the measurement tools as well as the system for collecting, analyzing, and then using the data must be customized to the unique context of a specific teamwork implementation. This section provides guidance for this development process by discussing the core questions that must be answered, including issues of purpose (why is measurement being conducted?), content (what should be measured?), locations of data collection (where should measurements occur?), timing (when should measurement happen?), and method (how is team performance measured?), as well as issues related to different roles in this process (who should measure, evaluate, assess, and diagnose team performance?).

Table 4.2 summarizes these questions and issues, potential options, and major considerations driving choices for each question. These issues are highly interrelated. Consequently, some unifying strategies are discussed in the following section.

WHY IS THE MEASUREMENT EFFORT BEING UNDERTAKEN?

The purpose of a measurement system plays an essential role in the development of that system. Data

are collected to answer questions. In the present context, these questions most commonly relate to the level of teamwork proficiency of team members, and the effectiveness of the improvement initiative. Answering these questions helps to guide the implementation in a systematic way to effect the desired changes. However, different measurement tools and approaches have different information yields[18] or utility for different purposes. Additionally, different approaches may be more or less demanding of various types of resources (e.g., staff time, complexity of analysis). Therefore, it is important to have a clear and explicitly articulated purpose for why the team performance measurement system is being developed. This purpose statement drives choices, sets priorities, and helps to manage the inherent tradeoffs among different measurement approaches. These tradeoffs are discussed in more detail throughout this chapter. There are two major categories of reasons to measure team performance during teamwork training initiatives: generating feedback for learners and implementing evaluation.

Feedback

Learning requires feedback, and measurement can provide a method for ensuring that feedback is consistent, timely, accurate, and focused on improving targeted processes and behaviors—all characteristics of effective feedback.[19,20] An important goal of a team training initiative is to develop a shared understanding of teamwork concepts, tools, strategies, and behaviors. If different trainers or coaches provide inconsistent feedback, this process of

Table 4.2   Overview of Key Decisions and Considerations in Developing Team Performance Measurement Systems

Type of Decision	Potential Options	Major Considerations
Why What is the purpose of the measurement?	• Feedback during acquisition • Feedback for continuous improvement • Evaluation of teamwork implementation	• Developing a clear and explicit purpose statement for the measurement effort will help to guide all future decisions. • Frequently it is useful to define different groups (e.g., staff members, administrators, implementers) that will need different information about the intervention.

What
What content needs to be captured by the measurement system?
	• Teamwork competencies (KSAs)
	  – Knowledge
	  – Behavior
	  – Attitudes
	• Multilevel Training Evaluation
	  – Reactions
	  – Learning
	  – Behavior change
	  – Results
		• The content of a team performance measurement system should be aligned with the content of the training program and goals of the change initiative.
		• Organizations are complex and a change or training initiative can be derailed in many different ways. Using a multilevel evaluation framework can help pinpoint where problems are in an implementation and provide information useful in correcting those problems.

Where
Where are measurements made?
	• Learning environment
	  – Classroom
	  – Simulation
	• On the job
	  – Unobtrusive field observations on the unit
	• Hybrid approaches
	  – Performance evaluations using in situ simulations; creates a compromise between control of simulation and robustness of on-the-job evaluation.
		Control over opportunities to measure teamwork vs. natural variation
		• Learning environments offer greater control over the demands placed on a team, and
		Typical vs. maximal performance
		• Typical performance (i.e., the level of team performance commonly displayed by staff) is what is of most interest. It is more likely to capture typical levels of performance in routine measurement in the work environment.
		• Maximal performance is more likely to be captured in contrived tasks and environments like simulations.

When
What is the best timing for measuring different constructs?
	• Relative to training sessions
	  – Pretraining
	  – During training
	  – After training
	• Frequency of measurement
		• A baseline measure is critical for interpreting most measures.
		• Different constructs will change at different rates and therefore should be measured at different frequencies.
		  – Behavior should be measured more frequently during the transfer phase to facilitate coaching and feedback. This can become less frequent over time, but should not go away completely.
		  – Results likely will change more slowly and can be measured less frequently.

(Continued)

Table 4.2   (Continued)

Type of Decision	Potential Options	Major Considerations
Who Who collects the data from whom, and who "makes sense" of it?	• Team members • Observers • Coaches	• Raters need expertise in the teamwork behaviors being trained and measured as well as an understanding of the clinical domain. • A system should be in place for developing observers (i.e., rater training and scoring guides). • A system should be in place for developing coaches to make use of team performance data (e.g., training in team facilitation skills). • Initially, team members may need external help in diagnosing and correcting team behaviors, but over time team members should take a bigger role in diagnosing their own performance.

How
What methods will be used?
	• Self-report
	• Observation
	  – Global rating scales
	  – Behaviorally Anchored Rating Scales (BARs)
	  – Behavior Observation Scales (BOSs)
	  – Frequency counts
	  – Event-based tools
		• Behavioral specificity
		  – How abstract or concrete are the measurement content and ratings scales?
		• Temporal resolution
		  – How much summating or collapsing across time are raters required to do?
		• Psychometric properties of the tools + rater training systems need to be established and monitored.

convergence is impeded. When feedback is the primary purpose, measurement must be able to help answer questions about a specific team and its members. If a team performed well, what specific behaviors were used appropriately? What needs to be reinforced? If a team performed poorly, what were the underlying reasons and what corrective feedback can be given or what additional learning activities are appropriate?

Implementation Evaluation

Team performance measurement plays an essential role in answering questions about whether or not a team training implementation is working, as well as what areas of that implementation need to be improved. Often, quality improvement initiatives require adaptation and fine tuning as they are implemented. Unforeseen problems arise, and having a measurement system in place to detect issues and help generate an understanding of why various aspects of the program may or may not be working is critical for rapid improvements. When implementation evaluation is the primary purpose, specific teams are no longer the focus (e.g., when providing feedback). Instead, trends in different aspects of teamwork across teams and across contexts (i.e., learning environment, on the job) must be understood. Measures used to provide feedback also can be used in an implementation evaluation, but a much broader view must be taken in the analysis and interpretation of the data.

WHAT CONTENT SHOULD BE MEASURED?

The content of a measurement tool is a representation of the attributes being measured; it is the "what you are measuring" aspect of the tool. This section deals with two aspects of content: teamwork competencies and multilevel training evaluation.

Teamwork Competencies

The content of a measurement tool used in team training should align as closely as possible to the content of the teamwork training program. That is, you measure what you are attempting to train or the behavior you are trying to change in the organization. This means that the teamwork competencies that form the content of the training program (i.e., the teamwork KSAs) also form the basis for measurement tool content. Consequently, clearly articulated teamwork KSAs and learning objectives facilitate the process of developing a teamwork performance measurement system.

There is a large and growing list of teamwork competencies. (For a recent and thorough review of the breadth of teamwork competencies, see Salas et al.).[13] Table 4.3 provides a brief overview of teamwork competencies and three general categories are described here.[21] *Team knowledge competencies* include shared mental models of the team, task, and environment; that is, team members should have a shared (or complimentary) understanding of the roles and responsibilities of other team members. This shared understanding helps team members coordinate their individual contributions. *Team skill competencies* include a wide variety of team process behaviors. Some prominent examples include communication, mutual performance monitoring, back-up behavior (or mutual support), and team leadership. *Team attitude competencies* include team orientation, mutual trust, and psychological safety. These competencies represent the emotions and attitudes that drive effective teamwork.

Multilevel Training Evaluation

To assess teamwork in the context of a training or change initiative, there are content areas to consider in addition to the teamwork KSAs. The multilevel training evaluation literature[22,23] offers a basic framework for the categories of content that should be attended to: reactions, learning, behavior, results, and return on investment. Measuring each of these levels represents a link in a chain of events that must occur to meet the overall objectives of increased quality and safety of care through teamwork. Each of these levels is briefly reviewed in the following.

Level 1—Reactions to training consist generally of what the learners thought of the training.[24] This content can be grouped into affective reactions (i.e., did the learners like or enjoy the training?) and utility judgments (i.e., did learners think that the training will be useful to them in their job?).[25] It has been shown that affective reactions to a training program do not correlate strongly with important outcomes such as learning and transfer.[25] That is, just because someone liked a training session, he or she may not apply what was learned or even have learned targeted competencies at all. However, utility judgments as well as ratings of self-efficacy (i.e., do learners feel confident in their abilities to perform the learned material?) do correlate with learning and behavior change.[25]

Level 2—Learning involves changes in the knowledge of trainees because of the training session. This includes immediate acquisition and retention of both declarative knowledge (e.g., how well did they learn the basic concepts or terminology?) and procedural knowledge or knowledge application (e.g., how well are they able to apply what they've learned appropriately?). For example, this includes assessments of how well people understand behaviors and principles of teamwork through traditional knowledge tests and demonstration of learned skills in various types of simulations. Of course, a training program will not be effective if the trainees do not acquire the basic knowledge; however, learning is necessary yet insufficient for producing behavior change on the actual unit. Consequently, transfer or behavior change must be measured.

Level 3—Behavior refers to transfer of the targeted competencies from the learning environment to the actual job. It is not just what the learners know or potentially *can* do, but the behaviors from the training that are *actually used on the job*.[23] This behavior change is the point at which many training implementations break down because organizational barriers can inhibit the transfer of learning to the workplace.[26]

Level 4—Results involve the final changes or impact the training program had on important organizational metrics such as efficiency, safety, and quality of care. In assessing the true effectiveness of a team training intervention, results are most frequently considered the gold standard (i.e., did the training improve safety and quality of care?). However, it is critical to assess the previous levels so

Table 4.3 Summary of Major Teamwork Competencies (KSAs)

KSAs	Description	Example Behavioral Markers	Example Citations
KNOWLEDGE			
Accurate and shared mental models (knowledge about team members and role structure, team task, and environment)	Organized knowledge structures of the relationships among task and team members	• Team members can recognize when other team members need information they have. • Team members anticipate and predict the needs of others. • Team members have compatible explanations of task information.	Cannon-Bowers & Salas, 1997; Klimoski & Mohammed, 1994; Artman, 2000; Stout, Cannon-Bowers, & Salas, 1996
Team mission, objective, norms, and resources	An understanding of the purpose, vision, and available means to meet team goals.	• Team members make compatible task prioritizations. • Team members agree on the methods adopted to reach their shared goals.	Cannon-Bowers, Tannenbaum, Salas, & Volpe, 1995; Marks, Mathieu, & Zaccaro, 2001
SKILLS			
Closed-loop communication	A pattern of information exchange characterized by three steps: a sender initiates a message, the receiver acknowledges the message, and the sender follows up to confirm that it was appropriately interpreted.	• Team members cross-check information with one another. • Team members give "big picture" updates to one another. • Team members proactively pass critical information to those that need it in a timely fashion.	Bowers, Jentsch, Salas, & Bruan, 1998; McIntyre & Salas, 1995; Smith-Jentsch, Johnston, & Payne, 1998
Mutual performance monitoring	Team members' ability to track what others on the team are doing while continuing to carry out their own tasks	• Team members recognize errors in their teammates' performance. • Team members have an accurate understanding of their teammates' workload.	McIntyre & Salas, 1995; Dickinson & McIntyre, 1997; Marks & Panzer, 2004
Backup/supportive behavior	The ability to shift and balance workload among team members during high-workload or high-pressure periods	• Team members promptly offer and accept task assistance. • Team members communicate the need for task assistance. • Team members redistribute the workload to members who are being underused.	Marks, Mathieu, & Zaccaro, 2000; McIntyre & Salas, 1995; Porter et al., 2003

Adaptability	The team's ability to adjust strategies to changing conditions.	• Team members replace or modify routine strategies when the task changes. • Team members detect important changes in their environment quickly. • Team members accurately assess the causes of important changes.	Burke, Stagl, Salas, Pierce, & Kendall, 2006; Entin & Serfaty, 1999; Kozlowski, Gully, Nason, & Smith, 1999
Conflict management/ resolution	Preemptively setting up conditions to prevent or control team conflict or reactively working through interpersonal disagreements between members	• Team members seek solutions to conflict wherein all members gain. • Team members discuss task-related conflict openly. • Team members find it acceptable to change positions and express doubts.	De Dreu & Weingart, 2003; Jordan & Troth, 2004; Simons & Peterson, 2000
Team leadership	Dynamic process of social problem solving involving information search and structuring, information use in problem solving, managing personnel resources, and managing material resources.	• Leaders develop plans and communicate them to the team • Leaders organize and delegate effectively based on the plan and changing work demands. • Leaders invite input from team members. • Leaders proactively facilitate the resolution controversy and conflict. • Team members accurately identify the person with the most appropriate skill set for leadership in a specific situation. • Team members shift leadership roles in response to task demands.	Burke, Stagl, Klein, Goodwin, Salas, & Halpin, 2006; Day, Gronn, & Salas, 2004
ATTITUDES Mutual trust	The shared belief among team members that everyone will perform their roles and protect the interests of their fellow team members	• Team members share information openly without fear of reprisals. • Team members are willing to admit mistakes. • Team members share a belief that team members will perform their tasks and roles.	Alavi & McCormick, 2004; Driskell & Salas, 1992; Jackson et al., 2006

(*Continued*)

Table 4.3 (Continued)

KSAs	Description	Example Behavioral Markers	Example Citations
Team/collective efficacy	The team members' sense of collective competence and their ability to achieve their goals.	• Team members share positive evaluations about the team's capacity to perform its tasks and meet its goals.	Bandura, 1986; Gibson, 2003; Katz-Navon, & Erez, 2005; Zaccaro et al., 1995
Team/collective orientation	Team members' preference for working with others as opposed to working in isolation	• Team members accept input from others and it is evaluated on its quality, not its source. • Team member value team goals over individual goals. • Team members have high levels of task involvement and participatory goal setting.	Alavi& McCormick, 2004; Eby & Dobbins, 1997; Mohammed & Angell, 2004
Psychological safety	The team members' shared belief that it is safe to take interpersonal risks	• Team members are interested in each other as people. • Team members are not rejected for being themselves. • Team members believe others on the team have positive intentions.	Edmondson, 1999

Source: Salas, E., Wilson, K. A., Murphy, C. E., King, H. B., & Salisbury, M. (2008). Communicating, coordinating, and cooperating when lives depend on it: Tips for teamwork. *Joint Commission Journal on Quality and Patient Safety, 34*(6). 333–41.

as to interpret the trends at Level 4 (e.g., are changes or lack thereof associated with true change in behavior or is something else happening on the unit?). A wide variety of organizational changes have been linked to teamwork training implementations, including changes in adverse event rates and composites of different adverse event rates (e.g., the Adverse Outcomes Index in Labor and Delivery; medication and transfusion error rates; staff perceptions of support; efficiency and reliability of processes).[27-31]

Level 5—Return on Investment (ROI) represents a "cost-effectiveness" estimate for the organization. That is, what are the financial benefits relative to the resources required to implement a training program? This is not frequently calculated; however, it can be powerful information for motivating hospital administrations. Given the high cost of medical errors, it is conceivable that avoiding just one high-cost medical error can justify the expense of an entire teamwork training implementation.

Other multilevel evaluation frameworks, such as Bloom's taxonomy or CIPP can be used in addition to or instead of the Kirkpatrick framework described in the preceding.[32,33] In addition to the described categories, it is useful to measure other factors associated with the effectiveness of a team training intervention (i.e., barriers and critical success factors) such as leadership support and opportunities to practice new behaviors[26] as well as other events on the unit that could potentially influence the effect of the training (e.g., staff turnover rates). Although these things do not directly measure teamwork, they can help to explain team performance measurement data. For example, if a multilevel training evaluation shows that trainee reactions are positive, learning was high, but there was no behavior change on the job, data on the presence or absence of critical success factors and barriers to implementation can generate insight into that pattern of results (e.g., was their front-line leadership support for the intervention?).

WHERE SHOULD PERFORMANCE BE EVALUATED?

Deciding where to evaluate performance is usually driven by the purpose of the measurement effort as well as practical considerations (e.g., available staff time, physical constraints of the space). Different locations can affect the measurement process in several ways. This section discusses two primary considerations for choosing locations and then describes three general types of locations and their impact on measurement.

Considerations for Choosing Locations: Control vs. Natural Variation, and Typical vs. Maximum Performance

First, different environments afford different levels of control and predictability of teamwork demands. For example, a simulation run in a dedicated simulation center allows for near-total control of the scenario and consequently highly predictable opportunities to observe teamwork behaviors.[34] This control can be leveraged into higher reliability (i.e., observers know when to look for what teamwork behaviors) and diagnostic capacity (i.e., scenarios can be designed to emphasize a specific teamwork competency) of observational measurement tools.[17] Often, the tradeoff with control is realism and natural variation; that is, in a controlled environment, you may not necessarily see the entire picture of how staff members are integrating teamwork into their daily routines.

Second, the location of measurement can influence whether typical or maximum performance is being measured.[35] Under certain circumstances (e.g., situations in which people know they are being assessed), people are more likely to perform at their highest level of ability (i.e., maximum performance) rather than the way they perform on a routine day-to-day basis (i.e., typical performance). It may be useful to know maximum performance during the initial acquisition of teamwork skills to ensure that team members have the capacity to perform as desired; however, it is ultimately the typical performance occurring every day on the unit that impacts safety and quality. Typical performance is more likely to be captured in unobtrusive observations on the job than in contrived performance episodes (e.g., simulations) or formal evaluations.

Types of Locations

Three general types of locations commonly used for team performance evaluation are discussed briefly in the following.

The *learning environment* includes class- or simulation-based activities. The defining feature is that the time and space are dedicated exclusively to learning and improvement activities. In general, learning environments offer the most control over the environment. Measuring trainee reactions and learning is appropriate in this setting. Although there has been no systematic research on this topic in healthcare, simulations may be particularly useful for assessing the maximum performance of team members and providing feedback. However, to assess behavior change on the job (i.e., typical performance), data collection must occur in other locations.

On the Job measurements of team performance can be methodologically challenging, but also provide the greatest opportunity for assessing the actual or typical level of teamwork being displayed on a day-to-day basis. The variation in teamwork demands (e.g., fluctuations in patient volume, complexity or difficulty of specific cases) complicates the process of assessing the effectiveness of a team. However, observation and self-report methods can be used to reliably detect team performance differences on actual clinical units.[36,37]

Hybrid approaches include in situ or in vivo simulations. These events create a compromise between the control of a pure simulation and the realism of on-the-job performance. These events can vary in how they are implemented, but essentially involve running a scripted simulation scenario in an actual clinical context.[38] There are tradeoffs with this approach as well. Most notably, there is less control over the environment in these sessions than in dedicated center–based simulation sessions. Additionally, the competing demands of patient care may call learners away from the activity before it is completed. However, in situ approaches provide a chance for team members to practice their new skills in on the unit *and* in a safe environment (i.e., patient safety is not at risk). Additionally, in situ events offer an opportunity for going beyond training teamwork competencies and identifying and correcting system issues on the unit.

WHEN SHOULD PERFORMANCE BE ASSESSED AND DIAGNOSED?

This section focuses on temporal issues in measuring teamwork to facilitate learning or evaluate implementations and change. Subsequently, some general temporal issues are discussed. More specifics on the timing of measurements are discussed in the general strategies section.

Facilitating Learning

When focusing on providing feedback to learners, decisions about when to assess and diagnose performance must be driven by considerations of how best to support learning. Timeliness (in addition to accuracy and specificity) makes feedback effective.[20] Consequently, the assessment and diagnosis of performance should be completed as quickly after a team performance episode as possible so that the experience is fresh in the minds of team members. Event-based measurement tools are helpful in simulation-based environments for this exact reason.[34,39] This approach to measurement design anchors opportunities of measure specific teamwork behaviors to simulation scenario events (critical or trigger events) that represent opportunities for team members to display the targeted behavior. Event-based tools provide a descriptive and process-focused way of capturing performance. Outside of a simulated environment, coaches need measurement tools that can help them structure observations and provide timely feedback. These protocols are more challenging and may involve more structured qualitative data collection as well.

Assessing Change and Implementation Evaluation

There are two main types of temporal decisions to make when designing an implementation evaluation: (1) when, relative to the actual training, should different constructs be measured? and (2) how frequently should different constructs be measured? Both of these questions rely on the purpose of measurement (i.e., what question is being asked?) as well as the nature of the construct being measured. Different constructs can be expected to change at different rates.[40]

Figure 4.1 provides an example timeline for the first four levels of a training evaluation relative to training actually being implemented. Conceptually, it only makes sense to measure Level 1 reactions immediately after a training session because learners

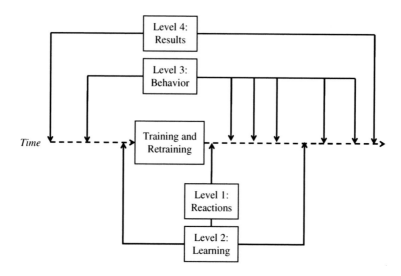

Figure 4.1
Example timeline for a team training implementation evaluation illustrating different times before and after training in which collecting different types of data can provide useful information.

have nothing to react to before that point in time. Level 2 learning can be assessed after a training session when compared with some standard (e.g., all learners should score above some criteria on a knowledge test) or the post scores can be compared with a measure of knowledge taken before training.

Three important aspects of measuring Level 3 are illustrated in Figure 4.1. First, a pretraining or baseline measure of teamwork behaviors is necessary to understand the impact of a training program; otherwise, it will be unclear the degree or type of changes in behavior a training produced on the unit. Second, the frequency of measuring Level 3 immediately after training should be high so as to generate the information needed to support coaching and facilitate transfer. However, as time progresses and after initial success of transferring teamwork skills to the unit, the measurement of Level 3 can become less frequent. However it should not drop off entirely because information will likely still be needed to detect and avoid skill decay or other issues that can erode the improvements achieved. Level 4 constructs usually change at a much slower rate than behaviors. Measures of things like safety culture, staff satisfaction, patient satisfaction, and quality and safety are: (1) influenced by levels of teamwork (among many other things), and (2) provide less detailed information

about what specific behaviors need to be improved. Consequently, these constructs can be measured less frequently than Level 3. Of course, training is usually not a single point in time as illustrated in Figure 4.1, but an ongoing process. However, the same framework illustrated in Figure 4.1 can be applied around multiple training sessions.

General Temporal Issues

Self-report measures of teamwork (e.g., attitudes toward teamwork, perceptions of teamwork) are susceptible to the referent or response shift bias,[41,42] as are all self-report measures used to assess training and learning. This means that changes in a learner's ratings may result from changes in his or her internal understanding of what is being rated rather than changes in the level of that construct. For example, if someone is asked to rate perceptions of teamwork before and after training, he or she may have a radically different understanding of what teamwork is at the separate rating times. In a sense, he or she would be rating two different things. Retrospective posttest measures are an alternative to using pre- and post-implementations of self-report measures; however, these methods are vulnerable to a different set of biases. Interested readers are referred to other sources for a more comprehensive review of these issues.[43]

HOW IS TEAM PERFORMANCE MEASURED?

Within the present context, there are two general categories of methods for gathering team performance data: self-report, and observation. Table 4.4 summarizes some of the main methods, including a description and discussion of strengths, challenges, and limitations as well as examples from the literature. These are described briefly in the following.

Self-Report

Self-report methods involve asking team members to provide ratings about themselves as individuals, the team, or the entire facility. These methods can be used to collect a broad range of measures of team performance–related constructs. It is well suited for capturing the attitude competencies (e.g., mutual trust, belief in the importance of teamwork, collective orientation, psychological safety) because these constructs are inherently subjective in nature. However, self-report methods are applied to perceptions of teamwork and team performance as well (e.g., the Mayo High Performance Teamwork Scale;[44] TeamSTEPPS Teamwork Attitudes Questionnaire, http://teamstepps.ahrq.gov/about-toolsmaterials.htm). The limitations of self-report methods for assessing performance or competence are broadly recognized.[45,46] Specifically, there is a tendency for self-perceptions of performance to be inflated (i.e., the "Lake Wobegon effect"), and this tendency is greater for novices in a domain than it is for experts.[47] This means that respondents with lower levels of competence with teamwork behaviors will be more likely to have inflated self-ratings. This creates challenges when attempting to detect change; that is, self-perceptions can shift downward as people increase in skill. (This is related to the response shift bias described in the preceding). However, survey-based knowledge tests are highly appropriate for evaluating team knowledge competencies such as knowledge about the team role structure.

Observation

Observation remains the primary method to obtain an objective measure of a team's level of performance.[48] There are four primary approaches to scoring team behaviors in observational measurement tools, each of which can capture some aspect of quality or quantity of teamwork behaviors. These include global rating scales, behaviorally anchored rating scales (BARSs), behavioral observation scales (BOSs), and event-based tools.[49,50] A description, summary of strengths and challenges, as well as examples from the literature are provided in Table 4.4. However, two properties of measurement scales can be useful in understanding the differences and deciding which tool to use: *behavioral specificity*, and *temporal resolution/granularity*. These factors greatly affect the psychometric properties of the tools as well as the utility of the data produced.

First, different approaches capture teamwork competencies at different levels of descriptive behavioral specificity, with some being highly abstract and others being much more concrete. For example, a global rating scale may ask a rater to score the team's overall level of communication on a Likert scale ranging from highly effective to highly ineffective. This represents the content in a very abstract way as it does not specify exactly what communication is or what effective and ineffective communication are. BARSs increase the behavioral specificity by using concrete descriptions of teamwork behavior as a part of the actual ratings scale.

Second, the temporal resolution or granularity of a tool refers to the degree of summation or collapsing across time that raters are required to undertake. For example, a global rating scale usually uses one rating per dimension to capture a team's performance in an entire performance episode. However, communication quality or quantity can vary greatly over the course of a single performance episode (e.g., one case). Ratings that collapse or summate across time like this can be thought of as having a low temporal resolution; that is, they do not provide insight into the variations in performance over time. In contrast, an event-based tool captures the level of performance at different points in time and consequently provides a more fine-grained view of how performance processes (e.g., communication) unfold

Table 4.4 Summary of Team Performance Measurement Methods

Measurement Tool Type	Description	Strengths/Challenges and Limitations	Example Citations
Self-report	Questionnaires administered to each team member individually and then aggregated in some manner to represent a team score	*Strengths* • Self-report methods are the best technique for capturing *affective teamwork competencies* (e.g., collective efficacy, mutual trust, etc.) as well as *knowledge teamwork competencies* (e.g., knowledge about role structure) *Challenges and Limitations* • Self-report of the perceptions of teamwork can be subject to a number biases (e.g., referent shift bias). • Aggregating individual responses to the team level can be challenging.	Malec et al., 2007; Smith-Jentsch, 2008
Global Ratings Scale	Observational protocol that asks raters to use a Likert scale to rate the quality of a given teamwork dimension	*Strengths* • This type of rating is familiar to people and on the surface is very simple to use. *Challenges and Limitations* • Can be difficult to achieve interrater reliability because the rating scales tend to be generic and abstract (e.g., rating "communication" as a whole). • Usually one score is given for an entire performance episode; however, performance fluctuates (i.e., sometimes things are done well, other times they are not) and raters must summate across time, which can create challenges for maintaining interrater reliability.	Hohenhaus, Powell, & Haskins, 2008
Behaviorally Anchored Ratings Scale	Observer rating protocol that provides brief descriptions of teamwork behaviors as anchors for each rating dimension	*Strengths* • The ratings scales are more concrete and descriptive than general Likert anchors (e.g., highly effective to highly ineffective), which helps to facilitate a common frame of reference for different raters. *Challenges and Limitations* • BARS require raters to summate over time; that is, they provide one rating of a team performance dimension (e.g., communication) for a specified period of time (e.g., an entire performance episode or phase of performance) even though performance may vary within that time period.	Kendall & Salas, 2003; Murphy & Pardaffy, 1989

(Continued)

Table 4.4 (Continued)

Measurement Tool Type	Description	Strengths/Challenges and Limitations	Example Citations
Behavior Observation Scale	Observer rating protocol using a Likert-type scale to rate the frequency of teamwork behaviors	*Strengths* • Produces a rating of a team's typical level of performance over time *Challenges and Limitations* • These tools require raters to estimate the frequency of teamwork behaviors and therefore may be susceptible to primacy and recency effects.	Salas et al., 2008; Tziner, Joanis, & Murphy, 2000
Frequency Counts	Observational protocol that requires the rater to count the number of times a specific team behavior occurs	*Strengths* • If the behaviors being looked for are specific enough, it is usually relatively easy to train observers to detect the targeted teamwork behaviors. *Challenges and Limitations* • It is difficult to develop and maintain interrater reliability of "misses" (i.e., instances in which a specific teamwork behavior should have occurred, but did not). The miss count is important for understanding the big picture of a team's performance.	Frankel et al., 2007; Weaver et al., 2010
Event-based Tools	Observational protocol consisting of behavioral checklists linked to simulation scenario "trigger events," learning objectives, and teamwork competencies	*Strengths* • Maintains linkages between opportunities to measure (i.e., scenario events), targeted teamwork behaviors, and learning objectives. • Focuses the observer's attention on predefined events and concrete behaviors. *Challenges and Limitations* • This method almost exclusively limited to use in simulation as it requires that observers be able to predict events in the environment. • Measurement tools are specific to each simulation scenario.	Fowlkes et al., 1998; Rosen et al., 2008; Lazzara et al., in press

Source: Rosen, M. A., Salas, E., Wu, T. S., Silvestri, S., Lazzara, E. H., Lyons, R., et al. (2008) Promoting teamwork: An event-based approach to simulation-based teamwork training for emergency medicine residents. *Academic Emergency Medicine, 15*(11), 1190–8.

over time. In general, higher levels of temporal resolution are useful for diagnosing performance and providing developmental feedback. Tools with lower temporal resolution are better suited for summative assessments such as overall effectiveness of a teamwork implementation. These tools can indicate the presence or absence of a problem, but do not provide much insight into the causes of those problems or how to correct them.

The different measurement approaches described here generally can be implemented in different ways: (1) global rating scales tend to be highly abstract when it comes to behavioral description and require raters to summate across time; (2) BARSs tend to be more behaviorally specific, but still require raters to summate across time to a large degree; (3) BOSs tend to have higher levels of both behavioral specificity and temporal resolution; and (4) event-based methods tend to be highly specific in terms of behavioral description and have a fine-grained temporal resolution as measurements are tied to specific events. Regardless of the specific method of capturing team performance, the basic psychometric properties of the tool should be established and monitored (i.e., reliability and validity evidence).

WHO SHOULD MEASURE, ASSESS, AND DIAGNOSE PERFORMANCE?

A broad range of people within a healthcare organization as well as external personnel are potentially capable of assessing and diagnosing team performance. When observational measurement tools are used, the reliability and validity of measurements are properties of both the tool *and* the observer. There are three basic issues to consider when selecting and preparing observers and raters of team performance in healthcare. First, they should have a deep understanding of the concepts of teamwork. They must understand the behaviors that are being measured. Second, they must be versed in the clinical domain in which the evaluation is taking place. They do not need to be clinical experts, but they need an understanding of the terminology being used and the tasks being performed. Third, they must be well trained in the specific measurement tools in use. Here rater training and other tools such as a scoring guide are essential to clarify the concepts and scoring rules.

All observers should be systematically trained and the reliability of their ratings assessed. Interrater reliability can be established using videos of team performance episodes.

GENERAL STRATEGIES FOR TEAMWORK IMPLEMENTATION

The preceding discussion represents a broad picture of the options and considerations involved in designing a team performance measurement system. Goal-oriented measurement is critical for improving team performance in a clinical setting. A teamwork training program is most effective if a few general measurement strategies are followed for each of the essential implementation phases of: (1) supporting *initial acquisition* of teamwork KSAs, (2) ensuring *transfer* of learned behaviors to the job, and (3) promoting *sustainment and continuous improvement* over time.

Initial Acquisition of Teamwork Knowledge, Skills, and Attitudes

Measurement can be a valuable tool in guiding staff members as they are first exposed to and develop basic teamwork competencies in didactic and practice-based learning activities. The following three strategies are particularly useful at this phase of implementation.

Root measures in the teamwork competencies targeted for acquisition and specific learning objectives. Clarity and specificity in the design of a team training program (i.e., clear teamwork competencies, specific learning objectives) translate into a clear specification of the content of the team performance measurement system. It defines both the competencies and the criteria for evaluation (i.e., the expectations for what good and poor team performance look like). By making the connections between training and measurement content, feedback to learners can be facilitated as well (i.e., the behavior targeted for change by the training is also the behavior captured by the measurement system driving feedback to learners).

Focus on measuring concrete teamwork behaviors. Focusing on concrete teamwork behaviors is critical for two main reasons. First, learning is greatly facilitated by the provision of timely, specific, and process-oriented feedback. This process is supported when measures are behaviorally descriptive and capture variations in performance over time (i.e., have a fine-grained temporal resolution). These types of measurement tools capture the team's performance in a way that can be quickly translated into feedback. Second, the process of building and maintaining high levels of interrater reliability for identifying specific teamwork behaviors requires less judgment on the part of the observers than more abstract ratings.

Take advantage of the high levels of control in learning environments. Simulation-based training is a critical delivery strategy and should be part of a team training program.[26] With a tightly controlled learning environment, measurement tools with high behavioral specificity and temporal granularity (e.g., event-based tools) can be developed in conjunction with low- and high-fidelity practice-based learning activities.[34] This provides the highest-level opportunities for practice-based learning and also provides important opportunities for high-quality assessment of the effectiveness of initial teamwork training.

Transfer

In addition to the previous strategies, the following three are useful for bridging the gap between the learning and work environments.

Measure behavior frequently enough to influence behavior. In contrast to many areas of science, in which the intent of measurement is to capture what happens without interfering or changing what is happening, measurement in change initiatives has the explicit purpose of influencing what is happening in the organization. This requires frequent measurement to provide specific feedback as well as to send the implicit message that the intervention is taken seriously by the organization. As behavior change is realized, the frequency of measurement can be adjusted as needed.

Measure the factors that influence transfer. In addition to actual team performance, a systematic assessment of the real and perceived barriers to transfer on the unit[13] should be generated. This information can guide other interventions (e.g., leadership engagement efforts, organizational culture on the unit, staff turnover) critical to realizing improvements in team performance on the unit.

Develop observers and coaches. In addition to the actual measurement instruments, the human components of the team performance measurement system require attention and development. Specifically, observers must be trained to reliably collect data. The impact of any measurement system is capped by the quality of the data, and, in the present context, observers play a large role in the quality of the data. Additionally, coaches must be developed so they can interpret and use the data to develop teams. This can include training in team facilitation.

Sustainment and Continuous Improvement

Making an initial improvement in the quality of teamwork and ultimately in patient care requires a substantial investment in time and resources by an organization. The following three strategies can help to ensure this investment is not lost over time.

Take a longitudinal approach. It can be difficult to maintain vigilance, attention, and interest in any given change initiative over time. Staff members are routinely confronted with new safety and quality programs. Sustained measurement, however, can both indicate to staff of the importance of the initiative as well as provide information on how to sustain and improve performance (e.g., are there any teamwork competencies that need refresher trainings?).

Make connections across levels. Connecting behavior change on the unit to important results (e.g., quality, safety, staff and patient satisfaction, culture change) can help maintain motivation and enthusiasm for the implementation. Additionally, drawing distinctions among individual, team, and unit-level performance and measuring at each of those levels provides insight into a broader range of factors that ultimately contribute to unit-level effectiveness (e.g., is a safety issue resulting from a lack of technical skill, a deficient work process, or team performance issues?). This information then can be used to guide the development of not only the team training intervention, but also other complimentary quality and safety initiatives.

Shift the "locus of assessment and diagnosis" over time from external to internal. As team members mature in their proficiency and understanding of teamwork, they should play a more central role in the measurement and diagnosis of their team's performance (i.e., they should become "self-learning" teams).[51] Staff resources external to the team (e.g., coaches, external observers) available for measuring and diagnosing team performance will always be limited. Consequently, team members themselves must engage in continuous improvement and coaching of their own team performance behaviors.

In addition to the three phases described in the preceding, team performance measurement can be highly useful in the developmental or preplanning phases of designing a teamwork training intervention. Here, observations of performance on the unit can be used to detect potential areas in which team training can be used to improve the unit's overall performance. These data should be combined with other sources of information collection in a training needs analysis.

CONCLUDING REMARKS

This chapter has attempted to cover a broad range of methods, applications, issues, and considerations in developing and implementing team performance measurement. In general, measuring team performance is complicated, especially within large dynamic organizations such as healthcare systems. However, it is a manageable task and an investment that can potentially pay off with more effective team training interventions and ultimately safer and higher quality care.

REFERENCES

1. Brannick, M. T., Salas, E., & Prince, C. (Eds.). (1997). *Team performance assessment and measurement: Theory, methods, and applications.* Mahwah, NJ: LEA.
2. Heinemann, G. D., & Zeiss, A. M. (Eds.). (2002). *Team performance in healthcare: Assessment and development.* New York: Kluwer Academic.
3. Kozlowski, S. W. J., & Ilgen, D. R. (2006). Enhancing the effectiveness of work groups and teams. *Psychological Science in the Public Interest, 7*(3), 77–124.
4. Salas, E., Cooke, N. J., & Rosen, M. A. (2008). On teams, teamwork and team performance: Discoveries and developments. *Human Factors, 50*(3), 540–7.
5. Salas, E., & Cannon-Bowers, J. A. (2000). The anatomy of team training. In S. Tobias & J. D. Fletcher (Eds.), *Training & retraining: A handbook for business, industry, government, and the military* (pp. 312–55). New York: Macmillan Reference.
6. Hackman, J. R., & Wageman, R. (2005). A theory of team coaching. *Academy of Management Review, 30*(2), 269–87.
7. Salas, E., Weaver, S. J., Rosen, M. A., & Smith-Jentsch, K. A. (2009). Managing team performance in complex settings: Research-based best practices. In J. W. Smither & M. London (Eds.), *Performance management: Putting research into practice* (pp. 197–232). San Francisco: Jossey-Bass.
8. Dyer, J. L. (1984). Team research and team training: A state of the art review. In F. A. Muckler (Ed.), *Human factors review* (pp. 285–323). Santa Monica, CA: Human Factors Society.
9. Salas, E., Dickinson, T., Converse, S., & Tannenbaum, S. (1992). Toward an understanding of team performance and training. In R. Swezey & E. Salas (Eds.), *Teams: Their training and performance.* Norwood, NJ: Ablex Publishing.
10. Humphrey, S. E., Morgeson, F. P., & Mannor, M. J. (2009). Developing a theory of the strategic core of teams: A role composition model of team performance. *Journal of Applied Psychology, 94*(1), 48–61.
11. Salas, E., Stagl, K. C., Burke, C. S., & Goodwin, G. F. (2007). Fostering team effectiveness in organizations: Toward an integrative theoretical framework of team performance. In R. A. Dienstbier, J. W. Shuart, W. Spaulding, & J. Poland (Eds.), *Modeling complex systems: Motivation, cognition and social processes, Nebraska Symposium on Motivation,* Vol. 51. (pp. 185–243). Lincoln, NE: University of Nebraska Press.
12. Salas, E., Wilson, K. A., Murphy, C. E., King, H. B., & Salisbury, M. (2008). Communicating, coordinating, and cooperating when lives depend on it: Tips for teamwork. *Joint Commission Journal on Quality and Patient Safety, 34*(6), 333–41.
13. Salas, E., Rosen, M. A., Burke, C. S., & Goodwin, G. F. (2009). The wisdom of collectives in organizations: An update of the teamwork competencies. In E. Salas, G. F. Goodwin & C. S. Burke (Eds.), *Team effectiveness in complex*

organizations: Cross-disciplinary perspectives and approaches (pp. 39–79). New York: Routledge.

14. Salas, E., Sims, D. E., & Burke, C. S. (2005). Is there a big five in teamwork? *Small Group Research, 36*(5), 555–99.

15. Hackman, J. R. (1987). The design of work teams. In J. Lorsch (Ed.), *Handbook of organizational behavior* (pp. 315–42). New York: Prentice-Hall.

16. Nunnally, J. C., & Bernstein, I. H. (1994). *Psychometric theory*, 3rd ed. New York: McGraw-Hill.

17. Salas, E., Rosen, M. A., Burke, C. S., Nicholson, D., & Howse, W. R. (2007). Markers for enhancing team cognition in complex environments: The power of team performance diagnosis. *Aviation, Space, and Environmental Medicine. Special Supplement on Operational Applications of Cognitive Performance Enhancement Technologies, 78*(5), B77–85.

18. Swing, S. R. (2002). Assessing the ACGME general competencies: General considerations and assessment methods. *Academy of Emerging Medicine, 9*(11), 1278–88.

19. Ericsson, K. A., Krampe, R. T., & Tesch-Romer, C. (1993). The role of deliberate practice in the acquisition of expert performance. *Psychological Review, 100*(3), 363–406.

20. London, M. (2003). *Job feedback: Giving, seeking, and using feedback for performance improvement*, 2nd ed. Mahwah, NJ: LEA.

21. Cannon-Bowers, J., Tannenbaum, S. I., Salas, E., & Volpe, C. E. (1995). Defining team competencies and establishing team training requirements. In R. Guzzo, & Salas, E. (Ed.), *Team effectiveness and decision making in organizations* (pp. 330–80). San Francisco: Jossey-Bass.

22. Kraiger, K., Ford, J. K., & Salas, E. (1993). Application of cognitive, skill-based, and affective theories of learning outcomes to new methods of training evaluation. *Journal of Applied Psychology, 78*(2), 311–28.

23. Kirkpatrick, D. L., & Kirkpatrick, J. D. (2006). *Evaluating training programs*. San Francisco: Berrett-Koehler.

24. Goldstein, I. L., & Ford, K. (2001). *Training in organizations: Needs assessment, development, and evaluation*, 4th ed. New York: Wadsworth.

25. Alliger, G. M., Tannenbaum, S. I., Bennett, W., Traver, H., & Shotland, A. (1997). A meta-analysis of the relations among training criteria. *Personnel Psychology, 50*, 341–58.

26. Salas, E., Almeida, S. A., Salisbury, M., King, H. B., Lazzara, E. H., Lyons, R., et al. (2009). What are the critical success factors for team training in health care? *Joint Commission Journal on Quality and Patient Safety, 35*(8), 398–405.

27. Mann, S., Pratt, S. D., Gluck, P. A., Nielsen, P. E., Risser, D., Greenberg, P., et al. (2006). Assessing quality in obstetrical care: Development of standardized measures. *Joint Commission Journal on Quality and Patient Safety, 32*(9), 497–505.

28. Deering, S., Rosen, M. A., Ludi, V., Munroe, M., Pocrnich, A., Leaky, C., et al. (2011). On the front lines of patient safety: Implementation and evaluation of team training in Iraq. *British Medical Journal, 37*(8), 350–6.

29. Morey, J. C., Simone, R., Jay, G. D., Wears, R. L., Salisbury, M., Dukes, K. A., et al. (2002). Error reduction and performance improvement in the Emergency Department through formal teamwork training: Evaluation results of the MedTeams project. *Health Services Research, 37*(6), 1553–81.

30. Nielsen, P. E., Goldman, M. B., Mann, S., Shapiro, D. E., Marcus, R. G., Pratt, S. D., et al. (2007). Effects of teamwork training on adverse outcomes and process of care in labor and delivery: A randomized controlled trial. *Obstetrics and Gynecology, 109*(1), 48–55.

31. Taylor, C. R., Hepworth, J. T., Buerhaus, P. I., Dittus, R., & Speroff, T. (2007). Effect of crew resource management on diabetes care and patient outcomes in an inner-city primary care clinic. *Quality and Safety in Health Care, 16*, 244–7.

32. Anderson, L. W., Krathwohl, D. R., Airasian, P. W., Cruikshank, K. A., Mayer, R. E., Pintrich, P. R., et al. (2001). *A taxonomy for learning, teaching, and assessing: Revision of boom's taxonomy of educational objectives*. New York: Longman.

33. Farley, D. O., & Battles, J. B. (2008). Evaluation of the AHRQ Patient Safety Initiative: Framework and approach. *Health Services Research, 44*(2), 628–45.

34. Rosen, M. A., Salas, E., Wu, T. S., Silvestri, S., Lazzara, E. H., Lyons, R., et al. (2008). Promoting teamwork: An event-based approach to simulation-based teamwork training for emergency medicine residents. *Academic Emergency Medicine, 15*(11), 1190–8.

35. Sackett, P. R., Zedeck, S., & Fogli, L. (1988). Relations between measures of typical and

maximum job performance. *Journal of Applied Psychology, 73*(3), 482–6.

36. Weaver, S. L., Rosen, M. A., DiazGranados, D., Lazzara, E. H., Lyons, R., Salas, E., et al. (2010). Does teamwork improve performance in the operating room? A multilevel evaluation. *Joint Commission Journal on Quality and Patient Safety, 36*(3), 133–42.

37. Undre, S., Healey, A., & Vincent, C. A. (2006). Observational assessment of surgical teamwork: A feasibility study. *World Journal of Surgery, 30*, 1774–83.

38. Forrest, F. C. (2008). Mobile simulation. In R. H. Riley (Ed.), *Manual of simulation in healthcare* (pp. 25–33). Oxford, England: Oxford University Press.

39. Fowlkes, J. E., Dwyer, D. J., Oser, R. L., & Salas, E. (1998). Event-based approach to training (EBAT). *The International Journal of Aviation Psychology, 8*(3), 209–21.

40. Mitchell, T. R., & James, L. R. (2001). Building better theory: Time and the specification of when things happen. *Academy of Management Review, 25*(4), 530–47.

41. Howard, G. S., & Dailey, P. R. (1979). Response-shift bias: A source of contamination of self-report measures. *Journal of Applied Psychology, 64*(2), 144–50.

42. Sprangers, M., & Hoogstraten, J. (1989). Pretesting effects in retrospective pretest-posttest designs. *Journal of Applied Psychology, 74*(2), 265–72.

43. Griner-Hill, L., & Betz, D. L. (2005). Revisiting the retrospective pretest. *American Journal of Evaluation, 26*(4), 501–17.

44. Malec, J. F., Torsher, L. C., Dunn, W. F., Wiegmann, D. A., Arnold, J. J., Brown, D. A., et al. (2007). The Mayo High Performance Teamwork Scale: Reliability and validity for evaluating key crew resource management skills. *Simulation in Healthcare, 2*(1), 4–10.

45. Dunning, D., Johnson, K., Ehrlinger, J., & Kruger, J. (2003). Why people fail to recognize their own incompetence. *Current Directions in Psychological Science, 12*(3), 83–7.

46. Hodges, B., Regehr, G., & Martin, D. (2001). Difficulties in recognizing one's own incompetence: Novice physicians who are unskilled and unaware of it. *Academic Medicine, 76*, S87–89.

47. Kruger, J., & Dunning, D. (1999). Unskilled and unaware of it: how difficulties in recognizing one's own incompetence lead to inflated self-assessments. *Journal of Personality and Social Psychology, 77*(6), 1221–34.

48. Cannon-Bowers, J. A., Burns, J. J., Salas, E., & Pruitt, J. S. (1998). Advanced Technology in Scenario-based Training. In J. A. Cannon-Bowers & E. Salas (Eds.), *Making Decisions Under Stress* (pp. 365–374). Washington, DC: American Psychological Association.

49. Kendall, D. L., & Salas, E. (2004). Measuring team performance: Review of current methods and consideration of future needs. In J. W. Ness, Tepe, V., & Ritzer, D. (Ed.), *The science and simulation of human performance* (pp. 307–26). Boston: Elsevier.

50. Salas, E., Rosen, M. A., Held, J. D., & Weissmuller, J. J. (2009). Performance measurement in simulation-based training: A review and best practices. *Simulation & Gaming: An Interdisciplinary Journal, 40*(3), 328–76.

51. Smith-Jentsch, K. A., Johnston, J. A., & Payne, S. C. (1998). Measuring team-related expertise in complex environments. In J. A. Cannon-Bowers & E. Salas (Eds.), *Making decisions under stress: Implications for individual and team training* (pp. 61–87). Washington, DC: American Psychological Association.

5

EDUCATING HEALTHCARE PROVIDERS TO PROMOTE TEAMWORK: ISSUES, REQUIREMENTS, AND GUIDELINES

Karen Frush, Gwen Sherwood, Melanie C. Wright, and Noa Segall

INTRODUCTION

The problem of unintended harm to patients who seek healthcare services, described by the Institute of Medicine (IOM) report a full decade ago, remains a major challenge.[1] Despite rigorous training and preparation of physicians, nurses, pharmacists and other healthcare professionals, thousands of Americans still suffer and die every year from preventable mistakes in their care.[2] These mistakes are often caused by systems failures, and the design of safer systems is critical to the prevention of medical errors in today's highly complex healthcare environment. In addition, mounting evidence suggests that healthcare culture plays a critically important role in the safety of patients, and effective teamwork has been linked to patient outcomes such as healthcare acquired infections and better surgical outcomes.[3-5]

Despite this evidence, there is a paucity of training in teamwork and communication throughout the curricula of the health professions. Most experienced clinicians never received formal training in teamwork, and many times they are not even aware of their own personal behaviors that impede effective communication. Students and young professionals,

who have not yet been influenced by the "traditional" healthcare culture of autonomy and individual expertise, may be ideal candidates for team training. The hope of leaders in teamwork and patient safety is that these "next generation" providers can then become change agents among more seasoned clinicians when they enter the health professions workforce.[6]

In this chapter, we will describe some current programs and efforts to provide teamwork training to practicing physicians, nurses, and other healthcare professionals. We'll also discuss efforts to integrate this training into the curricula of health professions schools, and describe competency requirements that support such training.

TEAM TRAINING FOR CLINICIANS

There is clear evidence of a link between good teamwork behaviors and effective team performance in a variety of work environments. In healthcare in particular, there is growing evidence to suggest a link between good teamwork behaviors and good clinical performance, and between good teamwork and improved patient outcomes.[3-5] In a recent simulation study at Duke University, for example, there was a positive correlation between behaviorally anchored observer ratings of medical student teamwork skills and performance of critical clinical tasks in an emergent care scenario.[7] Unfortunately, however, it is unclear whether or not we can truly influence teamwork behaviors through training and, if so, what forms of training are most effective.[8] Still to be answered are key questions such as what content to teach, what teaching methods have the most benefit, and how was it evaluated. Overall, there is still much to learn regarding how to implement a feasible training program that leads to measurable changes in clinicians' behavior and improvements in patient outcomes.[9]

It is tempting to simply initiate team training in a clinical area without thoroughly assessing the environmental context. To achieve lasting improvement, however, Salas et al. identified seven critical evidence-based success factors that should be considered when planning and implementing teamwork improvement training.[10] Leaders must match training goals with the organizations goals, assure organizational support, secure front line champions, prepare the environment, acquire resources, assure skills can be applied in the setting, and assess outcomes. Too often, training is initiated without addressing these factors, and despite the best efforts and hard work of trainers, the project's goals are not reached.

Some hospitals have implemented team training in the form of crisis resource management (CRM), using high fidelity human patient simulation.[11,12] Training in this environment provides a great deal of realism and interactivity that supports the development of teamwork skills such as leadership, assertiveness, and mutual support. Modern theories of adult learning highlight the value of interactivity, immediate feedback, integration of experience, and placing information in context.[13] Using high fidelity simulation, individuals can participate in crisis scenarios as multidisciplinary teams and undergo targeted individual instruction through video-taping of their performance and debriefing by qualified instructors. There is some preliminary evidence to support the effectiveness of simulation-based training of team coordination skills.[11]

The major problem with team training using high fidelity patient simulation is that it is both costly and time consuming. Programs are limited in the total

number of trainees who can participate and the specific medical topics they address. Teamwork and communication problems are prevalent throughout all of healthcare, in environments as varied as the operating room, intermediate-care hospital units, and the primary care setting. Individuals who would benefit from team training skills range from surgeons and anesthesiologists to nurse aids and technicians to medical and nursing students. In addition, some research suggests that for team training programs to be effective, they must be implemented on a recurrent basis.[14] Training programs that have instructor to trainee ratios on the order of 1 to 5 and can cost as much as $5,000 per day[11] are simply not feasible for the numbers of individuals that would benefit from training. Although simulation resources are expanding, the resources in terms of simulation center time and trained educators simply don't exist to accommodate the training need.

Because of these practical problems, programs are being developed in healthcare practices across the country, which implement more traditional didactic approaches to team training.[15–17] Within this movement, there is appreciation for the need to develop interactive and engaging training that allows trainees to practice teamwork behaviors.[18] Therefore, approaches to teaching larger groups of trainees also incorporate a wide variety of teaching techniques such as computer-based instruction, small-group sessions with role plays, analysis of video-taped teamwork scenarios, and workplace practice experiences.[16,19] Preliminary evaluations of these approaches provide some support for their effectiveness in improving trainees' knowledge and attitudes about teamwork.[16,19] Additionally, there is some evidence of improvements in behaviors and patient outcomes when the training program involves engaging individuals in the clinical unit, training clinicians in the unit as coaches for continued education, and incorporating process-related improvements identified by individuals being trained.[20]

Based on these experiences, key issues consistent with those described by Salas[10] may influence the success of training for clinicians. First, it is critical that leadership in clinical units be supportive of teamwork training. If leaders do not value and reinforce the principles being taught, success is unlikely. Second, teamwork training seems to have greater likelihood of success when there are local (e.g., on the unit) champions of the effort who will support and reinforce the lessons learned. And last, team training has the most positive impact when participants use principles of effective communication to make positive process changes to support effective teamwork locally. Examples may include ideas such as (1) the development of a "ticket to ride" with critical patient transfer details, (2) the use of white boards to share team member names, or (3) clarification of policies regarding key data to be communicated in hand-offs. Although it is not yet clear whether teamwork training is successful in changing personal generalizable behaviors (e.g., whether or not a person is able to recognize and demonstrate an appropriate level of assertion on a patients' behalf), it appears that teamwork training for clinicians can have a positive impact on the development of processes to facilitate effective communication. Of course, changing generalizable personal behaviors that support effective team coordination and communication continues to be a goal for educators and this is an area of ongoing research.

TEAMSTEPPS: A MODEL OF TEAMWORK TRAINING

One model for teamwork training that is used at a growing number of institutions across the country is TeamSTEPPS (*Team Strategies and Tools to Enhance Performance and Patient Safety*).[21] TeamSTEPPS, a widely accessible, evidence-based communication and teamwork curriculum, was developed by the Agency for Healthcare Research and Quality (AHRQ) and the Department of Defense (DoD) and is in use across the country. The curriculum is organized on five key principles. Team Structure provides the introduction and framework, followed by four key skills: Leadership, Situation Monitoring, Mutual Support, and Communication (Figure 5.1). Implementation of TeamSTEPPS is intended as a system change in which providers gain specific skills that support team performance principles through designated training requirements, behavioral methods, human factors, and cultural change. Team competencies required for high-performing teams

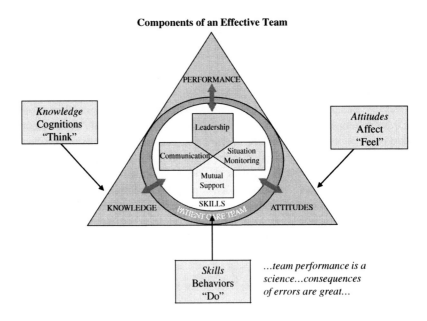

Figure 5.1
Components of an Effective Team. Logo of TeamSTEPPS®
Reprinted from Department of Health and Human Services, Agency for Healthcare Research and Quality, TeamSTEPPS®.

are grouped into measureable outcomes around Knowledge, Attitudes, and Performance (sometimes referred to as Knowledge, Skills, and Attitudes, KSAs). The dynamic interplay among the three outcomes and the four skills comprises the team effort to deliver safe, high quality care.

Recognizing that newly learned teamwork knowledge and behaviors have to be integrated into clinical practice, the TeamSTEPPS program includes several components devoted to Implementation, a multiphase process based on Kotter's model of organizational change.[22] Ideally, every unit or hospital that undertakes team training using the TeamSTEPPS curriculum will complete these phases, in order to optimize the potential for integrating and sustaining effective teamwork behaviors into daily practice.

In phase I, Assessment, organizational readiness for undertaking a TeamSTEPPS initiative is determined. In this phase, the hospital or clinical unit identifies leaders and key champions who will make up the "change team." The role of this change team is to determine specific opportunities for improvement that can be realized by employing a teamwork initiative, and to identify potential barriers to implementing change.[23]

Phase II is the planning and execution segment of the TeamSTEPPS Initiative. In this phase, members of the change team complete a 2-day intensive TeamSTEPPS train-the-trainer course consisting of core content modules, case studies, and interactive exercises. Culture change and coaching workshops that provide skills and strategies for implementing, sustaining, and spreading teamwork are introduced. Additionally, each unit or department produces an action plan: a tangible report detailing exactly how the initiative will be executed to best meet their unique circumstances. In some units, this will mean that a small number of individual tools from TeamSTEPPS will be introduced at specific intervals (a dosing strategy), whereas in other units or departments, change teams may elect to implement all the tools and strategies. This ability to customize the delivery of materials and contents has made TeamSTEPPS appealing to many institutions across the country.

In the final phase, phase III, the goal is to sustain and spread improvements in teamwork performance, clinical processes, and outcomes using a process improvement approach that entails monitoring and measuring the effectiveness of the intervention.

Sustainment is managed by the designated change team through coaching and active observation of team performance. It involves continuing training of the core curriculum through refresher courses and newcomers' orientation, conducting continual evaluations of teams throughout the organization, and providing meaningful, ongoing feedback to staff members in the workplace, where day-to-day healthcare is provided.[23] The goals of the implementation plan are to ensure that tools and strategies taught in the course are applied in the clinical setting, that clinicians practice and receive feedback on the trained skills, and that leaders continually reinforce the TeamSTEPPS principles in the unit or within the department.

To meet the demands for TeamSTEPPS, AHRQ and DoD established a national support network for TeamSTEPPS through the Centers for Medicare & Medicaid Services (CMS) Quality Improvement Organizations (QIOs). Following an agricultural extension model, the intent was for QIOs to serve as partners in the diffusion and adoption of TeamSTEPPS, further aiding healthcare entities in improving patient outcomes through the tracking of multiple performance metrics. QIOs were trained and supported via AHRQ funding through the American Institutes for Research (AIR), and five designated Team Resource Center training sites: Carilion Clinic, Creighton University Medical Center, Duke University Health System, the University of Minnesota Medical Center—Fairview, and the University of Washington. QIO staff and representatives from other healthcare organizations enrolled in regularly scheduled TeamSTEPPS Master Training Programs, comprised of 2½ day sessions that provide not only training but also demonstrations as to how TeamSTEPPS was effectively implemented at the host training center. Because each center is different in terms of capabilities, resources, size, and location, the five organizations provided a variety of training settings for addressing different needs, yielding a greater degree of flexibility in providing training and support to other organizations.

The TeamSTEPPS National Implementation is currently coordinated by the Health Research and Educational Trust (HRET) of the American Hospital Association. Several additional host training centers have been designated, and TeamSTEPPS Master Trainer courses continue to be offered across the country on a regular basis.

EDUCATING STUDENTS IN THE HEALTHCARE PROFESSIONS

The environment in which today's graduates of medical, nursing and other health professions schools will be practicing is rapidly evolving. Though young healthcare professionals will continue to require sound knowledge of disease management and good technical skills, they will also need to understand how systems problems contribute to risk and inadvertent harm to patients, how human factors impact their ability to provide good care, and how the clinical environment has evolved beyond the limitations of individual human performance. As evidence mounts supporting the link between effective teamwork behaviors and communication skills and the delivery of safe patient care, training to provide these skills needs to be integrated into the curricula of all healthcare professionals.

To send a strong message about the importance of teamwork in healthcare, some educational institutions are offering interdisciplinary training opportunities that integrate experiences for students in nursing, medicine, pharmacy and other healthcare professions. Although the logistics of offering such training can be quite challenging, this experience provides an opportunity for students to learn first-hand about each other's roles and training. Opportunities to clarify misperceptions and begin to form trusting relationships can help establish an environment of mutual respect before students work together in the clinical arena. This may help to mitigate poor working relationships, which are a known factor in nurse turnover and the growing national nursing shortage. Anecdotal feedback from some early experiences with interdisciplinary teamwork training suggests that students' awareness of the importance of other members of the healthcare team was enhanced by the experience of learning together.

As more and more medical schools and nursing schools have begun to introduce patient safety training (including a focus on teamwork and communication) into their curricula, a number of different teaching strategies have emerged. Approaches to delivering this education range from offering it as an elective experience[6] or an elective course,[24] to a full patient safety and quality improvement curriculum integrated into the existing curriculum.[25]

Whatever delivery approach is used, educating students about teamwork requires faculty who are knowledgeable about teamwork constructs and communication skills and who can also model teamwork behaviors in their interactions with other healthcare professionals. Pingleton et al, in describing residents' knowledge of quality and patient safety in academic medical centers,[26] suggested that "learning involves the transfer of knowledge through a formal curriculum consisting of learning objectives and curricular elements, and/or via an informal curriculum …where knowledge, attitudes and behaviors may be learned without overt intention or specific curriculum." With the current focus on culture change in medicine, students sometimes hear different information relayed through the formal curricular content on teamwork than they observe in the attitudes and behaviors of their faculty mentors. The behavior of faculty leaders, both clinical and administrative, sends strong messages to students about teamwork behaviors, and sadly this message is not always consistent with constructs they are taught "in the classroom."

EDUCATIONAL MODALITIES

As medical and nursing schools implement team training, a number of educational modalities are being used, ranging from traditional didactic approaches to teaching team coordination skills, to computer-based instruction, small-group sessions, analysis of video-taped team coordination scenarios, and workplace practice experiences.[16,19,27] Educational methods identified in an integrative review by Chakraborti et al. included lecture, case scenarios, teambuilding exercises, facilitated reflection, patient encounters, debriefing, role play, video-based discussion and mannequin simulation.[28]

Questions remain about the effectiveness of any of these strategies to achieve the necessary changes in student attitudes, knowledge, and skills, and there is little evidence for selecting particular methods. In one recent study, the TeamSTEPPS curriculum was adapted for presentation to nursing and medical students, and the effectiveness of four educational interventions to deliver this material was evaluated.[29] An interdisciplinary faculty team (nursing, medicine, human factors, psychometrics, safety, and high fidelity simulations experts) that designed and implemented the project was itself a model of team-work. This faculty team provided a lecture covering core teamwork concepts, and this was followed by one of four training sessions: further lecture, interactive lecture with an audience response system (ARS), low fidelity role play, and high fidelity human patient simulation.

Using an experimental design, 438 senior nursing students and fourth year medical students from two universities (Duke University and the University of North Carolina at Chapel Hill) were randomly assigned to the four cohorts, balanced according to profession. Students completed pre- and post-tests to measure changes in teamwork knowledge and attitudes. The control group ($N = 138$) received lecture only with a paper version of the common case scenario and no interactive learning activity. The three experimental groups were: Lecture with Audience Response System ($N = 140$), role play as low fidelity simulation ($N = 80$), and high fidelity human patient simulator ($N = 80$). To measure changes in knowledge and attitudes as a result of the training experience, students completed pre- and post-test versions of the validated 36-item Collaborative Healthcare Interdisciplinary Relationship Planning (CHIRP) scale[30] and a 10-item Teamwork Knowledge scale to measure changes in knowledge and attitudes after team training in the small groups. Evaluation of skill performance was done through interactions with standardized patients. All cohorts demonstrated significant improvement in knowledge based on the interventions, with no significant differences according to pedagogy. All cohorts likewise demonstrated significant improvement in attitudes toward teamwork, again with no significant differences by pedagogy.

Based on these outcomes, the Faculty team modified Year Two with a more concise 90 minute TeamSTEPPS lecture delivered via podcast (Duke) and webcast (UNC-CH). Modified instruments from Year 1 measured knowledge and attitudes pre- and post-lecture. Students ($N = 340$) were randomly assigned to interactive small groups with trained faculty facilitators for role play using two unfolding case studies, and a large group with no interactive exercise. A final exercise called for the students to watch a video of teamwork with opportunities for improvement and watch another video demonstrating successful team strategies, and use a rating instrument of team behaviors observed.

Results from the 2 years indicate low fidelity interactive exercises can produce improvements in student knowledge and attitudes related to team training. However, the evidence to support a transfer of gains in knowledge and attitudes to behavioral change in teamwork skills is lacking. Particularly when considering the potential for negative reinforcement by established clinicians who developed within a more hierarchical approach to teamwork, it is unclear whether demonstrating knowledge and attitudes regarding the appropriate behavior will translate into action when confronted with difficult team situations in patient care. Given the resource needs of high fidelity simulation, lack of faculty preparation to teach and model teamwork concepts, factors in retention and satisfaction, and implications for educating generation Xers, further study is warranted for evidenced based curricula changes to achieve the educational recommendations from the 2003 IOM report.[31]

A similar study at Florida Atlantic University implemented an educational intervention for nursing and medical residents to improve communication and collaboration.[32] Communication and collaboration demonstrated improvement, which in turn demonstrated improvement in patient outcomes and job satisfaction.

Many professional students lack opportunities to communicate across disciplines prior to graduating. Yet upon graduation, they are expected to communicate efficiently, having had limited instruction and opportunity to practice. Interdisciplinary team training can equip students with effective communication skills and empower them to communicate with confidence. Participating in educational experiences together contributes to professional role socialization amid developing an appreciation for the role of others. Cross-profession education is a key to improving patient care outcomes within a quality and safety context. The question remains whether changes can be sustained over time.

BUILDING A COMPETENCY BASED CURRICULUM IN TEAMWORK

Effective teamwork is often cited as "the most important competency" to improve quality and safety in healthcare. Today's complex healthcare environment requires teamwork skills across the disciplines to coordinate care,[33] and the inclusion of patients and families as team members can contribute to safer, more effective care.[34] Effective teams have a well-defined purpose relevant to patients and the organization and align goals with the purpose and outcomes.[35] Leaders influence activities to achieve goals, reach decisions, manage conflict, share ideas and information, coordinate tasks, provide feedback, listen and support, and trust across the team. Effective teams establish communication patterns, generate a sense of camaraderie from working together over time, and share pride in outcomes.

Teamwork training content often includes CRM principles such as effective leadership, communication skills, situational awareness and mutual support, and there are competencies that can be defined within each of these areas. Chakraborti et al. reviewed 13 studies reporting curricula for teamwork training interventions covering a variety of health professions.[28] Topics most frequently included were adaptability, team involvement in defining goals, and communication. Less frequently included principles were leadership, trust, team performance, monitoring, redistributing tasks by need, and ensuring team members are on the "same page."

The Accreditation Council on Graduate Medical Education (ACGME) requires Graduate Medical Education Programs (GME) to teach and assess six competencies for all residents and fellows, regardless of specialty. Although "patient safety" and "teamwork" are not explicitly discussed in any of the competencies, two of the six, *Practice Based Learning and Improvement* and *Systems Based Practice,* are inextricably entwined with safety, teamwork, and quality improvement.[36] These two competencies, however, have characteristically been the most challenging for individual residency programs to teach.[37]

The 2003 IOM report challenged the health professions community to overhaul clinician education by integrating core competencies including patient centered care, teamwork and collaboration, evidence based practice, quality improvement, safety, and informatics.[31]

Teamwork competencies are quite complex, but they can be defined by knowledge (cognitive), attitudes (affective), and performance (skills).[38,39] Integrating lessons learned from the literature and team training curricula, we propose five competencies all health professions students should achieve during their educational programs (Table 5.1) to build a safer, higher quality healthcare system.

ASSESSING AND MEASURING TEAM TRAINING

Various training methods have been discussed in this chapter. The implementation of these teaching methods and the interactive nature of teamwork may require new ways to assess how well students achieve teamwork knowledge, skills and attitudes. Assessing how clinicians and students master teamwork competencies is an important emerging area of study because of its complexity.[40] Team training is only useful when the behaviors are applied in practice so assessment may be multifaceted. Determining the purpose of the assessment will help determine how one measures training outcomes.

One comprehensive model that is being applied to team training programs begins with reaction to the training and moves upward to how well the participants learned the material and whether they can transfer the learning to their work. The most complex measure is the impact on the organization's performance. Kirkpatrick defines these measures in four levels that may help guide assessment methods in teamwork training programs.[41]

- Reaction: measures how well participants liked the experience (affective) and a secondly how useful it was (instrumentality)
- Learning: determines if participants developed new knowledge or skills
- Behavior: assesses if participants are able to transfer to the care environment
- Outcomes: examines the influence on the organizational performance

Reflection[42] is a strategy that can be used across the first three levels of assessment and was the most frequently cited strategy in Chakraborti et al.'s integrative review.[28] Team competencies require emotional intelligence to be able to examine one's own behavior in the context of others. Reflection is often expressed as combining the affective component with critical thinking. It is a form for expression of expectations, perceptions, and feelings of an experience and allows

Table 5.1   Teamwork Competencies (adapted from IOM, 2003; Cronenwett et al, 2007; Cronenwett et al, 2009)

Competency	Knowledge, Skills, and Attitudes (KSA's)
Individual: Manage self-awareness as a team member	*Knowledge:* Describe own strengths, limitations, and values in functioning as a member of a team *Performance/Skills:* Act with integrity, consistency and respect for differing views Initiate plan to develop one's strengths and limitations as a team member *Attitudes:* Recognize importance of own potential contribution to intra- and inter-professional collaboration to contribute to effective team functioning
Develop relationships with other team members, both in one's own discipline and interprofessionally	*Knowledge:* Describe scopes of practice, roles, and responsibilities of healthcare team members and manage overlaps Recognize contributions of other individuals and groups in helping patient/family achieve health goals *Performance:* Function competently within own scope of practice as leader or member of the healthcare team Initiate requests for help when appropriate to situation Clarify roles and integrate the contributions of others who play a role in helping patient/family achieve health goals *Attitudes:* Value and respect the perspectives, attributes, and expertise of all health team members including the patient/family.
Use effective communication	*Knowledge:* Analyze effective strategies and differences in style for communication among patients and families, and members of the health team. *Performance/Skills:* Adapt communication to the team and situation to share information; solicit input. Navigate conflict skillfully. *Attitudes:* Value teamwork and the relationships on which it is based. Value different styles of communication used by patients, families, and healthcare providers for effective care and conflict resolution.
Participate in teamwork behaviors that promote quality and safety	*Knowledge:* Describe examples of the impact of team functioning on safety and quality of care and how authority gradients influence teamwork and patient safety. *Performance/Skills:* Choose communication styles that diminish the risks associated with authority gradients among team members to accomplish care, assert one's own views, and minimize risks associated with handoffs among providers and across transitions in care. *Attitudes:* Recognize the risks across transitions in care and during handoffs among providers.

(Continued)

Table 5.1   *(Continued)*

Competency	Knowledge, Skills, and Attitudes (KSA's)
Participate in teamwork behaviors that contribute to a healthy work environment	*Knowledge:* Identify system barriers and facilitators of effective team functioning. Examine strategies for improving systems to support team functioning. *Performance/Skills:* Participate in designing systems that support effective teamwork. *Attitudes:* Value the influence of system solutions in achieving effective team functioning.

one to synthesize that experience (the personal way of knowing) with what one knows (cognitive way of knowing) to seek an improved performance in the future. The difficulty is in documenting that what one learned made a difference.

Reflective questions can include the affective domain (reaction, examine the knowledge for how one feels), cognitive domain (relevance, examine alternative views as well as how the competencies relate), and the psychomotor domain (responsibility, how the knowledge will be used). Facilitated reflection can guide structured feedback on performance. To use reflection as an assessment method, participants may be asked to write a 1 minute reflection on their experience in team training. The reflective writing rubric in Table 5.2 illustrates how guided reflective writing can be evaluated to determine integration of what was learned. Learners may use this as a self-guided assessment or it can be used by educators to assess learners and offer feedback.

- What was the most important skill related to teamwork you learned today? Why?
- When were you challenged by others on the team?
- How did the actions of the team affect safety?
- What impact will the actions of the team have on the organization's performance?

Other methods of assessment include participant survey instruments, knowledge tests, observational techniques, and simulation-based assessment of behaviors. A variety of surveys can be implemented including those that ask participants to assess confidence in their knowledge and skills and those that assess attitudes toward teamwork and patient safety. As an example, the CHIRP scale[30] uses a Likert scale to self-assess how one regards the interests and perspectives of other members of the healthcare team involved in care as well as the patient and family. Other items consider information sharing and communication. Knowledge tests generally include objective questions regarding effective team coordination and communication content.

Methods for assessing teamwork skills generally involve the use of observer-based rating scales, which often are specific to the healthcare task at hand.[43-46] Researchers have attained contradictory results with respect to the validity and reliability of these behaviorally anchored scales.[43,44,47-49] For example, Fletcher et al., in the evaluation of the anesthetists nontechnical skills (ANTS) rating scale, report moderate interrater agreement with correlation coefficients of between 0.55 to 0.67 at the level of individual elements of ratings and correlation coefficients of 0.56 to 0.65 at the level of teamwork categories.[42] Other research has reported high rates of interrater agreement but details of the analysis are unclear, and the high rate of agreement may only be at the level of an averaged overall teamwork score.[48] Morgan et al. presented less promising results associated with a general rating scale and advocate for the development of a domain specific scale for obstetrics.[49] Using simulated obstetric care scenarios, they evaluated the use of a human factors rating scale (containing 45 items representing 5 team skill constructs) and a global rating scale that uses a single 5-point rating of teamwork from unacceptable to acceptable. The single-rater intraclass correlation coefficient for external observers was 0.341

Table 5.2 Reflective Writing Rubric

Criteria	Advanced	Proficient	Basic	Below	Comments
How informative was the description of what was learned					
Level of synthesis in exploring and analyzing what was learned					
Application to practice and safety concerns					
Coherence and style of writing					

using the human factors rating scale and 0.446 for the global rating scale. Reliability of self-ratings was low and did not correlate highly with the observer ratings. Scores were not consistent across different scenarios. Malec et al. evaluated the "Mayo High Performance Teamwork Scale" in the context of self-assessment of performance in simulated teamwork scenarios.[47] Although they used psychometric techniques for the generation of the scale and established good internal consistency, construct validity, and sensitivity to improvement with repetition, they did not assess agreement between raters or between an external observer and the self-ratings.

Two recent experiences using team skill assessment tools in our research also underscore the limitations of current assessment techniques. In a previous study funded by the National Board of Medical Examiners, we evaluated a behaviorally anchored rating scale for interrater agreement (reliability) and correlation with clinical performance measures (validity).[40] In this study, nine teams of three or four first-year medical students were videotaped performing two classroom-based patient assessment tasks and two high-fidelity simulated emergent care tasks. On an average teamwork score across five dimensions of teamwork, we achieved moderate interobserver agreement between two observers in the classroom tasks: $r = 0.47$ for case 1 and $r = 0.58$ for case 2 and slightly higher agreement in the high fidelity simulation tasks: $r = 0.58$ for case 1 and $r = 0.73$ for case 2. However, when analyzed at the level of specific teamwork dimensions, interrater agreement failed to achieve significance

in 10 instances and Pearson correlation coefficients ranged from 0.35 to 0.58 in the other 10 instances. Another concern of this measure is that it lacked sensitivity. Participants generally scored high (the equivalent of 4.5 on a 5 point scale) and there was little variability in scores between participants. In general, because the medical students were working together, the teamwork dynamic did not adequately replicate the difficult teamwork scenarios that result in sentinel events such as those reported to the Joint Commission.[50]

In the previously referenced collaborative effort of Duke and UNC to train nursing and medical students, we compared methods of team training through a videotaped standardized patient (SP) encounter with teams of two medical students and two nursing students.[29] Preliminary assessment of interrater agreement of seven external raters scoring teams using a modified version of the Mayo High Performance Teamwork Scale[47] indicates a need for further tool development and rater training. Intraclass correlation coefficients were less than 0.4 for 5 of 10 scale items, ranged from 0.4 to 0.5 for 2 items, and were greater than 0.5 for 3 items. Intraclass correlation coefficients on a clinical behavior-based checklist were high, ranging from 0.68 to 1.0 for 9 of 10 checklist items. Another shortcoming of this approach is that the SP encounter did not foster an environment of rich teamwork interaction between participants. Although the scenario contained an embedded error that forced team members to share information, interaction between team members was limited and uncomplicated.

Although some successes in assessing team skill have been noted in the case of specialty-based tools for specific work environments, general team skill assessment tools intended to apply to a broader audience, or for the purpose of medical and nursing education, have not been strongly supported. Limitations of current assessment methods include: (1) a failure to attain high levels of interrater agreement with observer-based team skill rating scales, and (2) a failure to adequately assess teamwork skills with respect to managing difficult situations or difficult team members. Rosen et al. describe specific criteria for measuring team performance in simulation-based training:[51]

1. Ground measures in theory.
2. Design measures to meet specific learning outcomes.
3. Capture competencies.
4. Measure multiple levels of performance.
5. Link measures to scenario events.
6. Focus on observable behaviors.
7. Incorporate multiple measures from different sources.
8. Capture performance processes in addition to outcomes.
9. Create diagnostic power.
10. Train observers and structure observation protocols.

Current research in assessing team skills is exploring approaches more similar to those used for assessing patient interview skills using standardized patients. Using actors playing the role of team member care providers, it is possible to create difficult teamwork situations and to score individuals on objective, observable, teamwork dimensions,[52] meeting the criteria defined by Rosen et al.[51]

SUMMARY

Despite mounting evidence that effective teamwork is critical to patient safety and optimal clinical outcomes, little training in teamwork and communication has been integrated in the curricula of the health professions schools. Some academic centers are beginning to integrate training using lectures, interactive small group exercises and high fidelity simulation. Early studies suggest that all of these modalities may be effective in improving students' knowledge and attitudes about teamwork. Providing this education in real world multidisciplinary environments can be challenging. The benefits will outweigh real and perceived barriers such as the logistics of scheduling, but integrated training produces a rich educational milieu that can help achieve critical change in students' capacity to form effective healthcare teams. Longitudinal studies are needed to evaluate the most effective pedagogies for changing behavior in the clinical setting. Faculty development is a critical factor which has had little focus both for providing formal education and for coaching and modeling the competencies. Finally, with developing new educational models we must examine innovation in assessing how well learners master the competencies and develop ways to observe application in clinical practice. Change is happening albeit slowly, and continuing systematic examination of educational models will help us build an evidence based curriculum and pedagogy with the ultimate goal of improving patient outcomes.

REFERENCES

1. Kohn, L. T., Corrigan, J. M., Donaldson, M. S. (Eds.), Institute of Medicine. (2000). *To err is human: Building a safer health system.* Washington, DC: National Academies Press. Retrieved January 29, 2010 from: http://books.nap.edu/catalog/9728.html.
2. Leape, L. L., Berwick, D. M. (2005). Five years after To Err is Human: What have we learned? *JAMA, 293*(19), 2384–90.
3. Mazzocco, K., Petitti, D. B., et al. (2009). Surgical team behaviors and patient outcomes. *American Journal of Surgery, 197*(5), 678–85.
4. Sawyer M, Weeks K, et al. (2010). Using evidence, rigorous measurement and collaboration to eliminate central catheter-associated bloodstream infections. *Crit Care Med 38*(8Suppl), S292–8.
5. Pronovost P, Berenholtz SM, et al. (2008). Improving patient safety in intensive care units in Michigan. *Journal of Critical Care, 23*(2), 207–21.
6. Institute for Healthcare Improvement. Retrieved February 9, 2010 from: http://www.ihi.org/IHI/Programs/IHIOpenSchool/. Overview: What is the Open School. Page 1

7. Wright, M. C., Petrusa, E. R., Griffin, K. L., Phillips-Bute, B. G., Hobbs, G. W., & Taekman, J. M. (2009). Assessing teamwork in medical education and practice: Relating behavioural teamwork ratings and clinical performance. *Medical Teacher, 31*(1), 30–8.

8. Salas, E., Wilson, K. A., Burke, C. S., Wightman, D. C. (2006). Does crew resource management training work? An update, an extension and some critical needs. *Human Factors, 48*(2), 392–412.

9. Zwarenstein, M., Reeves, S., Barr, H., Hammick, M., Koppel, I, & Atkins, J. (2000). Interprofessional education: Effects on professional practice and health care outcomes. Cochrane Database of Systematic Reviews, Issue 3, Art. No. D002213. CO1:10.1002/14651858. CD002213.

10. Salas, E., Almeida, S., Salisbury, M., King, H., Lazzara, E., & Lyons, R., et al. (2009). What are the critical success factors for team training in health care? *The Joint Commission Journal on Quality and Patient Safety, 55*(8), 398–405.

11. Gaba, D. M., Howard, S. K., Fish, K. J., Smith, B. E., Sowb, Y. A. (2001). Simulation-based training in anesthesia crisis resource management (ACRM): A decade of experience. *Simul Gaming, 32*(2), 175–93.

12. Small, S. D., Wuerz, R. C., Simon, R., Shapiro, N., Conn, A, & Setnik, G. (1999). Demonstration of high-fidelity simulation team training for emergency medicine. *Academic Emergency Medicine, 6*(4), 312.

13. Ritchie, D., & Hoffman, R. (1977). Incorporating instructional design principles with the world wide web. In: Khan B (Ed.), *Web Based Instruction.* (pp. 135–8). Englewood Cliffs, NJ: Educational Technology Publications.

14. Hamman, W. R. (2004). The complexity of team training: What we have learned from aviation and its applications to medicine. *Quality and Safety in Health Care, 13*(Suppl 1), i72–9.

15. Leonard, M., Graham, S., Bonacum, D. (2004). The human factor: The critical importance of effective teamwork and communication in providing safe care. *Quality and Safety in Health Care, 13*(Suppl 1), i85–90.

16. Morey, J. C., Simon, R., Jay, G. D., et al. (2002). Error reduction and performance improvement in the emergency department through formal teamwork training: Evaluation results of the MedTeams project. *Health Services Research, 37*(6), 1553–80.

17. Wright, M. C., Luo, X., Richardson, W. J., et al. (2006). *Piloting team coordination training at Duke University Health System.* Proceedings of the HFES 50th Annual Meeting (pp. 949–53). San Diego: Human Factors and Ergonomics Society.

18. Hall, P., & Weaver, L. (2001). Interdisciplinary education and teamwork: a long and winding road. *Medical Education, 35,* 867–75.

19. Thurlow, S., Plant, M., & Muir, E. (2001). Making teamwork come alive: use of actors and multiprofessional co-leaders in small group teaching about teamwork. *Medical Education, 35*(11), 1081–2.

20. Meliones, J., Alton, M., Mericle, J., Ballard, R., Frush, K., & Mistry, K. (2008). Ten year experience integrating strategic performance improvement initiatives. AHRQ Advances in Patient safety: New Direction and Alternative Approaches, Vol 3. Performance and Tools. AHRQ Publication No. 08-0034-4. Rockville, MD: Agency for Healthcare Research and Quality.

21. Agency for Healthcare Research and Quality (2005). TeamSTEPPS®. Retrieved January 30, 2010 from: http://www.usuhs.mil/cerps/TeamSTEPPS.html. http://teamstepps.ahrq.gov/page 1 (home page)

22. Kotter, J., & Rathgeber, H. (2006). *Our Iceberg Is Melting: Changing and Succeeding under Any Conditions.* New York: St. Martin's Press.

23. King, H. B., Battles, J., et al. TeamSTEPPS: Team Strategies and tools to enhance performance and patient safety. 2008 Retrieved January 30, 2010 from: http://www.ahrq.gov/downloads/pub/advances2/vol3/Advances-King_1.pdf.

24. Rodriguez-Paz, J. M., Kennedy, M., et al. (2009). Beyond see one, do one, teach one: toward a different training paradigm. *Quality & Safety in Health Care, 18*(1), 63–8.

25. Varkey, P. (2007). Educating to improve patient care: Integrating quality improvement into a medical school curriculum. *American Journal of Medical Quality, 22,* 112–6.

26. Pingleton, S. K., Horak, B. J., et al. (2009). Is there a relationship between high-quality performance in major teaching hospitals and residents' knowledge of quality and patient safety? *Academic Medicine, 84*(11), 1510–5.

27. Shapiro, M. J., Morey, J. C., Small, S. D., et al. (2004). Simulation based teamwork training for emergency department staff: does it improve clinical team performance when added to an existing didactic teamwork curriculum? *Quality and Safety in Health Care, 13*(6), 417–21.

28. Chakraborti, C., Boonyasal, R., Wright, S., & Kern, D. (2007). A systematic review of teamwork training interventions in medical student and resident education. *Journal of General Internal Medicine, 23*(6), 846–53

29. Hobgood, C., Sherwood, G., Frush, K., et al, on behalf of the Interprofessional Patient Safety Education Collaborative (2010). Teamwork training with nursing and medical students: Does the method matter? Results of an interinstitutional interdisciplinary collaboration. *Quality and Safety in Health Care, 19*(6), 1–6.

30. Hollar, D., Hobgood, C., et al. (2007, November). *Validation of CHIRP, an instrument for assessing health professions teamwork attitudes.* Washington, DC: Association of American Medical Colleges Annual Meeting.

31. Institute of Medicine (2003). *Health Professions Education: A Bridge to Quality.* Washington, DC: National Academies Press.

32. McCaffrey, M. G., Hayes, R., Stuart, W., Cassell, A., Farrell, C., Miller-Reyes, C., et al. (2010). A program to improve communication and collaboration between nurses and medical residents. *Journal of Continuing Education in Nursing, 41*(4), 172–8.

33. Apker, J., Propp, K. M., Zabava Ford, W. S., & Hofmeister, N. (2006). Collaboration, credibility, compassion, and coordination: professional nurse communication skill sets in health care team interactions. *Journal of Professional Nursing, 22*(3), 180–9.

34. Sherwood, G., Thomas, E., Simmons, D., & Lewis, P. (2002). A teamwork model to promote patient safety. *Critical Care Nursing Clinics of North America, 14,* 333–40.

35. Micken, S. M., & Rogers, S. A. (2005). Effective health care teams. A model of 6 characteristics developed from shared perceptions. *Journal of Interprofessional Care, 19*(4), 358–70.

36. Joint Committee of the Group on Resident Affairs and Organization of Resident Representatives. (2003, February). *Patient Safety and Graduate Medical Education.* Association of American Medical Colleges.

37. Accreditation Council for Graduate Medical Education. *Educating Physicians for the 21st Century.* Retrieved January 30, 2010 from: http://www.acgme.org/acWebsite/home/home.asp. ACGME-Bulletin, Aug 2006; pp. 9–10.

38. Cronenwett, L., Sherwood, G., Barnsteiner, J., Disch, J., Johnson, J., Mitchell, P., et al. (2007). Quality and safety education for nurses. *Nursing Outlook, 55*(3), 122–31.

39. Cronenwett, L., Sherwood, G., et al.(2009). Quality and safety education for advanced practice nursing practice. *Nursing Outlook, 57*(6), 338–48.

40. Wright, M. C., Taekman, J. M., & Endsley, M. R. (2004). Objective measures of situation awareness in a simulated medical environment. *Quality and Safety in Health Care, 13*:65–71.

41. Kirkpatrick, D. L. (1994). *Evaluating Training Programs: The Four Levels.* San Francisco: Berrett-Koehler.

42. Horton-Deutsch, S., Sherwood, G. (2008). Reflection: An educational strategy to develop emotionally competent nurse leaders. *Journal of Nursing Management, 16*:946–54.

43. Fletcher, G., Flin, R., McGeorge, P., Glavin, R., Maran, N., Patey, R. (2003). Anaesthetists' Non-Technical Skills (ANTS): evaluation of a behavioural marker system. *British Journal of Anaesthesia, 90*(5), 580–8.

44. Healey, A. N., Undre, S., & Vincent, C. A. (2004). Developing observational measures of performance in surgical teams. *Quality and Safety in Health Care, 13*(Suppl 1), i33–40.

45. Thomas, E. J., Sexton, J. B., & Helmreich, R. L. (2004). Translating teamwork behaviours from aviation to healthcare: development of behavioural markers for neonatal resuscitation. *Quality and Safety in Health Care, 13*(Suppl 1), i57–64.

46. Frankel, A., Gardner, R., Maynard, L., & Kelly, A. (2007). Using the communication and teamwork skills (CATS) assessment to measure health care team performance. *Joint Commission Journal on Quality and Patient Safety, 33*(9), 549–58.

47. Malec, J. F., Tosher, L. C., Dunn, W. F., et al. (2007). Mayo High Performance Teamwork Scale (HPTS). *Simulation in Healthcare, 2,* 4–10.

48. Moorthy, K., Munz, Y., Adams, S., Pandey, V., & Darzi, A. (2005). A human factors analysis of technical and team skills among surgical trainees during procedural simulations in a simulated operating theatre. *Annals of Surgery, 242*(5), 631–9.

49. Morgan, P. J., Pittini, R., Regehr, G., Marrs, C., & Haley, M. F. (2007). Evaluating teamwork in a simulated obstetric environment. *Anesthesiolog, 106*(5), 907–15.

50. Joint Commission on Accreditation of Healthcare Organizations. (2005). *Sentinel Event*

Statistics. Oakbrook, IL: Joint Commission on Accreditation of Healthcare Organizations.

51. Rosen, M. A., Salas, E., Wilson, K. A., et al. (2008). Measuring team performance in simulation-based training: adopting best practices for healthcare. Simulation in healthcare. *Journal of the Society for Simulation in Healthcare, 3,* 33–41.

52. Segall, N., Wright, M. C., Hobbs, G., & Taekman, J. M. (2009). Validity and Reliability of the Skills Assessment for Evaluation of Teams (SAFE-Teams) Tool. *Anesthesiology,* A1065.

6

REGULATING AND MONITORING TEAMWORK AND TRAINING IN HEALTHCARE: ISSUES AND CHALLENGES

Karen Frush, Laura Maynard, Carol Koeble, and René Schwendimann

INTRODUCTION

Since the publication of the Institute of Medicine (IOM) report on patient safety a decade ago,[1] there has been a growing discussion about the role of teamwork and effective communication in patient safety and healthcare delivery. The IOM suggested that healthcare providers would benefit from inter-disciplinary team training to create a shared mental model for patient care and safety, and the Joint Commission reported in 2007 that communication errors are among the most common causes of sentinel events in US hospitals.[2] A number of studies have been published in the medical literature describing the importance of good teamwork in high acuity areas such as the operating room, the emergency department, intensive care units, and labor and delivery,[3-6] and several recent reports have shown a relationship between teamwork behaviors and patient outcomes.[3,5] The National Quality Forum (NQF) includes teamwork as one of its recommended safe practices for better healthcare and suggests that healthcare organizations must establish a proactive, systematic, organization-wide approach to developing team-based care through teamwork training,

skill building, and team-led performance improvement interventions that reduce preventable harm to patients (7).

The old, familiar picture of the solitary expert physician is giving way to a team-based approach to clinical care. Professional societies and national accrediting bodies are acknowledging the need for effective teamwork in today's highly complex healthcare environment. This trend from individual experts to expert teams was supported by Darrell Kirch in his presidential address at the 118th annual meeting of the Association of American Medical Colleges in 2007.[8] Dr. Kirch spoke passionately of the need for a dramatic cultural shift in academic medicine:

> [We need] a culture that is grounded in the values of collaboration, trust, and shared accountability. A culture that is reinforced through team-based structures and shared reward systems. A culture that encourages transparency and inclusivity, rather than exclusivity. A culture that is driven equally by our traditional commitment to excellence, and by service to others. A culture in which all learn and all

teach, and all experience great fulfillment in the process.

Despite growing interest, there remains ambiguity on teamwork in healthcare: What is the value of teamwork in healthcare? How is the impact of teamwork measured? How are teamwork behaviors encouraged or enforced? This chapter describes regulations related to teamwork (using aviation as a model), proposes a framework to embed teamwork within healthcare delivery, and discusses methods of monitoring teamwork among healthcare providers at the state and local levels.

A MODEL FOR TEAMWORK TRAINING: AVIATION

The IOM recommendation for interdisciplinary teamwork training for healthcare providers was based primarily on evidence of the positive impact of crew resource management (CRM) training in aviation. Crew resource management training encompasses a wide range of knowledge, skills, and attitudes, including communications, situational awareness, problem solving, conflict resolution, and teamwork. Crew resource management is best understood as a management system that makes optimum use of all available resources—equipment, processes, procedures, and human resources—to promote safety and enhance the efficiency of flight operations.[9]

Although technical knowledge and skills are needed for a pilot to operate an aircraft safely, CRM emphasizes the role of human factors and focuses on the nontechnical cognitive and interpersonal skills required to manage the flight within the aviation system.[10] In this context, cognitive skills are the mental processes used for gaining and maintaining situational awareness, solving problems, resolving conflict, and making decisions.[11] Interpersonal skills are comprised of a range of behavioral activities and communication techniques associated with teamwork. In aviation, as in other industries and professions, these skills often overlap with each other, and they also overlap with the required technical skills.[11] Although crew resource management is widely used to improve the performance of flight crews, there is no universal CRM training program. The Federal

Aviation Administration (FAA) mandates training, but allows air carriers to customize CRM training to meet the needs of their organizations.[12] Following the lead of the commercial airline industry, the US Department of Defense began formally training its air crews in CRM in the early 1990s.[13] Presently, the US Air Force requires all air crew members to receive annual CRM training, in an effort to reduce human error–caused mishaps.[13]

MONITORING TEAMWORK BEHAVIORS IN AVIATION

In the mid-1990s, leaders of several commercial airlines began to question whether concepts and skills taught in CRM training actually transferred to "front-line" pilots. Although routine front-line checks of pilots usually provided enough information to identify issues related to procedural compliance, they lacked information about pilots' actual performance during regular operations. Researchers from the University of Texas worked with the airlines to develop a CRM audit methodology that became known as the Line Operations Safety Audit (LOSA) (Table 6.1). [14] This methodology is based on the assumption that flight crews may commit errors and encounter threats (e.g., adverse weather, aircraft malfunctions) during ordinary flights, and these errors could potentially lead to an accident or adverse event. The importance of the threats and errors is not that they occur during normal operations, but rather how they are managed by the flight crew. The Threat and Error Management Model, which became known as LOSA, was designed to allow observations of pilots in the cockpit during normal operations by highly trained and calibrated observers. The observers record detailed narratives about the flight, and they also score teamwork behaviors such as communication techniques (callouts and structured language), situation awareness, and mutual support.[14] The observers are also trained to assess pilots' capacity to manage threats and errors that may occur, and data from these direct observations are analyzed and used to create a profile of safety strengths and weaknesses. This safety profile is then provided to the airlines, and it is their responsibility to use the data to prevent future accidents and adverse events, as well as to target further training needs.[14]

Table 6.1   Line Operations Safety Audit Criteria and Proposed Medical Model for Clinical Operations Safety Audit

LOSA Characteristic	LOSA Model	Healthcare Model
Jump seat observations during normal flight operations	Observation of normal flight operations to identify system strengths and weaknesses, not individual crew evaluations	Observation of normal clinical operations and activities for system evaluation. The Joint Commission's Tracer Methodology might fulfill this characteristic.
Anonymous and confidential data collection	Safeguards in place to protect any identifying information and ensure pilot's trust in the process	Anonymous and confidential data collection, clearly explained to all including physicians and senior leaders; de-identified data reported in aggregate
Voluntary flight crew participation	Provide education on the purpose LOSA to gain the crew's trust in the process; Pilots more open to observations but still an option to decline the LOSA	Voluntary participation by clinical area without direct or implied coercion
Joint management/ pilot association sponsorship	Formal agreement between airline management and pilot's associations to ensure confidentiality and anonymity of observation data	Joint administrative and clinical sponsorship of the audits. A formal compact between physicians and administration could be used to ensure confidentiality and anonymity, and to confirm joint commitment to the process.
Safety-targeted data collection form	LOSA Observation Form based on UT Threat and Management Model allows for a framework for collecting systemic factors that affect flight crew performance	A safety targeted and teamwork targeted data collection form would be necessary; one that is psychometrically sound, clear in meaning, and regularly shared with all being audited.
Trusted and trained observers	Trusted observers who are unobtrusive, nonthreatening, and highly trained	Trusted observers who are unobtrusive, nonthreatening, highly trained, and calibrated for interrater reliability using the audit tool
Trusted data collection site	Either a jointly appointed management/union representative or a third party can act as a data repository.	A trusted data collection site might include patient safety organizations or state level hospital associations. A third party data repository must be secure and trusted by both physicians and administrative leaders of healthcare organizations.
Data cleaning roundtables	Diverse group comprised of the data analyst and airline representatives look for inaccuracies and coding errors in the raw data and ensure correct data entry.	A PSO or hospital association could perform the data cleaning.

Table 6.1   (Continued)

LOSA Characteristic	LOSA Model	Healthcare Model
Data-derived targets for enhancement	Problematic data trends in noncompliance of operation standards are targets for improvement	Review at PSO or hospital association level to identify trends and target improvement needs
Results feedback to line pilots	Timely feedback to pilots including an audit summary and improvement strategies	Feedback of audit results to all clinical staff and physicians as well as to hospital administration

Klinert et al. have outlined ten operating characteristics of a successful LOSA, with each component being of equal importance.[14] These same ten principles could be applied to healthcare observations or audits of teamwork, to build a model for monitoring teamwork. If one substitutes "physician" for "pilot" in most cases this model is applicable, but it is costly, time consuming, and requires culture change to embrace it.

1. **Jump seat observations during normal flight operations. Healthcare: Observation of normal clinical operations and activities for system evaluation (i.e., Clinical Operations Safety Audit).** In aviation, the primary objective of a LOSA is to identify safety strengths and weaknesses in normal flight operations. The responsibility of LOSA observers is to complete a system evaluation related to safety, not an evaluation of individual members of the team.[14] There are some many similarities between this approach and the Joint Commission's current tracer methodology, which is used during the accreditation process. Such an approach, used by an objective body not associated with the accreditation organization, may provide an attractive model.

2. **Anonymous and confidential data collection. Healthcare: Anonymous and confidential data collection, clearly explained to all, including physicians and senior leaders. Develop structures to protect clinicians and administrators from any punitive action based on observation metrics.** "The difference between LOSA success and failure is *pilot trust* in the project. If pilots feel LOSA is a threat to their job or fear that an observation will find its way to management, they might be tempted to 'fake good performance' rather than normally performing. The

more pilots trust that LOSA will not identify individuals, the more likely observations will reflect the normal operational reality of the airline."[14] The culture of healthcare has traditionally been a punitive culture, as described in the 1999 IOM report.[1] Much work has been done in hospitals and healthcare organizations over the past decade, to transition from a culture of blame to a culture of accountability, but trust-building among physicians, administrators and a LOSA-type organization, would be critically important.

3. **Voluntary flight crew participation. Healthcare: Voluntary clinical area participation. A unit may refuse a clinical operations safety audit.** This is a way to build trust in the process. As noted here, it is essential to develop physician and nursing leadership trust in the process through education and discussion.

4. **Joint management/pilot association sponsorship. Healthcare: Joint administrative and clinical sponsorship of the audits.** An important safeguard to strengthen pilot trust is to require a formal agreement between airline management and the pilots' association. The agreement usually states that all LOSA data will be confidential, anonymous, and not used to discipline pilots.[14] In healthcare, a similar approach requiring a formal written agreement between administrative leadership and physician leadership would be critical to the success of an on-site audit/observation of clinical performance.

5. **Safety-targeted data collection form. Healthcare: A safety targeted and teamwork targeted data collection form would be necessary; one that is psychometrically sound, clearly**

understood, feasible, and regularly shared with all being audited.

6. **Trusted and trained observers. Healthcare: Trusted and trained observers who are unobtrusive, nonthreatening, highly trained, and calibrated for interrater reliability using the audit tool.** Traditionally, performance evaluations of healthcare providers have been heavily weighted toward cognitive assessment, or knowledge tests, rather than observations of actual performance. The advent of high-fidelity simulation and the creation of simulation centers across the country, however, have facilitated notable advances in the evaluation and assessment of clinical performance, including nontechnical skills such as communication techniques and teamwork behaviors. Observers who train and work in such centers could provide an important resource in the development of a national healthcare LOSA-type collaborative.

7. **Trusted data collection site. Healthcare: Trusted data collection site might include patient safety organizations or state level hospital associations.** A third-party data repository must be secure and trusted, by both physicians and administrative leaders, of healthcare organizations.

8. **Data cleaning roundtables. Healthcare: Same model of data cleaning and analysis.** A Line Operations Safety Audit employs strict data management procedures and consistency checks to assure quality data. After the observations are complete, a joint data cleaning roundtable is convened to review the raw data. The review team, comprised of an analyst and three to five representatives from the airline (flight ops, safety, or training) seek to identify and correct inaccuracies and coding errors in the data to ensure the correct database entry.

9. **Data-derived targets for enhancement. Healthcare: Data-derived targets for improvement.** During data analysis, it is possible that trends will emerge, indicating that certain errors occur more often, or that some processes are consistently defective. These patterns should become targets for improvement for the hospital, practice, or institution. A follow-up audit can measure whether the improvement strategies have led to better performance.

10. **Results feedback to line pilots. Healthcare: Results feedback to clinical areas.** On completing a LOSA, airline management and the pilots' association have an obligation to communicate LOSA results back to the line pilots. Pilots will want to see not only the results, but also management's plan for improvements. If this is done, pilots gain confidence in the process; if airlines wait too long before presenting results, line pilots will begin to believe nothing of value came from the project. A summary of the audit, including strategies on how they plan to use the data, is ideal.[14] In healthcare, audits and surveys are often conducted, but too often, results are not shared with those who participated in the assessment. Timely and transparent feedback to clinicians is critical to the success of performance-based monitoring in healthcare.

MONITORING AND REGULATING TEAMWORK IN HEALTHCARE

A LOSA, in the aviation world, provides an effective mechanism to evaluate teamwork competencies (knowledge, skills, and attitudes) that manifest as successful performance within (mainly) complex situations. This type of team performance model might also serve as a framework for monitoring and regulating teamwork in healthcare systems (e.g., measuring and monitoring the extent to which multidisciplinary teams of experts become multidisciplinary expert teams).[15] The competencies needed for teamwork could be evaluated by a variety of methods, including internal peer review and external inspection, such as at the time of accreditation. Such approaches are in line with the findings from a recent review,[16] in which it was found that reliable assessment of the quality of teamwork necessitates the identification of specific behaviors (i.e., collaboration, shared mental models, coordination, communication, leadership) and their interplay in relation to clinical performance and ultimately to patient outcomes.

A Model to Frame Teamwork Within the Healthcare System

Before procedural implementation of an approach such as LOSA in healthcare we propose to consider the use of a framework such as the Quality Health Outcomes Model (QHOM).[17,18] The QHOM posits reciprocal interactions among four constructs such as system characteristics, interventions, client or patient characteristics, and outcomes. Such a

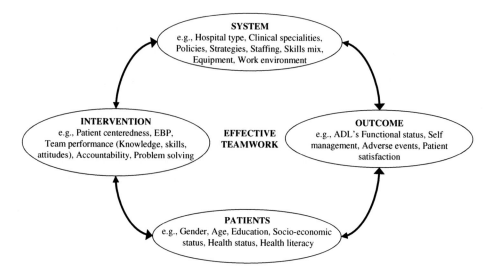

Figure 6.1
Quality Health Outcomes Model Characteristics

framework may help to reflect on the dynamics and complex interactions in which teamwork has to be performed (Fig. 6.1). In the model, the outcomes of healthcare interventions such as in hospitals (or other institutions) are mediated and moderated by characteristics of the care system and of the patients, with both patients and care system capable of being understood and measured at multiple levels (individual through population). Effective teamwork is a function of collaboration, coordination, leadership, and communication,[15,16] and as part of the intervention characteristics, it is obviously interdependent with the system and processes of care and its outcomes. The model has been used for instance in the context of care of women in labor,[19] and exemplified how to systematically organize collaborative efforts of physicians, nurses, and others toward achieving healthcare goals, which is in turn an essential of teamwork.

REGULATION OF TEAMWORK IN HEALTHCARE: CURRENT STATE

Although a LOSA-type approach may provide an attractive model for assessing and monitoring teamwork in healthcare, there is as yet no government or national mandate that requires team training. The Joint Commission, a leading national accrediting body for healthcare organizations, has embraced teamwork, but falls short of requiring teamwork training. Recent requirements do address the need for effective communication and teamwork behaviors among healthcare professionals through the National Patient Safety Goals.[20] Individual hospitals and healthcare organizations have developed a wide variety of methods to meet these goals, and their progress is most often monitored at the local (hospital) level or at the corporate (health system) level.

Similar to The Joint Commission's approach in the United States, the Council of Europe's Committee of Ministers has made recommendations for patient safety management and the prevention of adverse events to its member states.[21] Starting with the premise that patient safety is the underpinning philosophy of quality improvement, The Council stated that all possible measures should be taken to organize and promote patient-safety education. It recognized the need to promote open collaboration and coordination of national and international regulations concerning research in patient safety, and recommended that governments of member states develop a coherent and comprehensive patient-safety policy framework, making patient safety a leadership and management priority. Additionally, member states were asked to promote the development of educational programs for all relevant healthcare personnel, to improve the understanding of clinical decision making and appropriate approaches to patient-safety incidents. Although effective teamwork is not directly mentioned in the recommendations to the member states, the Council did include some basic expectations related to communication. They suggested that communication between individuals and teams, and across organizational levels, should be frequent, cordial, constructive, and problem oriented. Further, it was advised that in order to reduce and prevent patient-safety incidents, health professionals must understand their own behaviors, their decision-making process and their ability to cope with challenging situations in daily activities. Finally, the Council stated that interdisciplinary cooperation, a nonhierarchical structure and open communication are necessary for building a safety culture, and that in some specialties systematic training in team work is indispensable.[21]

The Swiss Academy of Medical Sciences provides another national model for patient safety and teamwork training through its Future of Medicine project. In this project, national leaders provided a series of recommendations and suggestions for patient safety education for healthcare professionals.[22] The general objectives of the project include "the ability to work across disciplinary boundaries in interdisciplinary teams," and address learning outcomes such as teamwork behaviors and effective communication between healthcare professionals. The recommendations include a focus on some specific team-leader skills such as briefing and debriefing, and underline the importance of additional elements of effective teamwork, such as conflict resolution and situation awareness.

On a global level, the World Health Organization (WHO) supports medical schools worldwide in implementing patient safety education by providing a comprehensive curriculum for patient safety. Topics such as human factors engineering, engaging with patients and families, and improving medication safety are included. Additionally, one of the main topics, being an effective team player, aims to support medical students' understanding of teamwork and how effective multidisciplinary teams improve care and reduce errors. Fortunately, the WHO curriculum guide is based on patient safety and educational principles that are applicable globally, and its delivery can be customized to local needs and culture.[23]

Despite the lack of a mandate for healthcare team training in the United States, there are numerous efforts to encourage and support such training. For example, the Agency for Healthcare Research and Quality (AHRQ) and the Department of Defense developed and released a national standard for team training in healthcare, called TeamSTEPPS® (Team Strategies and Tools to Enhance Performance and Patient Safety). This is a widely accessible, evidence-based communication and teamwork curriculum in the public domain.[24] Since 2005, TeamSTEPPS® has been implemented at numerous military treatment facilities across the United States. Additionally, through a national implementation program, training has been provided to representatives from all quality improvement organizations (QIOs), to facilitate the dissemination of team training in civilian healthcare facilities. These QIOs were required to provide team training as one component of the Centers for Medicare and Medicaid Services (CMS) 9th Scope of Work.

Although it is possible to monitor this training effort by counting the number of individuals and organizations that complete the TeamSTEPPS® course, there is currently no standard process or requirement for evaluating or monitoring the actual practice of teamwork within organizations once their clinical teams have been trained. Little research exists on the true effectiveness of TeamSTEPPS® or any other team training curriculum, because of the lack of validated evaluation measures. This dilemma is discussed in more detail in other chapters of this book. It is important to note that this lack of data underscores the difficulty in regulating training and monitoring the practice of teamwork in healthcare.

TRAINING AND MONITORING TEAMWORK AT A STATE LEVEL

State governments are accountable to ensure that healthcare organizations within the state provide safe patient care; however, no state legislative body has moved forward as yet with regulation that mandates systemwide initiatives. Therefore, statewide efforts to improve teamwork skills in healthcare organizations are often driven by grassroots efforts or private sector quality and safety organizations, working collaboratively with public entities. These efforts are often led by state organizations such as hospital associations, quality improvement organizations, patient safety organizations, or coalitions of several groups partnering together. In many states, QIOs have supported team training efforts of individual hospitals, as part of the CMS 9th Scope of Work. In a few states, team training initiatives are being led by the state hospital association, often in collaboration with other patient safety organizations. In North Carolina, for example, the NC Hospital Association's Center for Hospital Quality and Patient Safety provides team training courses using the TeamSTEPPS® program. Two TeamSTEPPS® courses, a Fundamentals and the Master Trainer course are offered regularly throughout the year. The courses are filled to capacity, which supports the need for statewide training and confirms the commitment of NC hospitals in optimizing team skills of their staff. The courses combine didactic and interactive team exercises to enhance learning. Additional instruction on how to implement TeamSTEPPS® tools at the organization level is included in the 2-day Master Trainer course. Participants are provided with TeamSTEPPS® pocket guides and DVDs. Finally, participants are offered the opportunity to participate in quarterly conference calls to follow up on training questions in addition to discussing successful strategies and challenges related to implementation.

Teamwork skills are also integrated into other NC Quality Center collaborative learning programs. Collaborative toolkits provide a resource for project team development, communication, and function, and TeamSTEPPS® tools are recommended and taught by improvement advisors, as appropriate, when coaching the hospitals' project teams on enhancing teamwork and communication among their staff. For example, hospitals' project teams participating in a NC Surgical Care Improvement Project collaborative received a half-day training focused on improving teamwork and communication in the operating room, as part of one of the regularly scheduled learning sessions for the collaborative.

Monitoring Teamwork at the Local Level

Numerous hospitals and healthcare systems across the country are supporting formal teamwork training of clinicians, especially those working in high acuity areas such as the emergency department, intensive care unit, labor and delivery, and perioperative services. A variety of training and implementation methodologies have been developed, ranging from simple educational efforts focusing on the use of SBAR,[25] to comprehensive training using all core components of the TeamSTEPPS® curriculum. Some hospitals are beginning to require that all healthcare providers complete teamwork training, but methods to regulate and monitor this training are lacking.

MEASUREMENT OF SAFETY CULTURE AS A METHOD FOR MONITORING TEAMWORK

There is a growing body of evidence to indicate that perceptions of teamwork, gathered through adequate group participation in a validated safety culture survey, predict actual teamwork behaviors, and even patient outcomes.[26] Although healthcare is far from applying a LOSA-type of direct observation to measure and monitor teamwork, a safety culture survey can be efficient and reasonably cost effective, and results can directly measure teamwork within clinical areas. The mandate then becomes a threshold teamwork climate score.[27,28] A number of hospitals and healthcare systems are using teamwork climate and safety culture scores to identify units in need of improved teamwork and communication, and to follow progress of units in response to improvement strategies.

Just as a hospital can gain knowledge about its culture through culture surveys, a state can do the same by using statewide culture surveys or healthcare organizations working collaboratively to share their survey data to a designated improvement organization. Analysis of the data provides healthcare organizations with standardized culture dimension summary scores that can be compared with statewide benchmarks. This aggregated data can be used by a state coalition to monitor improvement over time in

Table 6.2   Culture Survey Results

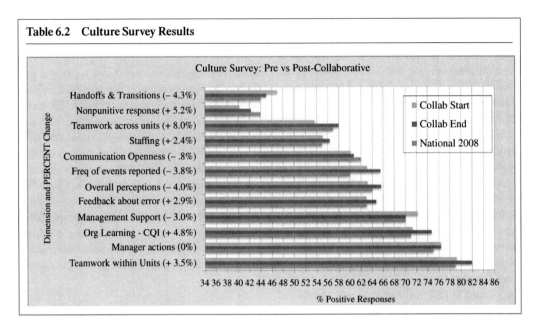

Culture Survey: Pre vs Post-Collaborative

the teamwork culture throughout the state, within a collaborative, and within certain categories of health-care facilities. It can provide guidance for teamwork training activities and initiatives, allowing these precious resources to be targeted to the organizations and culture dimensions with the greatest need. Table 6.2 displays the twelve roll-up dimensions of the AHRQ Hospital Survey on Patient Safety Culture. This is an example of an analysis that measures the percent change in survey responses before and after a state-level quality improvement collaborative.

To monitor and assess changes in the statewide teamwork culture, the NC Quality Center uses the AHRQ Hospital Survey on Patient Safety Culture. The Center encourages NC hospitals to use this survey to assess hospital culture and join the state initiative to use a dedicated vendor. Hospital-level reports include not only national benchmarks, but also state-level and peer group benchmarks. Hospitals participating in the initiative authorize the sharing of survey data with the NC Quality Center. The Center is then able to monitor changes in teamwork culture by specifically looking at the dimensions related to teamwork and communication. In the future the Center will use the data to target resources to organizations needing additional assistance.

It is reasonable to assume that a similar collaborative approach of providing training and support in

teamwork, aligned with measurement of teamwork culture, might be equally effective at a national level.

SUMMARY

Evidence from high reliability organizations such as commercial aviation and the military suggests that effective teamwork can lead to improved safety performance. Within healthcare, a growing body of literature supports a link between effective teamwork behaviors among healthcare providers and improved patient outcomes. As hospitals and healthcare organizations spend increasing amounts of time and resources to provide team training for their faculty, employees and health professions students, more research is needed to evaluate whether teamwork skills acquired in training are successfully integrated into the clinical setting and sustained over time. Additionally, more studies are needed to understand the link between effective teamwork behaviors and patient outcomes, so that appropriate monitoring and regulatory oversight can be established.

REFERENCES

1.   Kohn, L. T., Corrigan, J. M., Donaldson, M. S. (Eds.) (2000). Institute of Medicine. *To err*

is human: Building a safer health system.
Washington, DC: National Academies Press.

2. The Joint Commission. (2007). Sentinel event
    root cause and trend data. In *Improving America's
    hospitals: The Joint Commission's Annual
    Report on Quality and Safety 2007.* Oakbrook
    Terrace, IL: The Joint Commission.

3. Mazzocco, K., Petitti, D. B., et al. (2009). Surgical
    team behaviors and patient outcomes. *American
    Journal of Surgery, 197*(5), 678–85.

4. Morey, J. C., Simon, R., Jay, G. D., et al. (2002).
    Error reduction and performance improvement
    in the emergency department through formal
    teamwork training: Evaluation results of the
    MedTeams project. *Health Services Research,
    37*(6), 1553–80.

5. Pronovost, P., & Berenholtz, S. M., et al. (2008).
    Improving patient safety in intensive care units in
    Michigan. *Journal of Critical Care, 23*(2), 207–21.

6. Mann, S., & Pratt, S. D. (2008). Team approach to
    care in labor and delivery. *Clinical Obstetrics and
    Gynecology, 51*(4), 666–79.

7. National Quality Forum. (2010). *Safe Practices
    for Better Healthcare.* Retrieved January 30,
    2010 from: www.qualityforum.org/publications/
    reports/safe_practices_2009.asp

8. Kirch, D. (2007). *Culture and the Courage
    to Change.* AAMC president's address 2007.
    Retrieved January 30, 2010 from: http://www.
    ohsu.edu/xd/about/vision/upload/2007-20-
    AAMC-presidents-address.pdf

9. Lauber, J. K. Cockpit resource management:
    background and overview. In H. W. Orlady, &
    H. C. Foushee (Eds.), *Cockpit resource
    management training: proceedings of the NASA/
    MAC workshop.* Moffett Field, CA: NASA—
    Ames Research Center.

10. Helmreich, R. L., Merritt, A. C., & Wilhelm, J.
    A. *The Evolution of Crew Resource Management
    Training in Commercial Aviation.* Retrieved
    January 30, 2010 from: http://www.raes-hfg.com/
    reports/18octoo-RAWG-1/culture.pdf

11. *Crew Resource Management.* A Paper by the CRM
    Standing Group of the Royal Aeronautical Society
    (1999). London. Retrieved January 30, 2010 from:
    www.raes-hfg.com/reports/crm-now.htm

12. Pizzi, L., Goldfarb, N., & Nash, D. B. (2010).
    Crew Resource Management and Its Applications
    in Medicine. Retrieved January 30, 2010 from:
    www.ahrq.gov/clinic/ptsafety/chap44.htm

13. Air Force Instruction 11-290. Retrieved from:
    http://www.e-publishing.af.mil/shared/media/
    epubs/AFI11-290.pdf

14. Klinect, J. R., Merritt, A., & Helmreich, R.
    (2003). Line operations safety audit (LOSA):
    Definition and operating characteristics. In
    *Proceedings of the 12th International Symposium
    on Aviation Psychology* (pp. 663–8). Dayton, OH:
    Ohio State University.

15. Salas, E., Sims, D., Klein, C., & Burke, C. S.
    (2003). Can teamwork enhance patient safety?
    *Risk Management Foundation, Harvard Medical
    Institutions, Forum, 23*(3), 5–9.

16. Mansur, T. (2009) Teamwork and patient safety in
    dynamic domains of healthcare: A review of the
    literature. *Acta Anaesthesiologica Scandinavica,
    53,* 143–51.

17. Mitchell, P. H., Ferketich, S., & Jennings, B. M.
    (1998). Quality health outcomes model. American
    Academy of Nursing Expert Panel on Quality
    Healthcare. *Image: The Journal of Nursing
    Scholarship, 30,* 43–6.

18. Mitchell, P., & Lang, N. (2004). Framing the
    problem of measuring and improving healthcare
    quality. Has the quality health outcomes model
    been useful? *Medical Care, 42,* 2.

19. Mayberry, L. J., & Gennaro, S. (2001). Quality
    of health outcomes model for guiding obstetrical
    practice. *Journal of Nursing Scholarship, 33*(2),
    141–6.

20. National Patient Safety Goal 2a. Retrieved
    February 5, 2010 from: http://www.jcinc.
    com/2009-NPSGs-Gaol-2/

21. Council of Europe, Committee of Ministers.
    (2006). Recommendation Council of Europe
    Committee of Ministers. *Recommendation
    Rec(2006)7 of the Committee of Ministers to
    member states on management of patient safety
    and prevention of adverse events in healthcare.*
    Retrieved September 1, 2010 from: https://wcd.
    coe.int/ViewDoc.jsp?id=1005439&Site=CM&Ba
    ckColorInternet=C3C3C3&BackColorIntranet=E
    DB021&BackColorLogged=F5D383#Top

22. Aus- und Weiterbildung in Patientensicherheit
    und Fehlerkultur. Projekt "Zukunft Medizin
    Schweiz"—Phase lll. Schweizerische Akademie
    der Medizinischen Wissenschaften (SAMW)
    [Education and training in patient safety and
    medical-error culture. "The Future of Swiss
    Medicine" project, phase 3. Swiss Academy of
    Medical Sciences (SAMS)], Basel, 2007. http://
    www.samw.ch/en.

23. World Alliance for Patient Safety. (2009). WHO
    Patient Safety Curriculum. Guide for Medical
    Schools. A Summary. Geneva: World Health
    Organization. http://www.who.int/patientsafety/

education/curriculum/en/index.html. Accessed
May 4, 2012.

24. Agency for Healthcare Research and Quality.
(2005). TeamSTEPPS®. Retrieved January
30, 2010 from: http://www. usuhs.mil/cerps/
TeamSTEPPS.html

25. Haig, K., Sutton, S., & Whittington, J. (2006).
SBAR: A shared mental model for improving
communication between clinicians. *Journal of
Quality and Safety, 32,* 167–75.

26. Sexton, J. B., Thomas, E. J., & Helmreich, R. L.
(2000). Error, stress, and teamwork in medicine
and aviation: Cross sectional surveys. *British
Medical Journal, 320,* 745–9.

27. Sexton, J. B., Grillo, S., Fullwood, C., &
Provonost, P. (2009) *Assessing and Improving
Safety Culture. The Essential Guide for
Patient Safety Officers.* Washington, DC: Joint
Commission of Accreditation of Healthcare
Organizations and the Institute for Healthcare
Improvement.

28. Sexton, J. B., & Thomas, E. J. (2008). The
Safety Climate Survey: Psychometric and
Benchmarking Properties. The University of
Texas Center of Excellence for Patient Safety
Research and Practice. *Journal of Critical Care,
23,* 188–96.

PART THREE

INSIGHTS FROM PRACTICE IN HEALTHCARE

7

TEAM TRAINING IN LABOR AND DELIVERY

Susan C. Mann and Stephen D. Pratt

INTRODUCTION

Reducing medical errors and improving patient safety are important goals for all healthcare providers. Crisis management simulation and team training based on the concepts of crew resource management (CRM) have been proposed as potential ways to achieve these goals. Labor and delivery (L&D) units offer specific challenges to the implementation of team-based training. Unlike the operating room environment, clinicians may be caring for multiple patients at one time. Unlike medical/surgical wards, clinicians must perform highly invasive and potentially life-threatening medical interventions. Unlike most medical arenas, clinicians and patients may be directly competing for limited resources, and the decisions made by one clinician may directly and negatively affect the care available for another patient. Finally, unlike any other place in medicine, two patients (mother and baby) are affected by every medical decision and negatively impacted by each medical error. These challenges in providing safe care can cause breakdowns in care of individual patients or the workflow of the entire L&D environment. It is understandable how adverse outcomes can occur in the high-stress obstetrical (OB) environment, when providers may care for patients only during the episode of the birth and antenatal information may not always be available to providers.

COMMON LABOR AND DELIVERY CULTURE

The culture of most L&D units has evolved slowly over time, and many behaviors have developed for the benefit of those providing the care and not necessarily those who are receiving the care. For far too long, we have operated in "silos" in which we mainly communicate within our individual disciplines of care. Plans are not shared or reviewed for safety. Work load variations can stress the ability of individuals to safely care for their patients, and yet no system generally exist to identify or correct these workload variations.

Conflicts can readily occur; for example, an elective cesarean delivery may be in progress when the same obstetrician is also needed to cover an emergent case involving a delivering patient in L&D. Obstetrical providers usually make an effort to get the bulk of their work done during daylight hours which is complicated by the competing concerns of laboring patients, office patients, operating room schedules, fatigue and the interest of the physician's family.

Despite the challenges outlined in the preceding, team training and simulation may be powerful tools in the efforts to decrease medical error in obstetrics. A growing body of literature is helping to validate this position.

WHAT DOES TEAM TRAINING LOOK LIKE IN OBSTETRICS?

The translation of CRM-based teamwork to the labor and delivery environment is a growing art and science. Salas suggests that there is a set of "big five" team behaviors necessary for successful teamwork:[1]

- Leadership;
- Mutual performance monitoring;
- Back-up behaviors;
- Adaptability; and
- Team orientation.

These behaviors are supported by shared mental models, closed loop communication, and mutual trust. However, the specific factors needed to successfully translate these concepts to the clinical environment have not been fully elucidated. The literature and the authors' experience suggest that the following are necessary:

1. A team structure;
2. Specific team behaviors;
3. Specific team skills that individuals can learn and perform, including methods for conflict resolution; and
4. Tools to help the behaviors and skill take root.

This chapter reviews each of these based on the available literature and the work done the authors' own institution over the past decade. We developed specific teams on the unit to support the teamwork behaviors and improve role clarity and communication processes, based on MedTeams and TeamSTEPPS®.[2,3] These teams were the core team, coordinating team, and a contingency or rapid response team. The core team includes the obstetricians, anesthesiologists, midwives, nurses, residents, scrub technicians, and unit secretaries (where applicable). They provide direct patient care and inform the coordinating team regarding the status of their patients. The coordinating team is composed of the charge (resource) nurse, a dedicated obstetrical anesthesiologist, an

obstetrician, and the chief OB resident. The coordinating team is charged with the overall management of workflow for an L&D unit. This group prioritizes cesarean deliveries, elective and nonelective, induction of labor patients and may make recommendations regarding use of labor stimulants based on the volume and acuity of the patients. The contingency team is a rapid response team that responds to obstetrical emergencies such as stat cesarean deliveries, deliveries complicated by emergent cesarean delivery, and postpartum hemorrhage. The members are preassigned, come from the core team, and have specific roles and responsibilities.[4] The expectation is that these teams meet regularly to ensure a "shared mental model" (in which everyone is on the same page), workloads are evenly distributed, and plans are progressing and still appropriate.

We developed a classroom-based course again based on the MedTeams emergency medicine curriculum and TeamSTEPPs®.[3,5] The course uses clinical vignettes, videos, educational scenarios, and role-playing to help teach teamwork concepts.[2] Four content areas are covered:

- Leadership
- Communication
- Situation Monitoring
- Mutual Assistance

These modules help staff learn specific team behaviors (Table 7.1) and individual skills (Table 7.2) to improve communication and resource management, the important role of leadership in ensuring that communication and teamwork behaviors occur, ways to develop shared mental models or shared vision, and error prevention strategies. Using unit-based scenarios provides greater buy-in and allows participants to gain an understanding of how communication or teamwork behaviors break down, and if members commit to practicing in a safety-based culture how similar situations could be prevented.

TRANSLATION OF CURRICULUM CONTENT TO AN IN SITU ENVIRONMENT

The leadership module stresses the facilitation of communication events, management of resources,

Table 7.1   Team Behaviors

	Definition	Frequency
Team Meeting	Multidisciplinary meeting designed to discuss the patients on the unit, expected workload (C-sections, inductions), potential problems (staffing shortage, equipment malfunction, patient concerns), and other issues that might affect the care of patients. See Figure 7.1 for Template.	Once a shift and ad hoc as needed to maintain a safe environment
Preprocedure Briefing	A multidisciplinary meeting of those to be involved in a medical procedure (c-section, extraction of placenta, operative vaginal delivery, etc). Operative and anesthesia plans, safety plans, and medical concerns are openly discussed. See Figure 7.2 for Template.	Before operative procedures. May be abbreviated or skipped during emergencies
Debriefing	Structured discussion of relevant *teamwork* events after a procedure, shift, or adverse event. The purpose is to improve teamwork behavior. Care must be taken to ensure peer review protection and to only discuss teamwork issues.	As needed
Huddle	A brief update between two or more team members to ensure maintenance of situation awareness and shared mental model.	As clinical conditions change

Table 7.2   Individual Teamwork Skills

Behavior	Definition
SBAR	Structured technique for presentation of relevant patient information consisting of *S*ituation, *B*ackground, *A*ssessment, *R*ecommendation
DESC Script	Structured technique for conflict resolution in which speaker *D*escribes their concerns, *E*xplains why this is a problem, *S*uggests alternative approaches, and seeks *C*onsensus
2-Challenge Rule	Concept that patient safety concern must be verbalized at least twice if behavior is not corrected. This ensures that concerns is heard and understood.
Check Back	Orders and clinician needs must be repeated back to the sender to ensure that the receiver has understood the message correctly.
Call Out	Important events are called aloud, especially during rapidly changing situations. Facilitates anticipation of next steps (e.g. "The patient is intubated, you can make the incision.")
Situation Monitoring	Actively scanning the unit to assess patients and their plans of care, team member performance, and the environment; looking for potential errors
Situation Awareness	The state of knowing one's surroundings and work condition
Patient Advocacy	Actively working to ensure patient safety at all times
Resource Management	Appropriately re-allocating resources or work load to ensure that no patient is at risk because of overworked staff
Feedback	A form of verbal support that help colleagues to improve their teamwork. Specific techniques are employed to assist with learning and minimize defensiveness.

Pertinent Patient Information

Plan of Care

Provider Availability

Resource Management

Staff Workload

Elective and Non-elective work

Figure 7.1
Team Meeting Template

and assistance with conflict resolution. The communication events include multidisciplinary team meetings, physician–nurse huddles, pre-procedural briefings, and event debriefing. Templates are developed to facilitate each communication event (Figs. 7.1 and 7.2). Leaders create the expectation that team members participate in team behaviors, and hold members accountable. Members also hold one another accountable, because it is everyone's responsibility to participate in these communication events.

The ability to provide information to one's team members for huddles or team meetings requires the development of situation awareness through situation monitoring. Thus, it is important to come to a team meeting understanding the status of one's patients, progress of labor and plans of care, any safety concerns regarding one's patients (e.g., previous postpartum hemorrhage or shoulder dystocia), any fetal heart rate abnormalities, and potential needs for additional resources at delivery. Medical concerns, physician availability, scheduled work (inductions, c-sections), and staffing issues should all also be discussed at a team meeting. Sharing this type of precise, patient and provider-specific information for each patient on the L&D unit allows staff to understand the acuity and volume of the entire unit, and all caregivers are able to develop a shared mental model about both specific patients and the unit as a whole at a given time. For instance, in a situation in which several patients might be experiencing abnormal fetal heart rate patterns, this information is discussed and a decision to delay elective cases may be made to allow all the patients on the unit the safest care possible.

- Introduce Team Members

- Patient Name

- Procedure to be done (CS [primary or repeat] with or without tubal)

    o Side/site marked if ovarian cystectomy planned

- Indication for CS (repeat, breech, etc)

- Planned anesthetic (spinal/epidural/CSE/GA)

- Allergies

- Antibiotics to be given and when

- Pertinent Medical/Surgical history

- Blood availability

- Any issues or extra personnel/equipment necessary (e.g. NICU)

- OB H&P and Consent (dated and timed) in chart

- Anesthesia Assessment and Consent (dated and timed) in chart

- Encourage open communication of any concerns when in OR

Figure 7.2
Preprocedural Briefing Template

Using templates for briefings before operative procedures, a template for timeout and a checklist sign-out process at the end of cases has been shown to reduce morbidity and mortality by 36% in operative patients using the World Health Organization's Safe Surgery Checklist.[6] The preoperative surgical briefing allows the anesthesiologist to prepare for any safety concerns regarding hemorrhage and for discussion to occur regarding mode of anesthesia as well as any other particular safety concerns. At times conflict can arise among healthcare team members. Team members learn conflict resolution techniques, and leaders assist members by modeling behaviors or role-playing the difficult conversations that allow team members to resolve issues without harboring ill feelings. Moreover, it has been our experience that conflict occurs with much less frequency when members create shared mental models regarding patient care. Creating an environment in which information is shared freely helps staff to perform other error-reduction strategies, including checkbacks regarding completed tasks and callouts for information transfer (such as when it is safe to make an incision for a cesarean delivery). Using closed-loop communication and Situation, Background, Assessment and Response (SBAR) information transfer are additional error reduction strategies. Having clear handoff strategies for team members, with the opportunity to ask questions is important for patient safety and has been a Joint Commission National Patient Safety Goal.[7]

INSIGHTS LEARNED FROM TRAINING AND IMPLEMENTING TEAMWORK IN LABOR AND DELIVERY

What follows is a series of insights into the ways that team training can improve patient care in obstetrics, and important lessons learned in the successful implementation process.

Insight 1: Resources Are Limited.

Clinicians in all areas of medicine must work with finite resources. However, perhaps in no other arena do the decisions of one clinician so directly impact that availability of resources for others as in obstetrics. Anesthesia personnel and operating room (OR) space are frequently limited on L& D units, especially during off hours. The decision to "push the pit" may be reasonable in an effort to facilitate delivery of an individual fetus. However, if this leads to fetal heart rate compromise and an urgent cesarean delivery, this may preclude others from having a cesarean delivery because no anesthesiologist or OR is available. If this is done at a time when other fetal heart rate patterns are concerning, clear safety concerns can arise. Even the simple decision of when to place a labor epidural, or when to send a labor nurse to lunch can dramatically affect the safety of the labor unit.

The coordinating team, as described, can help ensure that limited resources are used effectively and thoughtfully. When this team is appropriately informed of labor plans, it can help direct care and minimize risk.

Insight 2: There Are Inherent Risks When a Patient Does Not Have a Clear Plan of Care That Is Shared with All Providers.

The delivery of a child is an inherently personal and private activity. Although respecting the family's wishes for privacy is important, it can create risk. Plans are literally made behind closed doors, and too often they are not shared with others on the unit. The safety of these plans cannot be assessed when they are hidden within the private labor room. Creating a shared vision for all members of the patients' care teams is vital for the safe functioning of an L&D unit. When there are limited human resources, as described in Insight #1, it is prudent to understand which patients are at imminent risk. In addition, physicians often leave an L&D unit without indicating their availability to the charge nurse or the nurses caring for their patients. This scenario can then create a situation in which a nurse is reluctant to push an oxytocin-augmented labor when there is a concerning fetal heart rate pattern because she is unaware of the availability of the covering physician. When the physician returns to reevaluate the patient and the oxytocin drip has been shut off, the reaction is usually anger because the physician's plan all along was to deliver the patient, and if the labor could not progress because of pattern issues, then a cesarean delivery would be performed, but this message was never conveyed to the staff. Having a team meeting in which one of the care providers states the plan of care for the patient and the availability of the providers aids in managing expectations and resources and results in safer care for patients, averting emergent situations when avoidable.

Insight 3: Conflict Is Common in Obstetrics, and Conflict Resolution Is Difficult.

Patient safety is predicated on trust, open communication, and effective interdisciplinary teamwork.[8] Some physicians undermine the atmosphere of trust with disruptive or abusive behavior. A Joint Commission Sentinel Event Alert indicated that "intimidating and disruptive behaviors can foster medical errors, contribute to poor patient satisfaction and to preventable adverse outcomes, increase the cost of care, and cause qualified clinicians, administrators and managers to seek new positions in more professional environments."[9] It has been estimated that 3%–5% of physicians present a problem with disruptive behavior.[10] Rosenstein et al. demonstrated the negative effects that aggressive and disruptive behaviors have on patient safety and staff retention in the perioperative setting.[11–13] Similar behaviors have been described in obstetrics. Veltman found that 60.7% of labor and delivery units noted disruptive behavior, generally occurring at least monthly; 41.9% indicated that adverse patient outcomes had occurred as a direct result of these behaviors; and 39.3% stated that nurses had left the unit because of intimidation.[14] In another survey, 34% of nurses stated that they had been concerned about a physician's performance, but only 1% actually shared these concerns.[15] Obstetrical nurses have described explicit episodes of aggressive behavior: "I would be petrified if at 7 a.m. they [the physicians] walked in and I didn't have the pit going. They'd yell at me."[8]

Physicians can help create an open and trusting communication atmosphere by asking other team members to raise safety concerns, and expressly giving them permission to question unclear orders or challenge apparently dangerous actions. Openly communicating in this way during a briefing before surgery (e.g., cesarean delivery) can set the tone for better communication throughout the procedure.[16] Physicians should thank staff who question their behavior, even if the questioner is wrong, because the act of questioning done for patient safety and should be encouraged.

Insight 4: Physician Coverage Arrangements Are Not Clear at All Times and Often Are Not Communicated to Essential Staff.

Obstetricians work in different environments within a given week or even a given day (e.g., labor and delivery, office, operating rooms). Although the perception is often that the on-call physician is always readily available, this is simply not true if he or she is performing surgery. Most physicians are willing to help out in a clear emergency or when asked to specifically cover an event. The precise identification of another physician who is capable of covering a labor patient's needs when the identified physician is unavailable (e.g., in the operating room or an office several miles away) is frequently not communicated to all parties caring for a patient. Having an identified place to indicate the covering physician and the culture that it is the physician's responsibility to identify the back-up doctor, and that the person's identity is shared with the charge nurse and nurse carrying for a labor patient during the time that the primary physician is not available. We use the multidisciplinary team meeting to understand the workload of other physician staff and engage in conversations of availability for coverage if the need arises.

Insight 5: Unevenly Distributed Workload Among Providers Can Put Patients at Risk.

The L&D workplace is a dynamic environment. Cesarean deliveries and elective induction of labor are usually scheduled in the morning, causing an increase in workflow. At the same time, discharges are needed to free up postpartum beds. Elective cesarean sections are often scheduled when the obstetrician is on call in L&D, and he or she may also need to cover unscheduled gynecological cases in the main operating rooms during the same time period. When multiple patients arrive and/or the acuity suddenly shifts it is important to have a clear understanding of resources available. An environment in which providers feel that they are either "too busy to ask for help" or would appear "weak" in doing so can be an impediment to good patient care. The multidisciplinary team meeting is a good place for nursing to balance workload and having a quick meeting during an emergency (e.g., significant postpartum hemorrhage) allows physicians to understand the magnitude of the emergency and prioritize the care of the other patients on the unit.

Insight 6: A Structured Process for Prioritization of Care Does Not Usually Exist or Is Not Recognized by Staff.

A lack of structure that identifies and empowers leaders on the L&D unit can lead to ineffective and or inaccurate triaging of patient care. Physicians often advocate strongly for their own patients, and the triaging function can fall on the shoulders of the single charge nurse. Developing a coordinating team allows for joint decision making regarding the triaging of cesarean deliveries when there are limited and competing resources. If an emergency is ongoing, the coordinating team may decide to stop oxytocin infusions in patients having an augmented labor or in delaying elective work such as labor inductions or initiating nonemergent procedures. In addition, if there is a provider who is straying from the established plan of care and there are safety concerns, the coordinating team can discuss the concerns with the individual and help with any ensuing conflict issues.

Insight 7: Poor Communication Is Common in Obstetrics.

Substandard care contributes to approximately 50% of maternal deaths, with poor communication or teamwork being the primary factors in the substandard care.[17] Poor communication and coordination of care has been identified in 43% of closed malpractice claims in obstetrics.[18] The Joint Commission identified poor communication as a root cause in 72% of perinatal deaths.[19] Improving communication may be the single most important factor in the effort to improve patient safety in obstetrics. Data exist demonstrating that obstetrical care providers frequently communicate ineffectively in both simulated and clinical environments. Using *in situ* simulated eclampsia drills, Thompson et al. found that timely communication with senior obstetrical

staff was a recurrent problem.[20] Similarly, Daniels et al. demonstrated that obstetrical residents communicated poorly with their pediatric team members during a simulated emergent delivery. Although 63% called for pediatric help during the simulated maternal cardiopulmonary arrest, and only 10% gave helpful information to the pediatricians when they arrived.[21]

More concerning, interdisciplinary communication may be lacking in the clinical care of the parturient. Simpson et al. used focus groups to describe the communication patterns between the obstetricians and obstetrical nurse in four L&D units. The authors found that the communication processes were frequently not consistent with effective teamwork.[8] The nurses at one site often communicated with obstetricians only for admission orders and delivery, amounting to only two to four minutes of interaction during the entire labor process. Across the sites, nurses described having to use catch phrases or code words to get the obstetricians to listen to their recommendations. They even purposely withheld information from physicians so as to influence their interactions. This need to play the "physician–nurse game" clearly has the potential to undermine trust between team members and lead to patient harm.

Team behaviors (e.g., team meetings and preprocedure meetings) create structured opportunities for interdisciplinary communication. Crew resource management-based teamwork also teaches specific teamwork skills to improve communication. These include the use of check-backs (closed-loop communication), structured hand-offs (SBAR), and the two-challenge rule.

Insight 8: Handoffs of Care Are Frequently Inadequate.

The transfer or hand-off of patient care from one provider to another is common. Generally, these hand-offs occur within specialties (OB to OB, nurse to nurse, etc). Rarely are all providers together to share plans or safety concerns. This may lead to an incomplete picture of the risks to the patient and her baby. The multidisciplinary team meeting allows all providers to come together and share their safety concerns about all the patients in labor and delivery, providing situation awareness for all providers and a chance for providers to cross-monitor plans of care.

The handoff of a patient from the operating room after a cesarean delivery to the postanesthesia care area can be variable because it may include a completely different set of providers. In addition, it can cause confusion as to who the patient care leader is when a patient has pain concerns or hypotension. Should the obstetrician be called to evaluate for possible post-partum hemorrhage, or should the anesthesia provider be called to assess for possible complications related to regional anesthesia. Identifying a leader of care and expectations for communication during this period is helpful for safe patient care.

Insight 9: The Impact of Team Training Can Be Measured in Obstetrics

Although various outcomes measures are used in obstetrics, at least three tools can be used for measuring process and outcomes related to changing to a teamwork culture. These tools include: (1) the Adverse Outcome Index (AOI) for measuring outcomes of mothers and neonates, a series of process measures that can be beneficial for identifying improvement in the short term, (2) patient satisfaction scores using tools such as Press-Ganey, and (3) surveys focusing on teamwork and safety attitudes using questionnaires such as the AHRQ HSOPS (hospital survey of patient safety culture) or the Safety Attitude Questionnaire (SAQ), developed by Sexton.[22–24] The AOI was developed as part of a trio of measures to assess obstetrical outcomes. The AOI is a composite measure of 10 significant adverse maternal or neonatal outcomes designated in Figure 7.3. The AOI is defined as percentage of deliveries complicated by one or more of the identified outcomes. A scoring system was developed in conjunction with the American College of Obstetricians and Gynecologists' Quality Improvement and Patient Safety Committee to assess the severity of the outcomes. Two other measures were developed with the AOI to further assess severity and acuity of the care on an L&D unit. The Weighted Adverse Outcome Score describes the acuity of the care and is the total score of all adverse events identified in the table divided by the number of deliveries. The Severity Index describes the severity of cases with an adverse outcomes. It is the sum of the adverse

Maternal death	750
Intrapartum & neonatal death > 2500 gm	400
Uterine rupture	100
Maternal admission to ICU	65
Birth trauma	60
Return to OR / labor & delivery	40
Admission to NICU > 2500g & for > 24 hours	35
APGAR < 7 at 5 minutes	25
Blood transfusion	20
3° or 4° perineal tear	5

* ICU, intensive care unit; OR, operating room; NICU, neonatal ICU.

Data adapted from Mann S., et al.: Assessing quality in obstetrical care: Development of standardized measures. *Jt Comm J QualPatient Saf* 32:497–505, Sep. 2006.

Figure 7.3
Adverse Outcome Index.
Data adapted from Mann S., et al. (2006). Assessing quality in obstetrical care: Development of standardized measures. *Joint Commission Journal on Quality and Patient Safety, 32,* 497–505.

outcome scores divided by the number of deliveries with an identified adverse outcome. The AOI and WAOS outcome measures have recently been used in studies evaluating interventions in labor and delivery and in describing a comprehensive patient safety initiative involving team training.[25–27]

Insight 10: Teamwork Appears to Improve Outcomes in Obstetrics.

A large, prospective, randomized trial evaluating the impact a classroom-based CRM course based on the MedTeams curriculum failed to demonstrate improvements in patient outcomes. The authors did find a 10-minute (~33%) improvement in the time from decision to incision in emergent cesarean deliveries.[2] However, others have demonstrated improvements in patient outcomes associated with both classroom and simulation-based team training. Pratt et al. trained more than 220 in a classroom-based CRM teamwork course. In addition, the authors described a structured implementation process involving the use of templates, structured language, coaches, and three types of formal teams that helped to translate the

behaviors to the clinical environment. They found that obstetrical complication rates decreased by 23% after the implementation of teamwork.[4] Pettker described a multistep process designed to improve safety on their L&D unit, including clinical protocols, fetal monitor certification, a safety committee, and classroom-based team training (Fig. 7.4). The entire process required nearly 2 years. The adverse event rate decreased by nearly 28%.[25] CRM-based teamwork as part of large, multi-step patient safety initiatives has been shown to decrease adverse events and the associated medical malpractice costs.[28,29] Similar data have been demonstrated in the private practice obstetrical setting. Shea-Lewis described a 43% reduction in the rate of adverse obstetrical events after the implementation of a CRM-based team training curriculum in an intermediate-sized community hospital.[26] Riley found that the inclusion of teamwork-based simulation along with TeamSTEPPS training was associated with dramatic improvements in the WAOS compared to TeamSTEPPS alone or no team training at all.[27] Finally, Draycott et al. developed a 1-day course that combined didactic and simulation training in both teamwork behaviors and obstetrical

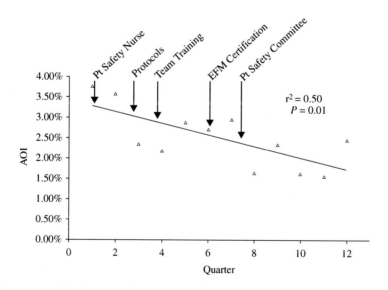

Figure 7.4
Change in Adverse Outcomes Index with implementation of safety initiatives.
Reprinted from Pettker, C. M., Thung, S. F., Norwitz, E. R., et al. (2009). Impact of a comprehensive patient safety strategy on obstetrical adverse events. *American Journal of Obstetrics and Gynecology, 200*(5), 492, with permission from Elsevier.

crisis management. All obstetrical care providers at a large urban center were required to attend the course in multidisciplinary sessions. Evaluation of more than 19,000 deliveries demonstrated a 50% reduction in the rate of neonatal hypoxic ischemic encephalopathy after the training.[30]

Insight 11: The Implementation of Team Behavior Requires Leadership

Different types of hospitals, whether teaching, community, or military, pose different challenges to the implementation of any culture change. Similarly, different disciplines within the practice of medicine also respond to change with varying enthusiasm. The overriding principle for successful implementation and sustainment of the behaviors is that leadership, from the executive suite to department chairpersons to nursing managers, must be involved in and support the safety culture for change to occur. In military hospitals, providers of care are usually more accustomed to accepting change and not questioning hierarchy if the case for change is made and a plan is rolled out with leaders holding staff accountable for defined behaviors. Most teaching hospitals today are hybrids of resident physicians, employed hospital-based attending physicians, and private practice attending physicians working side by side. Often there is respect for leadership in academic institutions; however, decisions made regarding changes in practice are sometimes met with resistance from resident staff or private attending staff. In military institutions the challenge is not usually in leadership involvement and respect for leadership but the high rate of turnover of staff and need for frequent training of new staff. In community hospitals the leadership is usually more amorphous, with the department chair being an elected or rotated position for a period of 1–2 years and often not a desired position. The chief of the medical staff is sometimes the one who holds staff accountable for agreed-on behaviors.

The chairperson or the chief medical officer may have some success changing behavior, but it is important to have the clinical champions of the department involved from the onset. These champions should be identified as trainers and subsequently coaches. Ideally, when initially implementing behaviors it is best if the coaches have no other clinical responsibilities. Coaches can use team meetings as a teaching tool demonstrating where staff are gaining situation awareness regarding their patients, developing shared mental models, and how this information may modify care. Similarly, if a conflict arises regarding a plan of care or an interpersonal exchange, the coach can help staff members navigate conflict in a constructive way. Nurses generally accept changes in practice without as much difficulty as physicians. Nurses who work the night shift may already feel that they work together as a team as there is less of a presence of physician staff at night requiring a more cohesive working environment. However, a shared mental model may still be lacking, regarding a particular patient or clear designation for coverage of patients and their plans of care. Anesthesia providers often find this collaborative model useful, because they are frequently consulted for cases of emergent cesarean delivery, or when there is a deviation from the plan of a routine vaginal birth. The ability to plan, prepare, and share safety concerns regarding airways or preexisting medical conditions can be invaluable.

There is a problem in the patient safety movement of change fatigue, which describes what happens to staff when the work environment is in constant flux in an attempt to improve care for patients. Frequent change can lead to a failure of acceptance of the change and the provider burnout.[31] Managing the resistance of providers is required if efforts to change culture are to succeed. Different approaches such as presenting at staff meetings and getting buy-in before initiation of training, one-on-one meetings, and mandating training but providing some form of incentive to busy staff may be helpful. Using process measures (e.g., percent of elective cesarean deliveries that start on time) for short-term feedback and patient outcome and staff satisfaction for long-term sustainability are very useful tools to support culture changes.

Insight 12: Team Training May Lead to Other Patient Safety Improvements

The successful implementation of teamwork in an L&D unit can reap benefits not directly related to the teamwork training. Improved staff satisfaction has been linked to the implementation of CRM-based behaviors.[4,25,32] Many environments are experiencing nursing shortages, and improved satisfaction can help decrease sick calls and staff turnover.[33] Education of new staff may also improve. New nurses on L&D

units traditionally shadow an experienced nurse for a predetermined period, and then are given full clinical duties. They are thus exposed to only those clinical situations that their mentors experience during the orientation process. Within a teamwork environment, both the mentor and trainee will be expected to know about the history and management plans for all patients on the unit. Team meetings can serve as educational opportunities to learn about all the patients on the unit, thus increasing the depth and breadth of their clinical exposure during orientation. Finally, the climate of trust and "teamliness" may help with other performance improvement efforts. When the entire unit is working together as a team in an effort to improve patient safety, systems issues, latent errors, communication weaknesses, and other potential safety problem can be more easily identified. The process improvements for these problems can then have input from multiple specialties and new systems put into place in an effective and well-coordinated fashion.

CONCLUSION

The L&D setting is complex, with multidisciplinary teams caring for patient dyads with high expectations and varying acuity and volume. It is often difficult for providers to obtain and share critical information needed to ensure consistently safe care for patients and a desirable work environment for colleagues. The competing demands on obstetricians and anesthesiologists may make their immediate availability a challenge, leaving the unit without adequate supports or planning. Team training offers the supports and framework to assist in such a complex and challenging milieu. Considerable research on team training in obstetrical and other medical settings has been done and is ongoing. Although we may not have yet identified the best method to teach the concepts of CRM and successfully change culture, the combination of a didactic course and structured implementation of the teamwork behaviors into daily work processes to facilitate a culture change, combined with simulation to provide an arena to practice the skills of teamwork, especially in crisis situations, may emerge as the desired approach. With the introduction of team training and simulation in obstetrics we have certainly seen improvements in patient outcomes and improved staff satisfaction regarding safety that can be beneficial to patients, their families, and providers.

REFERENCES

1. Salas E SD, Burke CS. (2005). Is there a "big five" in teamwork? *Small Group Research 36*, 555–99.
2. Nielsen PE, Goldman MB, Mann S, et al. (2007). Effects of teamwork training on adverse outcomes and process of care in labor and delivery: a randomized controlled trial. *Obstetetrics and Gynecology, 109*, 48–55.
3. TeamSTEPPS. Retrieved April 9,2012 from http://teamstepps.ahrq.gov
4. Pratt SD, Mann S, Salisbury M, et al. (2007). Impact of CRM- based training on obstetric outcomes and clinicians' patient safety attitudes. *Joint Commission Jouranl on Quality Patient Safety, 33*, 720–5.
5. Morey JC, Simon R, Jay GD, et al. (2002). Error reduction and performance improvement in the emergency department through formal teamwork training: evaluation results of the MedTeams project. *Health Services Research, 37*, 1553–81.
6. Haynes AB, Weiser TG, Berry WR, et al. (2009). A surgical safety checklist to reduce morbidity and mortality in a global population. *New England Journal of Medicine, 360*, 491–9.
7. Handoffs and Signouts. Agency for Healthcare Research and Quality. Retrieved April 9, 2012.
8. Simpson KR, James DC, Knox GE. (2006). Nurse-physician communication during labor and birth: implications for patient safety. *Journal of Obstetrics and Gynecology, Neonatal Nursing, 35*, 547–56.
9. Sentinel Event Alert, Issue 40: Behaviors that undermine a culture of safety. Joint Commission, 2008. Retrieved at http://www.jointcommission.org/sentinel_Event_alert_issue_40_behaviors_that_undermine_a_culture_of_safety/
10. Leape LL, Fromson JA. (2006). Problem doctors: is there a system-level solution? *Annuals of Internal Medicine, 144*, 107–15.
11. Rosenstein AH, O'Daniel M. (2006). Impact and implications of disruptive behavior in the perioperative arena. *Journal of the American College of Surgeons, 203*, 96–105.
12. Rosenstein AH, O'Daniel M. (2005). Disruptive behavior and clinical outcomes: Perceptions of nurses and physicians. *American Journal of Nursing, 105*, 54–64.

13. Rosenstein AH, et al. (2002). Disruptive physician behavior contributes to nursing shortage. Study links bad behavior by doctors to nurses leaving the profession. *Physician Executive, 28,* 8–11

14. Veltman LL. (2007). Disruptive behavior in obstetrics: a hidden threat to patient safety. *American Journal of Obstetrics and Gynecology, 196,* 587 e1–4.

15. Maxfield, D., Grenny, J., McMillan, R., et al. *Silencekills; The seven crucial conversations for healthcare.* Retrieved April 9, 2012 from: http://www.silencekills.com/PDL/SilenceKills.pdf

16. Lingard L, Regehr G, Orser B, et al. (2008). Evaluation of a preoperative checklist and team briefing among surgeons, nurses, and anesthesiologists to reduce failures in communication. *Archives of Surgery, 143,* 12–17.

17. Crofts JF, Ellis D, Draycott TJ, et.al. (2007). Change in knowledge of midwives and obstetricians following obstetric emergency training: a randomised controlled trial of local hospital, simulation centre and teamwork training. *British Journal of Obestrics and Gynecology, 114,* 1534–41.

18. Gardner R, Walzer TB, Simon R, Raemer DB. (2008). Obstetric simulation as a risk control strategy: course design and evaluation. *Simulation Healthcare, 3,* 119–27.

19. Preventing infant death and injury during delivery. Retrieved April 9, 2012. http://www.jointcommission.org/Sentinel_Event_Alert__Issue_30_Preventing_infant_death_and_injury_during_delivery_Additional_Resources

20. Thompson S, Neal S, Clark V. (2004). Clinical risk management in obstetrics: Eclampsia drills. *Quality and Safety in Healthcare, 13,* 127–9.

21. Daniels K, Lipman S, Harney K, Arafeh J, & Druzin M. (2008). Use of simulation based team training for obstetric crises in resident education. *Simulation in Healthcare, 3,* 154–60.

22. Mann S, et al. (2006). Assessing quality obstetrical care: development of standardized measures. *Joint Commission Journal on Quality Patient Safety, 32,* 497–505.

23. Press Ganey. Retrieved April 9, 2012, at http://www.pressganey.com/index.aspx.

24. Hospital Survey on Patient Safety Culture. Agency for Healthcare Research and Quality. Retrieved April 9, 2012. http://www.ahrq.gov/qual/patientsafetyculture/hospform.pdf

25. Pettker CM, Thung SF, Norwitz ER, et al. (2009). Impact of a comprehensive patient safety strategy on obstetric adverse events. *American Journal of Obstetrics and Gynecology, 200,* 492.

26. Shea-Lewis A. (2009). Teamwork: crew resource management in a community hospital. *Journal of Healthcare Quality, 31,* 14–18.

27. Riley W, Davis S, Miller K, et.al. (2011). Didactic and simulation nontechnical skills team training to improve perinatal patient outcomes in a community hospital. *Joint Commission Journal on Quality and Patient Safety, 37,* 357–64.

28. Grunebaum A, Chervenak F, Skupski D. (2011). Effect of a comprehensive obstetric patient safety program on compensation payments and sentinel events. *American Journal of Obstetrics Gynecology, 204,* 97–105.

29. Clark S. (2008). Improved outcomes, fewer cesarean deliveries, and reduced litigation: results of a new paradigm in patient safety. *American Journal of Obstetrics and Gynecology, 199,* 105, e1-.e7.

30. Draycott T, Sibanda T, Owen L, et al. (2006). Does training in obstetric emergencies improve neonatal outcome? *British Journal of Obestetrics and Gynecology, 113,* 177–82.

31. Making Change Last: How To Get Beyond Change Fatigue. *Ivey Business Journal,* Retrieved April 9, 2012, at http://www.iveybusinessjournal.com/topics/innovation/making-change-last-how-to-get-beyond-change-fatigue.

32. Haller G, Garnerin P, Morales MA, et al. (2008). Effect of crew resource management training in a multidisciplinary obstetrical setting. *International Journal of Quality Health Care, 20,* 254–63.

33. Mann S, Pratt SD. (2008). Team approach to care in labor and delivery. *Clinical Obstetrics and Gynecology, 51,* 666–79.

8

TEAMWORK IN THE OPERATING AND RECOVERY ROOMS

Shilo H. Anders, Daniel J. France, and Matthew B. Weinger

In February 2003, a prestigious US medical center made international news headlines when a young girl died there after receiving a heart–lung transplant that was incompatible with her blood type.[1] The breakdown in team processes, especially inadequate checks and rechecks of organ–blood match, were to blame. Media reports, case studies, and research findings have highlighted the role of human and organizational failures in adverse events occurring in the perioperative environment (i.e., presurgical through postoperative). Increasing reports of wrong-site surgeries and other communication-related incidents prompted The Joint Commission (which accredits US hospitals) to designate the elimination of these types of errors as a National Patient Safety Goal,[2] and the Accreditation Council for Graduate Medical Education (ACGME), which accredits American physician specialty training, to designate interpersonal skills, communication, and systems-based practice as core competencies.[3]

This chapter provides an overview of the structure and nature of teamwork and teamwork training in the operating room. The chapter begins by describing the perioperative environment, defining the clinical roles required to provide and support care in this setting, and concludes with specific insights from practice about perioperative and surgical teamwork. Eight insights are presented and discussed to highlight current knowledge about operating room (OR) teamwork, the state of teamwork training, and the impact of effective teamwork on operational and clinical outcomes. Although this chapter provides general information on how teamwork affects perioperative patient care in real-life situations, current knowledge is incomplete and further research is needed to enhance teamwork in this patient care environment.

THE PERIOPERATIVE ENVIRONMENT

Perioperative care involves an interdisciplinary team of anesthesia, surgical, nursing, and ancillary healthcare personnel providing care before, during, and after surgery. Each team member has his or her own specialized skill set and expertise. In the OR, there are anesthesia professionals (e.g., anesthesiology attendings, anesthesiology resident physicians, certified registered nurse anesthetists), surgical professionals (e.g., surgery attendings, surgery resident physicians, surgical physician assistants or nurse practitioners), nursing professionals (e.g., circulating nurse, scrub nurse, technician), and medical or nursing students. Other professionals also commonly found in the OR include anesthesia, radiology, and pharmacy technicians, neurophysiologists, and cardiopulmonary perfusionists. Besides the patient, the OR may contain 12 or more individuals at any given time. Preoperative and postoperative care occurs in adjacent units such as the postanesthesia care unit (PACU) and involves other specialized healthcare professionals including nurses and technicians. Additional members may join the team as patient care requirements dictate (e.g., respiratory therapist in the PACU if the patient requires ventilator support).

These perioperative clinicians work in a complex, rapidly changing, time-constrained, and stressful environment. This domain is similar to aircraft cockpits, air traffic control rooms, and combat information centers in that effective performance requires expert knowledge, appropriate problem-solving strategies,[4] fine motor skills, and effective teamwork. The safe administration of anesthesia requires vigilance (e.g., the ability to detect sudden changes in patient condition), situation awareness,[5] time sharing among multiple tasks, and the ability to rapidly make decisions and take actions with life-or-death consequences.[4-7]

Essentially, the anesthesiologist manages a single highly interactive system composed of the patient, anesthesia equipment, surgeons, nurses, and the broader OR environment. Primary management goals include protecting the patient from harm and facilitating the surgery. Like an airplane flight, anesthesia has an initial take-off (called "induction") and a landing ("emergence" from the anesthetic state). The time in between, during which surgery occurs, is called the "maintenance" phase. During maintenance, the anesthesiologist's job becomes primarily one of monitoring the patient and the surgeon's activities, and supervising the anesthesia delivery system and other devices. The anesthesiologist must constantly anticipate and be prepared for both routine and non-routine events. Data about system status are obtained by querying multiple sources. The anesthesiologist verifies the information's validity and formulates a hierarchy of data in terms of importance at the moment. An assessment is made concerning the patient's current status that is compared with the desired system state. An action plan is then formulated and executed. The anesthesiologist monitors the outcome of the intervention, thereby returning to the beginning of this iterative cycle.

The surgeon's task starts outside the OR with initial decision making about the operative plan, preoperative patient preparation, communicating the plan to the rest of the perioperative team, and assuring that all necessary instruments and other materials are available for the procedure. In the OR after induction of anesthesia, the surgeon focuses on the technical aspects of the procedure including real-time decision making as unexpected conditions arise (e.g., abnormal anatomy, excessive bleeding). There are usually two surgeons on each case, the primary (or operating) surgeon and an assisting surgeon. Surgical needs must be communicated effectively and efficiently to the entire OR team. For example, the surgeon may request more muscle relaxation (to the anesthesia provider) or a different instrument (to the nurses). At the end of the case, the surgeon needs to communicate (and often orchestrate) the patient's postoperative care.

The OR nurses typically divide their work into two categories. One nurse or technician (or sometimes more) is "scrubbed in" and hands sterile instruments to the surgeons. The circulating nurse performs all nonsterile surgical tasks (e.g., adjusting equipment settings), makes sure that the surgeons, scrub, and anesthesia providers have all of the equipment and supplies they need, manages workflow and crowd control, and performs the voluminous required patient care documentation.

The nuances of the perioperative environment contribute to the challenges of effective team performance. These individuals come together on a relatively ad hoc basis for each patient's surgery (or for one OR day). The team has a shared responsibility for the outcome regardless of whether team members have worked together before. Past research in aviation suggests that ad hoc teams are less effective than more stable "fixed" teams and less likely to identify potential safety issues.[8] Additionally, the OR is a very dynamic environment in which time pressure abounds. Not only is the team faced with stressors relating to patient care; it also faces pressures to finish cases on time and manage competing demands (especially for surgeons) outside the OR. The surgical patient represents an ill-structured problem because no two people react the same to the anesthesia and surgery. It is unlikely that any one team member will have complete information and, more commonly, conflicting information will be present. The environment is further complicated by high levels of task uncertainty.

TEAMWORK IN THE PERIOPERATIVE ENVIRONMENT

A team is a small number of individuals, each with specific complementary expertise, who work together toward a common goal for which they are accountable. Effective teamwork in the OR includes commitment, competence, common goals, communication, collaboration and coordination, and a supportive culture.[9] The OR team is formed on the basis of commitment to a common goal. Each member aims for competence in their roles; however, individual factors (e.g., sleep deprivation, fatigue, stress, workload), environmental factors (e.g., noise, crowding), and technological factors (e.g., malfunctioning machines) may contribute to less than optimal individual and team performance.[7,10,11]

Communication, both verbal and nonverbal, is an essential component of teamwork, especially in the OR. Studies of communication failures in the perioperative setting have documented adverse consequences such as case delays, tension among team members, and adverse patient outcomes.[12,13] Lingard et al. (2004) found communication failures in 129 of 421 observed communications; 36.4% of these had a visible effect such that an inefficiency or redoing of a procedural step occurred.[12] Communication is critical for coordination and collaboration. Additionally, the culture of the perioperative environment must be responsive to team members' needs and supported by the organization. Anesthesiology was the early adopter of team training programs and, as a result, has produced much of the published research on the topic, although surgeons are increasingly getting involved in these efforts. The following insights have resulted from research in the perioperative environment.

INSIGHTS FROM PRACTICE

Insight 1: Surgeons, Anesthesiologists, and Nurses Differ in Their Perceptions of Operating Room Teamwork.

Research on safety culture in perioperative settings has shown that significant provider-level differences in the perceptions of teamwork and team communication likely undermine team cohesion and performance. The results of cross-sectional surveys of clinicians showed that the level of teamwork perceived among individual surgeons, anesthesiologists, and nurses working together in an OR varies significantly. Surveys of teamwork climate in large samples of US ORs and labor and delivery units, respectively, showed that surgeon and anesthesiologists were more satisfied with physician–nurse collaboration than nurses.[14,15] Older caregivers have also been found to rate teamwork climate more positively than younger providers in the same job class.[16] Only 40% of anesthesiologists surveyed at 11 Scottish hospitals felt that team briefings and debriefings were important for safety and teamwork.[17] Helmreich reported that surgeons were less likely than anesthesiologists to use team-briefing techniques.[18] Training programs that focus on implementing tools and processes that facilitate open communications among the OR team will be the more likely to succeed in improving perioperative teamwork behaviors.

Insight 2: Measuring the Culture of the Operating Room Helps Diagnose Teamwork Climate.

Organizational culture has been identified as a significant determinant of safety performance in high-risk industries. A positive safety culture is widely considered the foundational requirement of high-reliability organizations, whereas its absence has been cited as a contributor to many large-scale system failures and catastrophes. Numerous survey instruments have been developed to measure organizational safety climate, but few include specific survey items that measure teamwork. These instruments broadly assess individuals' perceptions of communication culture within a work unit.[19] The Safety Attitudes Questionnaire (SAQ) is a 60-item instrument that includes a six-item teamwork climate scale in addition to scales for safety climate, stress recognition, perceptions of management, working conditions, and job satisfaction.

The Hospital Survey on Patient Safety Culture, developed by the Agency for Healthcare Research and Quality (AHRQ), measures teamwork at both the unit and hospital (i.e., across units) levels.[20] Both surveys have undergone extensive validation and reliability testing, have been shown to have sound psychometric properties, and have been used widely in patient safety research and quality improvement initiatives to measure the impact of safety interventions on safety culture and its domains.[20,21] The teamwork scales from these surveys have been frequently used to assess teamwork at the unit level and inform process improvement initatives.[14,22]

Insight 3: Formal Training Programs Can Improve Team Behaviors in the Perioperative Environment.

Anesthesia Crisis Resource Management (ACRM) and TeamSTEPPS® (Team Strategies and Tools to Enhance Performance & Patient Safety) were developed to improve teamwork skills in the OR environment. Anesthesiologists from the Veterans Administration Palo Alto Health Care System and Stanford University developed ACRM from aviation's CRM model in the early 1990s to begin addressing the issue of human error as a threat to patient safety.[23,24] A typical ACRM course would incorporate didactic instruction, video analysis of a reenacted medical or nonmedical incident, and simulation-based training followed by video-facilitated debriefing sessions.

More recently, military clinicians and training experts developed a healthcare surgical teamwork training curricula that is now provided through AHRQ as TeamSTEPPS®.[25] Recent studies of TeamSTEPPS® revealed a favorable reaction by staff and significantly higher scores on the Hospital Survey on Patient Safety Culture, and significant increases in the quantity and quality of presurgical briefings.[25–27]

Insight 4: A Multidisciplinary Effort Results in Better Teamwork Training.

Surgeons, anesthesiologists, and OR nurses each receive specialized training to prepare them for their respective professional roles. These training programs (i.e., medical/nursing school, residency) emphasize different technical and behavioral skills and attitudes. An unintended consequence of the specialization of healthcare professional training has been the formation of a hierarchical organizational structure in the OR that fosters the development of distinct and sometimes divisive group cultures along functional roles. There are strong cultural and attitudinal differences among surgeons, anesthesiologists, and OR nurses that can create

barriers to effective communication, teamwork, and care quality.[15]

One solution to this challenge is to educate OR teams collectively about these culture differences and equip them with the nontechnical skills to work together more effectively as a team. A substantial multidisciplinary effort is necessary to create a unified culture and improve team behaviors in the OR. For example, the Veterans Health Administration's National Center for Patient Safety (NCPS) developed a Medical Team Training (MTT) program that requires each participating VA to form an interdisciplinary implementation team before the start of training. Implementation team training includes an NCPS-facilitated 1-day learning session using didactic instruction and clinical video vignettes to demonstrate CRM principles in the OR setting. The implementation team then provides the hands-on training to clinicians and managers in their local work setting. OR training includes the use of preoperative briefings (e.g., checklists) and postoperative debriefings, interdisciplinary administrative briefings, and standardized patient handovers.[28,29]

Insight 5: Scripts, Checklists, and Memory Aids Can Improve Team Communications in the Operating Room.

Changing the teamwork and communication cultures of the OR is difficult and takes time. Many medical and nursing schools have revised their curricula to emphasize multidisciplinary learning and teamwork. Many hospitals have created quality improvement programs that routinely measure safety indicators. More are requiring clinical staff to participate in team training programs. Experts hope with time that a culture of open communication and teamwork will become an inherent part of healthcare. To facilitate the adoption of OR team behaviors an array of tools has been developed to guide and support clinicians during this learning process. These tools include scripts for calling pre-procedural timeouts, checklists, and memory aids such as posters, laminated pocket-sized cards, and electronic whiteboards. Some of the tools that have been integrated into the OR are described in the following.

Starting in 2003, an interdisciplinary team at Vanderbilt University Medical Center, implemented team training principles and work processes into the perioperative environment after all OR personnel had completed an introductory 8-hour course.[30] The team worked directly with surgeons, anesthesiologists, and nurses to create a toolkit that included poster- and pocket-sized checklists and briefing scripts as memory aids. Additionally, "communication whiteboards" in the holding rooms and ORs displayed patient, procedural, and staff information. The tools were iteratively refined to be usable in all sites and case types. Operating room personnel took a multimedia webinar to learn about the initiative. The checklists (Table 8.1) were designed to assure that the team communicated about critical patient and procedural elements throughout the perioperative process.

Other hospitals have developed targeted interventions to improve surgical safety. A multidisciplinary team at Kaiser Permanente used human factors principles to develop a surgical preoperative safety briefing designed to improve OR team communication, collaboration, teamwork, and situational awareness.[31] Nundy et al. (2008) used in-service training sessions to implement a preoperative briefing at a tertiary academic center. The attending surgeon used a standardized tool during a 2-minute preoperative briefing to review the operative plan, identify and mitigate patient hazards, and ensure that required equipment was available.[32]

The World Health Organization's "Safe Surgery Saves Lives" surgical checklist includes questions to be answered at three points in time: before induction, before incision, and before leaving for recovery.[33] The goal of this type of checklist has been to improve safety, standards compliance, and communication among providers. The addition of the checklist into the OR in eight diverse hospitals worldwide improved adherence to standards and significantly decreased surgical complications.[29] This study found that the use of the checklist significantly reduced mortality from 1.5% to 0.8% and inpatient complications from 11% to 7%.

Insight 6: There Are Reliable Methods to Measure Teamwork Behavior in the Operating Room.

The proliferation of team training programs in response to healthcare's increased emphasis on

Table 8.1   Checklist Items Added to Operating Room Process

Holding Room Checklist (before going to OR)	Preprocedural Briefing (before incision)	Postoperative Debriefing (before surgical site close)
Patient verification (correct patient)	Critical patient information (name, MRN, age, allergies, etc.)	Performance feedback from those involved in surgical case
Procedure verification (correct procedure)	Procedure verification	Assessment of safety performance
Correct side and site verification	Surgeon's expectations about the surgery	Status of surgical counts
Marking of surgical site by operating surgeon	Marking of the surgical site	Verification of the counts
Administration of ordered medications	Potential challenges related to the surgery	Review of final procedure and diagnosis
Verification of DVT prophylaxis	Status of the induction (how initial anesthesia procedures went)	Patient's status and disposition
	Needed preparation for potential problems	Summary of all inputs
	Antibiotics administered 10–60 minutes before incision	"Thank you" to team for assisting in case
	Room, equipment, and staff requirements	

improving teamwork and patient safety has created a need for methods to measure teamwork behaviors in clinical settings. In the last decade, there has been appreciable progress in developing and applying behavioral marker systems for the OR.

Carthey et al. (2000) developed a qualitative framework of individual, team, and organizational markers of surgical excellence.[34] Pediatric cardiac surgeons who had the highest procedural excellence scores were characterized by more of the positive behavioral markers than did surgeons with low performance scores. Limitations of the use of behavioral markers include: Some behaviors are not observable or observed behaviors may not accurately reflect underlying thoughts or intentions; human reviewers are inherently subjective and prone to bias; there is no "gold standard" against which to validate the results; and reviewer training time can be significant.

Fletcher et al. (2003) developed the Anesthetists' Non-Technical Skills (ANTS) behavioral marker system to describe the primary nontechnical skills believed to be important for good anesthesia practice.[35] Anesthetists' Non-Technical Skills system groups behavioral markers into four major categories: (1) task management; (2) team working; (3) situation awareness; and (4) decision making. Positive team behaviors are exemplified by coordination with team members, exchanging information, appropriately using authority and assertiveness, assessing capabilities, and supporting others. The ANTS system appears to have satisfactory validity, reliability, and usability. The ANTS system was used to demonstrate that simulation-based CRM training improved the nontechnical skills of anesthesiology residents.[36]

The Observational Teamwork Assessment for Surgery (OTAS) tool developed at Imperial College London by Healey, Undre, and Vincent assesses teamwork during the perioperative process using two observers.[37] The first observer monitors specific tasks carried out by the surgical team and categorizes them based on their relevance to the patient, environment, equipment, supplies, and communications. The second observer uses a behavioral observation scale to rate team behaviors categorized as cooperation, leadership, coordination, awareness, or communication. The OTAS tool has adequate construct validity, as evidenced by consistent scoring differences between expert and novice team members.[38]

The Oxford Non-Technical Skills (NOTECHS) scale was developed based on a validated aviation instrument to assess teamwork and cognitive skills in surgical teams.[39] The NOTECHS scale is structured along four behavioral dimensions: leadership and management, teamwork and cooperation, problem solving and decision making, and situation awareness. The NOTECHS scale has been refined to allow separate analyses of surgical subteams (e.g., anesthesia, surgery, nursing). The NOTECHS scale was validated based on observations of teams performing laparoscopic cholecystectomies but may be limited in its wider application because of significant observer training requirements and poor scalability.[39]

Guerlain and colleagues developed the Remote Analysis of Team Environments (RATE) to digitally record, score, annotate, and analyze surgical team performance.[40] The mobile system allows for prospective analysis of operative performance, intraoperative errors, team performance, and communication. The system can also support postoperative discussion and review of critical events and performance feedback. The RATE tool has been used to assess a small sample of surgical teams performing laparoscopic cholecystectomies, but may be limited because of technological and training requirements.[40]

There are a number of methods to measure teamwork behaviors in the OR; however, many of these are limited because of the significant amount of time required to train evaluators. Although the current tools help to measure teamwork in the OR, they have been limited in scope. Rating tools that require minimal training, timely process improvement feedback, and are comprehensive for all types of surgeries are needed to further refine how teamwork is measured in the OR.

Insight 7: Medical Teamwork Can Be Improved Through Realistic Patient Simulation Training and Evaluation.

Simulation has been touted as an effective tool to enhance medical teamwork[9,41,42] because one can: (1) recreate the actual work domain and all of its contextual factors; (2) present standardized and replicable clinical events; (3) conduct sessions at mutually convenient times; (4) videotape the simulation to facilitate debriefing and more reliable evaluation; and, most important, (5) *never* put a patient's life at risk during clinician training or evaluation. Realistic patient simulators are plastic mannequins embedded with a wide range of physical and computer-based features to emulate an acutely ill patient.[41]

Patient simulation courses were initially provided to anesthesia and emergency medicine trainees, but have expanded to other domains, including intensive care and perinatal medicine.[43] The more effective courses tend to emphasize teamwork (or behavioral) skills. Failures of technical performance by surgical teams are less likely to lead to major morbidity and mortality than do behavioral OR communication failures.[44] In fact, a recent study showed that the primary difference between high and low surgical mortality hospitals was not the incidence of technical complications, but the failure to recognize and manage those complications effectively.[45] The expansion of surgical simulation has provided a viable platform to improve

these behavioral skills.[46,47] Simulation-based team training is effective when the scenarios are guided by learning needs and outcomes, and performance is measured at the individual and team level.[48]

Insight 8: Improving Team Behaviors Can Improve Operating Room Efficiency and Patient Outcomes.

Perhaps the biggest challenge facing researchers and hospital administrators in this era of patient safety and quality improvement is quantifying the impact of interventions on hospital performance and patient outcomes. Although the data are still limited, there is increasing evidence that teamwork training improves operational and safety outcomes in the OR. For example, of 18 participating rural Norwegian hospitals, 17 modified their trauma protocols after

Table 8.2   Studies Examining Patient Outcomes as a Result of Changed Teamwork Behaviors

Author(s)/ Year	Site	Intervention	Findings/Outcomes
Awad et al. (2005)	OR offered to surgical service	Team training session	Significant increase in the number of patients who received timely intragenative prophylactic antibiotics and deep venous thrombosis (DVT) prophylaxis[28]
Nielsen et al. (2007)	Obstetrics	Completion of MedTeams Labor & Delivery Team Coordination Course	Adverse outcome indices remained similar to control hospitals, significant decrease in amount of time between the decision to perform an immediate cesarean delivery to the incision.[50]
Pratt et al. (2007)	Labor and delivery unit	CRM-based team training program	Based on malpractice claims, there was a significant decrease in severe events (13–5 per 20,000 deliveries)[51]
Mazzocco et al. (2009)	OR	Observed for presence of nontechnical behaviors	Patients had increased odds of complications or death when specific teamwork behaviors (i.e., information sharing, briefing during handoff phase) were exhibited less frequently.[52]
Haynes et al. (2009)	8 worldwide hospital's ORs	Surgical Safety Checklist	Significant reduction in mortality rates and inpatient complications[29]
Wolf et al. (2010)	OR team	Medical Team Training course	Significant reductions in surgical case delays[53]
Neily et al. (2010)	Veterans Health Administration OR teams	Medical Team Training course	18% reduction in annual mortality 1 year after enrollment in team training program[54]

Table 8.3 Summary of Insights about Teamwork in the Perioperative Environment

1. Surgeons, anesthesiologists, and nurses differ in their perception of teamwork in the OR.
2. Measuring the culture of the OR can be a means to diagnose team climate.
3. Training programs have been developed to improve team behaviors in the perioperative environment.
4. A multidisciplinary effort results in better teamwork training.
5. Scripts, checklists, and memory aids have been demonstrated to improve team communications in the OR.
6. Methods have been developed to measure teamwork behaviors.
7. Medical teamwork can be improved through realistic patient simulation training and evaluation.
8. Improving team behaviors improves operational efficiency and surgical outcomes.

---

a damage control course.[49] A post-course phone survey revealed 12 cases of lifesaving rural damage control operations by course participants with an estimated associated cost savings of $15,075 per life saved. Table 8.2 summarizes additional studies that have seen significant improvements in mortality or other variables after the implementation of team training programs.

FUTURE DIRECTIONS

This chapter has highlighted essential points to consider when trying to improve teamwork in the perioperative environment (Table 8.3). Increasing evidence suggests that interventions targeting enhanced OR teamwork, behavioral skills, and communication can improve surgical patient outcomes.

Nonetheless, research is still needed to determine the most effective interventions, how best to implement them in the OR, and to measure their effects on teamwork and safety outcomes. More specific questions still to be addressed include the details of what, when, how, and to whom should team training be offered. For example, medical students may be more receptive to teamwork training, especially simulation-based training. But then, how often would those principles need to be refreshed to assure excellent team practices when they are surgeons or anesthesiologists? Furthermore, the role of informatics in teamwork has yet to be explored. What is the role of support tools beyond simple checklists? Implementing and long-term ongoing teamwork initiatives are nontrivial, and

a sustainable model for the perioperative environment is yet to be realized.

REFERENCES

1. Grady D. (2003). Donor mix-up leaves girl, 17, fighting for life. *The New York Times.*
2. The Joint Commission. (2006). *Facts about the 2006 patient safety goals.* Washington, DC: The Joint Commission.
3. Stewart, M. (2009). Core Competencies. *Accreditation Council for Graduate Medical Education.* Retrieved July 14, 2009 from: http://www.acgme.org
4. Seamster, T. L., Redding, R. E., Cannon, J. R., Ryder, J. M., & Purcell, J. A. (1993). Cognitive task analysis of expertise in air traffic control. *International Journal of Aviation Psychology, 3,* 257–83.
5. Gaba, D. M., Howard, S. K., & Small, S. D. (1995). Situation awareness in anesthesiology. *Human Factors, 37,* 20–31.
6. Gaba, D. M., Fish, K. J., & Howard, S. K. (1994). *Crisis management in anesthesiology.* New York: Churchill Livingstone.
7. Weinger, M. B., & Englund, C. E. (1990). Ergonomic and human factors affecting anesthetic vigilance and monitoring performance in the operating room environment. *Anesthesiology, 73,* 995–1021.
8. Woody, J. R., McKinney, E. H., Barker, J. M., & Clothier, C. C. (1994). Comparison of fixed versus formed aircrews in military transport. *Aviation and Space Environment Medicine, 65,* 153–6.

9. Barach, P., & Weinger, M. B. (2007). Trauma team performance. In: W. C. Wilson, C. M. Grande, & D. B. Hoyt (Eds.), *Trauma*. Vol. 1. *Resuscitation, Anesthesia and Emergency Surgery*. (pp. 101–13). New York: Taylor & Francis.

10. Mills, P., Neily, J., & Dunn, E. (2008). Teamwork and communication in surgical teams: Implications for patient safety. *Journal of the American College of Surgeons, 206*(1), 107–12.

11. Weinger, M. B., & Ancoli-Israel, S. (2002). Sleep deprivation and clinical performance. *Journal of the American Medical Association, 287,* 955–7.

12. Lingard, L., Espin, S., Whyte, S., et al. (2004). Communication failures in the operating room: an observational classification of recurrent types and effects. *Quality and Safety in Health Care, 13,* 330–4.

13. Morris, J., Carrillo, Y., Jenkins, J., et al. (2003). Surgical adverse events, risk management, and malpractice outcome: Morbidity and mortality review is not enough. *Annals of Surgery, 237,* 844–52.

14. Sexton, J., Makary, M., Tersigni, A., et al. (2006). Teamwork in the operating room: Frontline perspectives among hospitals and operating room personnel. *Anesthesiology, 105,* 877–84.

15. Sexton, J. B., Helmreich, R. L., Neilands, T. B., et al. (2006). The Safety Attitudes Questionnaire: psychometric properties, benchmarking data, and emerging research. *BMC Health Services Research, 6,* 44.

16. Carney, B., Mills, P., Bagian, J., & Weeks, W. (2010). Sex differences in operating room care giver perceptions of patient safety: A pilot study from the Veterans Health Administration Medical Team Training Program. *Quality and Safety in Health Care, 19,* 128–31.

17. Flin, R., Fletcher, G., McGeorge, P., Sutherland, A., & Patey, R. (2003). Anaesthetists' attitudes to teamwork and safety. *Anaesthesiology, 58,* 233–42.

18. Helmreich, R. L., Schaefer. H-G. (1994). Team performance in the operating room. In: Bogner MS, ed. *Human Error in Healthcare*. Mahwah, NJ: LEA.

19. Colla, J., Bracken, A., Kinney, L., & Weeks, W. (2005). Measuring patient safety climate: A review of surveys. *Quality and Safety in Health Care, 14*(5), 364–6.

20. Hospital Survey on Patient Safety Culture. Retrieved May 2009 from:http://www.ahrq.gov/qual/patientsafetyculture/hospsurvindex.htm

21. Schaefer, H., & Helmreich, R. (1993). The operating room management attitudes questionnaire (ORMAQ). Austin, TX: NASA/University of Texas at Austin.

22. Thomas, E. J., Sexton, J. B., & Helmreich, R. L. (2003). Discrepant attitudes about teamwork among critical care nurses and physicians. *Critical Care Medicine, 31,* 956–9.

23. Gaba, D. (1989). Human error in anesthetic mishaps. *International Anesthesiology Clinics, 27*(3), 137–47.

24. Howard, S., Gaba, D., Fish, K., Yang, G., & Sarnquist, F. (1992). Anesthesia crisis resource-management training: Teaching anesthesiologists to handle critical incidents. *Aviation, Space, and Environmental Medicine, 63,* 763–70.

25. TeamSTEPPS®. *National Implementation.* Retrieved August 7, 2009 from: http://teamstepps.ahrq.gov/index.htm

26. Weaver, S., Rosen, M., DiazGranados, D., et al. (2010). Does teamwork improve performance in the operating room? A multilevel evaluation. *Joint Commission Journal on Quality and Patient Safety, 35*(8), 398–405.

27. Davis, S., Miller, K., & Riley, W. (2008). *Reducing patient harm through interdisciplinary team training with in situ simulation.* Paper presented at: Improving Patient Safety Conference. Cambridge, UK: Robinson College.

28. Awad, S., Fagan, S., Bellows, C., et al. (2005). Bridging the communication gap in the operating room with medical team training. *American Journal of Surgery, 190,* 770–4.

29. Haynes, A. B., Weiser, T. G., Berry, W. R., et al. (2009). A surgical safety checklist to reduce morbidity and mortality in a global population. *New England Journal of Medicine, 360,* 491–9.

30. France, D., Stiles, R., Gaffney, E., et al. (2005). Crew resource management training: Clinicians' reactions and attitudes. *Association of periOperative Registered Nurses Journal, 82*(2), 214–24.

31. DeFontes, J., & Surbida, S. (2004). Preoperative safety briefing project. *Permanente Journal, 8*(2), 21–7.

32. Nundy, S., Mukherjee, A., Sexton, J., et al. (2008). Impact of preoperative briefings on operating room delays. *Archives of Surgery, 143*(11), 1068–72.

33. *Surgical safety checklist.* (2009). Geneva: World Health Organization.

34. Carthey, J., de Leval, M., & Reason, J. (2000). *Understanding excellence in complex,*

dynamic medical domains. Paper presented at International Ergonomics Association and Human Factors Society Triennial Conference. Santa Monica, CA.

35. Fletcher, G., Flin, R., McGeorge, P., Glavin, R., Maran, N., & Patey, R. (2003). Anaesthestists' non-technical skills (ANTS) evaluation of a behavioural marker system. *British Journal of Anaesthesiology, 90*(5), 580–8.

36. Yee, B., Naik, V., et al. (2005). Nontechnical skills in anesthesia crisis management with repeated exposure to simulation-based education. *Anesthesiology, 103*(2), 241–8.

37. Healey, A., Undre, S., & Vincent, C. (2004). Developing observational measures of performance in surgical teams. *Quality and Safety in Health Care,* 13, i33–40.

38. Sevdalis, N., Lyons, M., Healey, A., Undre, S., Darzi, A., & Vincent, C. (2009). Observational teamwork assessment for surgery: Construct validation with expert versus novice raters. *Annals of Surgery, 249*(6), 1047–51.

39. Mishra, A., Catchpole, K., & McCulloch, P. (2009). The Oxford NOTECHS system: Reliability and validity of a tool for measuring teamwork behavior in the operating theatre. *Quality and Safety in Health Care, 18,* 104–8.

40. Guerlain, S., Adams, R., Turrentine, F., et al. (2005). Assessing team performance in the operating room: Development and use of a "black-box" recorder and other tools for the intraoperative environment. *Journal of the American College of Surgeons, 200*(1), 29–37.

41. Gaba, D. M., Howard, S. K., Fish, K. J., Smith, B. E., & Sowb, Y. A. (2001). Simulation-based training in anesthesia crisis resource management (ACRM): A decade of experience. *Simulation Gaming, 32,* 175–93.

42. Morgan, P., Pittini, R., Regehr, G., Marrs, C., & Haley, M. (2007). Evaluating teamwork in a simulated obstetric environment. *Anesthesiology, 106,* 907–15.

43. Harris, K., Treanor, C., & Salisbury, M. (2006). Improving patient safety with team coordination: Challenges and strategies of implementation. *Journal of Obstetric, Gynecologic, & Neonatal Nursing, 35,* 557–66.

44. Chopra, V., Bovill, J., & Spierdijk, J. (1992). Reported significant observations during aneasthesia: A prospective analysis over an 18-month period. *British Medical Journal,* 68, 13–7.

45. Ghaferi, A., Birkmeyer, J., & Dimick, J. (2009). Variation in hospital mortality associated with inpatient surgery. *New England Journal of Medicine, 36,* 1368–75.

46. Moorthy, K., Munz, Y., Adams, S., Pandey, V., & Darzi, A. (2005). A human factors analysis of technical and team skills among surgical trainees during procedural simulations in a simulated operating theatre. *Annals of Surgery, 242*(5), 631–8.

47. Powers, K., Rehrig, S., Irias, N., et al. (2008). Simulated laparoscopic operating room crisis: An approach to enhance the surgical team performance. *Surgical Endoscopy 22,* 885–900.

48. Salas, E., Wilson, K. A., Burke, C. S., & Priest, H. A. (2005). Using simulation-based training to improve patient safety: What does it take? *Journal of Quality and Patient Safety, 31*(7), 363–71.

49. Hansen, K., Uggen, P., Brattebo, G., & Wisborg, T. (2007). Training operating room teams in damage control surgery for trauma: A followup study of the Norwegian Model. *Journal of the American College of Surgeons, 205*(5), 712–6.

50. Nielsen, P., Goldman, M., Mann, S., et al. (2007). Effects of teamwork training on adverse outcomes and process of care in labor and delivery: A randomized controlled trial. *Obstetrical and Gynecological Survey, 62*(5), 294–5.

51. Pratt, S., Mann, S., Salisbury, M., et al. (2007). John M. Eisenberg Patient Safety and Quality Awards. Impact of CRM-based training on obstetric outcomes and clinicians' patient safety attitudes. *Joint Commission Journal on Quality and Patient Safety, 33*(12), 720–5.

52. Mazzocco, K., Petitti, D., Fong, K., et al. (2009). Surgical team behaviors and patient outcomes. *American Journal of Surgery, 197*(5), 678–85.

53. Wolf, F., Way, L., & Stewart, L. (2010). The efficacy of medical team training: Improved team performance and decreased operating room delays: A detailed analysis of 4863 cases. *Annals of Surgery, 252*(3), 477–85.

54. Neily, J., Mills, P., Young-Xu, Y, et al. (2010). Association between implementation of a medical team training program and surgical mortality. *Journal of the American Medical Association, 304,* 1693–700.

IMPLEMENTING TEAM TRAINING IN THE EMERGENCY DEPARTMENT: THE GOOD, THE UNEXPECTED, AND THE PROBLEMATIC

Shawna J. Perry, Robert L. Wears, and Sandra S. McDonald

The introduction and implementation of team training into any work domain is a significant undertaking. To varying degrees, it engenders culture change for all individuals within a work system. Commercial aviation is one of the most widely publicized industries to adopt team training in the form of crew resource management (CRM) over 30 years ago. This came in response to overwhelming evidence that the rigidly hierarchical human–human interactions within this domain were infusing added risk of failure into the high stakes endeavor of flight. The evolution and impact of teamwork in aviation has been well documented in the literature[1] and there is increasing evidence of its potential benefits within the domain of healthcare.[2-4] Little has been written about the nature of the cultural impact of its implementation on the sharp end of clinical work. This chapter will discuss good, unexpected, and problematic secondary effects associated with the introduction of teamwork training into an emergency department (ED).

MEDTEAMS™: TEAM TRAINING FOR THE ED

One of the earliest introductions of team training into the healthcare setting was the MedTeams™ Project in the late 1990s.[5] This multicenter quasiexperimental research project was developed to test the translation of CRM teamwork principles into the ED setting with subsequent assessment of its impact on error patterns, performance, and emergency care cost.[6] The curriculum was developed by behavioral scientists and emergency care subject matter experts, trained in CRM teamwork principles, after an assessment of emergency medical teamwork and the potential impacts of improved medical teamwork on emergency care cost and performance. Based on over 250 hours of ED observations, ED teamwork processes were categorized into five dimensions: (1) maintain team structure and climate, (2) apply problem solving strategies, (3) communicate with the team, (4) execute plans and manage workload, and (5) improve team skills.[5] Forty-eight specific teamwork behaviors were associated with these five team dimensions and detailed behaviorally anchored rating scales (BARS) were developed to assess teams performance. Using a model of evaluation-driven instructional development, the BARS served as the basis for the Emergency Team Coordination Course (ETCC™) curriculum and evaluation instruments. Expert panels of emergency medicine physicians and nurses representing 12 hospitals of various sizes from across the United States and representatives from professional medical and nursing societies guided curriculum review and refinement. Draft curriculum was taught to over 150 ED staff members at a tertiary care facility, which continued to serve as a teamwork "laboratory" to help refine the course content and translation into implementation.

The final teamwork curriculum implemented consisted of an 8-hour block of classroom instruction organized with an introduction, the five main learning modules, and an integration unit supplemented by video material depicting examples of good and poor teamwork within the ED.[7] A physician-nurse pair from each participating hospital was trained as instructors to teach the entire ED staff at their institution. Practicums, coaching, mentoring, and review sessions provided further learning experiences subsequent to classroom instruction.

Upon completion of training, the teamwork implementation phase was initiated on an established date. This phase was characterized by (1) forming teams by shift and delivering care in a team structure, (2) completing a 4-hour practicum with each staff member during which teamwork behaviors were practiced and critiqued by an instructor, and (3) coaching and mentoring of teamwork behaviors by instructors and associate instructors during normal shifts. The basic team structure is shown in Figure 9.1.[6] One or more core teams delivered direct care to patients, the coordinating team managed resources and workflow, and *ad hoc* resuscitation teams were formed for emergent events.

A total of 1,054 ED physicians, nurses, and technicians participated in the project across five civilian and four military hospitals; five academic settings, and four community hospitals. These same facilities participated in a prospective, quasiexperimental untreated control group experiment with one pretest and two posttests to examine the effectiveness of the ETCC course and teamwork implementation.[8] Three outcome constructs were assessed: team behaviors, attitudes and opinions, and ED performance. Further details of the training and assessment can be found in Risser, Rice, Salisbury, et al.[6] and Morey, Simon, Jay, et al.[8]

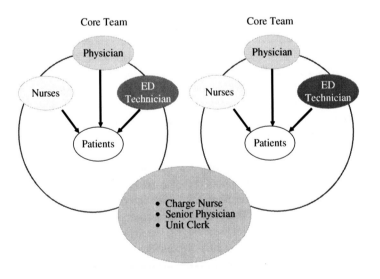

Figure 9.1
Coordinating Team

One Facility's Experience:

The University of Florida Health Sciences Center/ Jacksonville was one of the largest academic medical centers to participate in the project with 760 beds 220,000 patient visits per year and 30,000 annual admissions. The ED and associated Level I trauma center averaged 90,000 annual visits at the time, including 27,000 children. The ED was staffed by 28 attending physicians, 47 emergency medicine residents in postgraduate training years 2 to 4, 4 fellows, 5 physician assistants, and roughly 140 nursing and technical staff. The ED acuity was quite high as the regional safety net facility, providing 61% of all hospital admissions.

Participation in the MedTeams™ training classes was deemed mandatory for all faculty, residents, and staff with 25 classes of 16 to 20 students taught over 6 weeks. New team structures were implemented in the ED that consisted of 2 care teams (blue and orange) each with a physician resident leader, 2 nurses, 1 to 2 ED technicians and 1 to 2 medical students. Each treatment area also had an administrative team that consisted of an ED attending, a senior emergency medicine resident/chief of the day; charge nurse/ nurse of the day and unit secretary.

The Good:

- The small class size with a maximum of 16 participants integrated by skill set (e.g., ED attending sitting next to a housekeeper sitting next to a nurse) provided a unique opportunity for leveling the hierarchy in the institution. This was further supported by the requirement to use first names in the class. The result was a number of episodes in which the staff traditionally without a voice gained an opportunity to be heard. For instance, during a module related to the use of team resources for managing workload, one of the nurses stated that she had stopped attempting to assist the unit secretaries because they consistently refused. A very shy unit secretary spoke up and stated that that was because the nurses "try to tell us our job and what we need help with rather than asking how could they help us. They treat us like children." The room became very still as everyone reflected on a previously unrecognized

paternalistic climate these staff members perceived. The nurse who made the initial statement paused and quietly acknowledged her understanding and apologized, as it had never occurred to her that she was behaving in this manner.

- There were also a number of "ah-ha" moments in which participants gained insight into pretraining interactions that had resulted in strained relationships, especially between physicians and nurses. In one such occurrence, a resident was awed as she realized the source of persistent tension with one of the nurses was likely caused by a failure to create a shared mental model of what the treatment plan was for a difficult patient. The structure of the MedTeams™ training and curriculum provided an opportunity for uninterrupted reflection of factors that impact clinical work and the establishment of a team climate.

- Following implementation, the effects of leveling the hierarchy could be seen quite readily, as in the case of Dee, an ED housekeeper. During implementation, housekeeping staff were given the additional task of transporting patients to the floor in an attempt to connect the support staff more closely to clinical care. Following a recent transport, Dee approached the ED attending, a shy and quite reserved professor who had worked there for many years and who was often misperceived as aloof. She told him about how she was attempting to improve her status in life and one way was by reading the patients charts that she transported upstairs (this was prior to the Health Insurance Portability and Accountability Act known as HIPAA). Dee had noticed that several of the patients she transported over the week had a diagnosis of meningitis and that these patients had the same address as a public housing complex near the hospital. She wanted to bring this to someone's attention because she wondered if this was something to be worried about. The ED attending, also post his team training, was pleased (and a bit surprised) to have been approached. He praised Dee for bringing this information to him so he could follow it up. Interactions such as these illustrate the improved engagement of the ED staff with one another and greater empowerment by all skill sets required for the ED to function.

The Unexpected:

- There was significant reticence about the project among the ED physicians and staff but not from the expected quarters. Pushback had been anticipated from the most senior and experienced physicians and staff (those with more than 20 years professional experience, and a high level of expertise—some identified as "crusty"). This, however, turned out not to be the case. Skepticism toward the use of CRM in the clinical setting was strongest among those with the least clinical experience (e.g., residents and recent nursing and ED technician graduates). This appeared to be the result of differences in experiential reserves from which to measure the benefits of teamwork behaviors. The least experienced ED clinicians and staff were less likely to have been involved in situations where teamwork failure resulted in near misses and injury to patients. The more experienced staff voiced significant frustration in their work because "good teams" had always seemed to be more a matter of luck and having "good people." The classes provided an opportunity for seasoned staff to share anecdotes of difficult shifts with high acuity in which they were "glad to have a good team on"; however, now they were able to label the teamwork behaviors in play during those high risk situations. These same veteran "crusty" clinicians and staff surprisingly became vocal advocates, as well as volunteer and ad hoc coaches for the use of team training once implemented in the ED.
- The actual implementation of the team behaviors into the ED following the training was highly iterative, requiring extemporaneous refinement for the first several weeks, at times on an hourly basis. For example, the core teams were on occasion overwhelmed by the patient volume and associated workload, especially in the late afternoon and early evening. In response, staff on duty created an ad hoc team from the administrative team of each area (lead resident and charge nurse) who would pick up low workload patients together to balance out the patient assignments across the established teams. Such real-time adjustments were encouraged by ED leadership, who were cognizant of the need for input from those trying to embed team behaviors into their work in a highly dynamic clinical environment. Tools that supported open communication about teamwork in the ED included walk rounds by MedTeams™ champions 3 to 4 times per day in the ED and the availability of "MedTeams™ consults," a standing pager for asking questions or relaying ideas. Being responsive and visible to the staff (even to MedTeams™ pages from overnight shifts) were important acknowledgments of the value of team members' input to the success of the project.
- Another interesting phenomenon was the contraction of key concepts and scripts from the training to meet the time constraints of the ED. Two examples are the Two-Challenge rule and the DESC (Describe, Express, Specify, Consequences) script. The former, which requires an individual, acting as an advocate for the patient, to assert his or her opinion twice when it differs substantially from that of the decision-maker, was contracted to "I'm Two-challenging you" or "I'm being an advocate." The later, DESC script which provides a four-line guide for communicating behavioral concerns to a team member, was truncated to "I need to DESC script you." These examples demonstrate that the core concepts had been understood and that explicit recitation was not necessary or supportable in a time-pressured work environment.
- Unexpected spillover of some team behaviors was demonstrated by other disciplines or ancillary support to the ED. For instance, EKG techs, food service workers, and others extemporaneously began to use (and on occasion write on) the manual whiteboard to obtain and provide situational awareness to the ED. These boards also supported large-scale coordinated work of less tightly coupled groups such as the ambulance and fire rescue units seeking to support their situational awareness about the likelihood of ED overcrowding resulting in ambulance diversion.

- One method for maintaining situational awareness across and within teams, small team briefings or "huddles," was quite difficult to engrain into the clinical work of the ED. The dynamic nature of the work requires ED staff to be in almost constant motion (e.g., moving between patients performing tasks, documenting, obtaining supplies, answering phones), making it difficult to carve out periods for planned interactions for short updates or briefings. One reason appeared to be a distorted sense of the passage of time during these huddles periods. The staff was uncomfortable stopping and standing to talk as a team, no matter how briefly, because of an overwhelming sense that they were "losing time" and "falling behind" on caring for their patients and tasks were continuing to accumulate.

- Additionally, there were latent features of the ED work system that made finding the ideal time for updates across and within teams difficult to identify. It became evident that there was a lack of synchronization of the work between the skill groups making up the ED teams. Unlike in the cockpit, where the pilot and copilot have predictable episodes of synchronous work (i.e., take-off and landing procedures), the workloads of nurses, physicians, and ED technicians occur in parallel, were more often asynchronous (except in dire emergencies like cardiac arrest), and each peaks at different times. Contributors to this included: (1) the nature of shift work and different times for change of shift (physicians were on 8- and 10-hour shifts, nurses and techs on 12-hour shifts) resulting in variable "wrap up" times for each, (2) the unplanned nature of emergency care (the only thing certain is that one's shift will eventually end), and (3) variation in the type of tasks being performed by each team member. For example, each order given by a physician translates into a number of discrete tasks for the nurse or technician to perform. An order to "start an intravenous line" translates into tasks such as (1) gathering of materials, (2) preparing the patient, (3) hanging intravenous fluids, (4) updating the family, etc. Each of these tasks has a number of steps that need to be completed (i.e., verify patient identity, locate site to start line, place tourniquet, clean with alcohol, etc.) Many orders are written on each patient the staff member is assigned to, therein exponentially increasing the workload because of the number of steps required to complete them and exacerbating the staff's sense of losing momentum when asked to stop for a briefing or huddle.

The Problematic:

- The person-hours of investment needed for the teaching and implementation were significant. The physician and nurse instructors invested 200 hours each in just the classroom portion alone, which did not include preparation and setup. The implementation was even more time intensive, requiring a great deal of nonclinical "time on the floor" coaching and translating curriculum into the real-time work. This at times included defusing staff who were experiencing periods of frustration while trying to "learn to ride a bike in a hurricane." The bulk of this time investment by instructors was volunteered, because it far outstripped the salary support provided by the project.

- Sustainment was a remarkably problematic feature of the implementation; not only after the project ended but in maintaining the behaviors to the changing clinical context and workflow during the project. Multiple vehicles were utilized in support of both types of sustainment (e.g., microrefresher courses, pocket reminders, on the job training) that required instructor support. With the loss of external funding at the end of the training, on-the-job training was decided to be the most economical because it would not require removing staff from the clinical area. It proved to be very difficult in the dynamic and unpredictable ED setting, often interrupted by more immediate clinical needs.

- These same characteristics of the ED also undermined assumptions that feedback and reinforcement of concepts from other team members would occur in support of a team culture. All of these methods were likely less effective because they added to the existing myriad of competing goals faced by ED staff working with multiple patients simultaneously (e.g., start this IV, see the new patient with chest pain, document in the record, talk to the family of Bed 3). There was little to no time in the busy setting for additional teaching; only enough time to provide examples in support of the teamwork themes and concepts. Simulation would have provided an opportunity for reinforcing of the teamwork behaviors in the face of the changing landscape of emergency care (i.e., higher acuity, boarding of patients, high staff turnover); however, funding was not available for its development.

SUMMARY AND CONCLUSION

A decade later, remnants of the MedTeams ™ project can still be seen at this site but many of the behaviors have eroded. The fundamental core teams with physician leaders still exist. The manual whiteboards (in parallel with electronic status boards) track work assignments to teams and the flow of clinical work. During high-risk time-pressured events, such as cardiac resuscitation and endotracheal intubations, call outs and checkbacks are still used and physician leaders are expected to communicate out loud with the resuscitation teams in a way that will support shared mental modeling and situation awareness. These tools and behaviors have become engrained in the culture, although there are few individuals remaining that know their origin.

The status of this ED team training project in the other participating healthcare organizations is not known to the authors. During the project, some sites experienced differing impediments to implementation. At some study sites, the physical layout of the ED made team interactions more effortful, especially if there were separate workstations for physicians and nurses. This was even more consequential if these areas were walled off. Our large, open ED layout with a single combined work station supported situational awareness by encouraging cross-monitoring and extemporaneous interactions, as well as allowing staff to overhear or "eavesdrop" on conversations. The number of staff available per shift was also an obstacle for some of the smaller EDs, requiring them to creatively define and establish teams because their staffing numbers only allowed for more than one ED core team a few hours per day. Implementation sites were also impacted adversely by a lack of senior management buy-in and limited vision of the effect of the program on the organization as a whole. Key insights from our experience are summarized in Table 9.1.

Teamwork training can be both well-received and effective in healthcare. An ED is not like a cockpit, so directly importing aviation team training into emergency medicine would likely not have been as effective. But, the approach of abstracting general principles of importance from aviation team training to the emergency setting, and then

---

Table 9.1   Insights of Team Training in the Emergency Department

Teamwork training and its subsequent implementation and sustainment in the ED should be viewed as fluid, reactive, and dynamic phenomena that mirror the clinical work of emergency care.
Reduction of barriers across skill sets and the authority gradient were best overcome in integrated informal small group sessions with participants on a first name basis.
Expected users of the teamwork behaviors must feel a sense of ownership of the material and be allowed to tailor their clinical work in ways that will support distributed work teams and the desired behaviors.
The physical environment of the ED can influence the success of team training; identifying environmental barriers or facilitators is important in implementation.
Team training and implementation in the ED are only the beginning. Along with the sustainment phase, all must be adequately resourced for success in the face of staff turnover and changes in clinical context.
Long- term multilevel organizational buy-in is critical, not only for implementation but also sustainment. Senior management's strategic vision for ED teamwork training should be as an important entrée for these behaviors into the organization, as part of a scheduled diffusion of teamwork training to the great clinical environment.

developing the training based on how those principles play out in the ED setting, was a successful strategy for moving team training from aviation into emergency medicine. Teamwork performance should be treated as a part of basic clinical competency—not taken for granted that it will be picked up and maintained by osmosis. After customizing teamwork principles and behaviors to the ED setting in general, effective implementation requires fitting them into a specific workplace and culture in a specific way; ideally led by the front-line workers most affected.

REFERENCES

1. Helmreich, R. L., Merritt, A. C., & Wilhelm, J. A. (1999). The evolution of crew resource management in commercial aviation. *International Journal of Aviation Psychology, 9,* 19–32.
2. Thomas, E. J., Sherwood, G. D., Mulhollen, M. A., Sexton, J. B., & Helreich. R. L. (2004). Working together in the neonatal intensive care unit: Provider perspective. *Journal of Perinatology, 24,* 552–9.
3. Stead, K., Kumar, S., et.al. Teams communicating thru STEPPs. (2009). *Medical Journal of Australia,190,* S128–32.
4. Sundar, E., Sundar, S., Pawlowski, J., Blum, R., Feinstein, D., & Pratt, S. Crew resource management and team training. *Anesthesiology Clinics, 25*(2), 283–300.
5. Morey J, Simon R, Jay GD, & Rice MM. (2003). A transition of aviation crew resource management to hospital emergency departments: the MedTeams story. In the *Proceedings of the 12th International Symposium on Aviation Psychology.* (pp. 826–31).
6. Risser, D. T., Rice, M. M., Salisbury, M. L., Simon, R., Jay, G. D., Berns, S. D., and The MedTeams Consortium. (1999). The potential for improved teamwork to reduce medical errors in the emergency department. *Annals of Emergency Medicine, 34,* 373–83.
7. Morey, J. C., & Salisbury, M. (2002). Introducing teamwork training into healthcare organizations: Implementation issues and solutions. In *Proceedings of the Human Factors and Ergonomics Society 46th Annual Meeting* (pp. 2069–73), Santa Monica, CA: Human Factors and Ergonomics Society.
8. Morey, J. C., Simon, R., Jay, G. D., Wears, R. L., Salisbury, M., Dukes, K. A. (2002). Error reduction and performance improvement in the emergency department through formal teamwork training: Evaluation results of the MedTeams project. *Health Services Research, 37*(6), 1553–81.

10

COLLABORATIVE CARE FOR CHILDREN: ESSENTIAL MODELS FOR INTEGRATING AND OPTIMIZING TEAM PERFORMANCE IN PEDIATRIC MEDICINE

Nana E. Coleman, Sheila K. Lambert, and Anthony D. Slonim

INTRODUCTION

It is clear that the integration and optimization of clinical teams in pediatric medicine is a complex, but necessary process. We cannot expect to improve medical outcomes, even in the face of scientific advancement, without a true commitment to the improvement of the function and structure of pediatric medical teams. We will here first consider the value of teamwork in pediatrics—to patients, healthcare providers, and medical systems. Subsequently, we will present key insights for successful pediatric team development and performance measurement in the context of specific pediatric zones of practice. Last, we will provide a brief discourse on the best practices and models for team efficiency in this unique medical care environment.

VALUE OF TEAMWORK IN PEDIATRICS

When asked to identify characteristics of successful teams, even across disciplines, there are several recurring themes. Communication, mutual respect, reliability, cooperation, and creativity are among the qualities that arise most often. Similarly, experience,

honesty, patience, and compassion are regarded as necessary attributes of well-performing teams. Cultivating these characteristics requires practice, because although some of these behaviors are innate, if not utilized, they will not develop further. When pediatric teams confront medical illness, they are charged with an exceptional responsibility—to deliver the highest quality of medical care to the patient, all while balancing the personal and professional challenges such as task can bring. When executed well, however, there is no match for the satisfying and gratifying outcomes that cohesive and productive pediatric teams can affect (Fig. 10.1).

Value of Teams to Patients and Families

Imagine having your child or that of a loved one emergently and unexpectedly hospitalized. Your world as once known has changed. The onset of medical illness in a loved one generates sadness, anger, frustration, fear, and uncertainty even in the most stoic of individuals. These feelings are only enhanced when the individual is a young, seemingly helpless person—a child. At such a time, the understanding and support of strangers, as well as family can entirely shape the medical experience. By providing families with the opportunity to participate in their child's care, through rounds, their presence at the bedside or when possible, assisting with care, pediatric teams empower and bring comfort to families during what is often the worst time in their lives.

Family-centered care, which includes several of the initiatives noted above, represents a practice paradigm designed to involve parents and families more directly in their child's medical care (Fig. 10.2). It is assumed that by providing families with the opportunity to participate directly in their child's care, they will have a more satisfying, cohesive, and safe medical experience. Although this holds true in most instances, this principle can quickly evolve to "family-directed" care if pediatric practitioners are not careful to maintain the boundaries of practitioner and patient. What may have begun as a collaborative, well-intentioned endeavor soon generates an antagonistic and uncomfortable practice environment.

When skilled pediatric providers learn to work closely with patients and their families in a mutually rewarding way, the results can be significant. Countless medical errors are averted each year, simply by family members who ask for information about medications being administered to their child. Similarly, medical history and information from parents is invaluable, particularly when a patient is unknown to the medical facility and care team. Families who are engaged with the medical team are typically more satisfied with and less distrusting of the medical experience. Likewise, children thrive in medical environments where their needs are both anticipated and met with the support of their families.

Value of Teams to Providers

As we have acknowledged, the care of pediatric patients requires special commitment and unique skills. What is often forgotten is the impact that continued work with a demanding and challenging patient population may have on the providers. Strong pediatric teams provide a mechanism of support and rejuvenation for their members. The sense of camaraderie and mutual understanding that specialty teams provide to each other is what enables them to survive.

No matter how much they try, even loved ones often cannot understand the true scope of their family or friend's work, given the limitations of patient confidentiality and medical knowledge that surround pediatric medical care. Thus, coworkers and teammates provide a source of comfort and reliability that other individuals cannot provide for pediatric health providers. The shared burden of healthcare is great, but made lesser by the strength of successful medical teams.

Professional teams can also be a source of motivation and self-improvement for their members. By providing a consistent group of individuals with

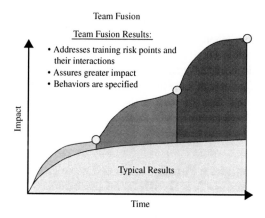

Figure 10.1
Progression of Team Performance Improvement Initiatives over Time

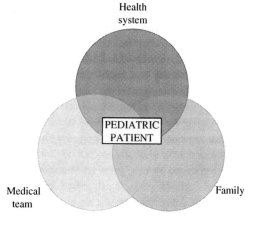

Figure 10.2
Schematic of Teams in Pediatric Medicine

common goals to the team member, medical teams serve as a forum for academic enrichment and personal growth. Team members wish to improve their knowledge base and skills not only for their patients, but also for the team members with whom they work. Pediatric team participants across varied settings report great professional satisfaction when they are considered an integral part of their work team. Team members feel a sense of pride and responsibility for the child's well-being and outcomes, and thus perform to the highest of their ability. Such diligence and drive, although alone not sufficient to eliminate mistakes, is most certainly a solid starting ground for improvement and success.

Value of Teams to Systems

Besides the professional and personal benefits that pediatric teams bring to patients, families, and care providers, their value to healthcare systems is indisputable. A well-functioning medical team can serve to reduce medical error, increase revenue, improve reputation, and facilitate better health outcomes in almost any medical environment. What distinguishes facilities with strong teams is not their lack of medical errors or inefficiencies; rather, a strong team will promote recognition and acknowledgment of mistakes, but also work to devise constructive means of performance improvement. Without organized and efficient teams, health systems become disorganized and unproductive; their performance and reputations suffer.

Ultimately, although patient care drives much of quality improvement, financial motivations cannot be ignored. The difference in cost savings and revenue between healthcare facilities with strong teams in place versus those without is significant. For example, team structures that encourage a questioning attitude by all team members exhibit fewer adverse events, and in turn fewer resources must be allocated toward paying for mistakes. Likewise, team members that are motivated and supported within their institutions remain loyal and committed "investors" in the healthcare system. Even reimbursement for healthcare expenditures is, in part, based on preventable medical errors that cohesive teams are likely to avoid.

Successful teams continue to reap many rewards of their efforts both at individual and system-wide level. Performance incentives may help to encourage pediatric team success, but sustainability is cultivated through consistent and frequent positive reinforcement. Formal reviews, debriefings, and quality improvement sessions highlight opportunities for change and advancement. Acknowledgment of both individual and group achievements promotes maintenance of the core principles of accomplished pediatric medical teams.

The benefit of unified and reliable pediatric medical teams to patients, families, providers, and health systems is multifaceted, yet certain. The medical team is at the core of the healthcare experience, and solid team performance correlates positively with successful health outcomes for children. Whether in rural settings or large academic centers, what matters most for pediatric teams is their openness toward and commitment to the distinctive principles that underlie pediatric medicine. We cannot emphasize enough the need for continued initiatives to promote skilled and dedicated clinical teams across all pediatric medical environments.

ZONES OF PEDIATRIC TEAMWORK: INSIGHTS FROM PRACTICE

The scope of pediatric healthcare is broad; accordingly pediatric healthcare providers serve in multiple capacities and require specialized training. We will present a variety of clinical settings in which children are cared for, and discuss the optimal role of an integrated medical team in each environment (Table 10.1). In many of these settings, the care is both complex and tightly coupled, implying that there is a high degree of interdependency to prevent errors and advance the care of patients. At the same time, complex and tightly coupled systems are error prone, thus the work of the interdisciplinary team is even more essential for the successful care of the patient and family.

Insight 1: Family-centered care cannot become family-dictated practice.

The most acutely ill children in any hospital will be cared for in the intensive care unit, with premature and newborn infants found in the neonatal intensive care unit (NICU) and older children managed

Table 10.1   Key Insights for Pediatric Team Performance

Key Insights for Pediatric Team Performance	Guidelines for Goal Achievement
Family-centered care cannot become family-dictated practice.	Include families in as many aspects of care as possible, but do not be afraid to set boundaries.
	Set realistic expectations for families, e.g., that although there may be multiple medical collaborators, there is a central team responsible for their child's care.
	Encourage open and consistent dialogue between patient, family and providers.
	Educate the clinical team in advance about the role of family in care delivery.
	Provide opportunities for clinical team to speak confidentially about concerns.
A clearly defined shared mental model of care is essential for goal achievement.	Define shared mental "roadmap" early in the treatment course.
	Emphasize situational awareness for all team members.
	Review progress regularly.
	Encourage team members to function in parallel, not in series.
	Promote individual accountability for actions and performance.
Successful teams must strengthen both their adaptability and efficiency across clinical situations.	Emphasize the need for timely triage and disposition of patients.
	Remain sensitive to the risk of "burnout" and fatigue among providers in "high risk, high-stress" zones.
	Encourage sensitivity to unpredictable and varied patient populations.
	Utilize protocol-driven and goal-directed care strategies to maximize efficiency.
Medical errors will occur: how teams deal with mistakes matters most.	Foster a culture of trust and constructive improvement by sharing facts openly.
	Denounce punition and encourage education.
	Normalize process improvement by providing routine forums for self-analysis and discussion.
	Address mistakes promptly and without judgment.
Practice may not make perfect, but makes better.	Identify "leaders of change" within the clinical team and encourage their participation.
	Define regular processes for performance improvement.
	Perform risk-assessments and modify goals of care with these risks in mind.
	Provide consistent educational opportunities, not only in response to adverse events.
	Utilize educational technology to review best practice and areas of weakness.

in the pediatric intensive care unit (PICU), where available. In few other environments than in the ICU is there greater stress, intensity, and propensity for errors. Likewise in this unique medical environment, discussions of medical futility, end of life care, and ethical practice are commonplace. Correspondingly, a strong therapeutic relationship between the patient, family, and healthcare team is essential. A typical medical team structure in the PICU or NICU may consist of an attending physician, trainees such as postgraduate fellows and residents, clinical nurses, pharmacists, respiratory therapists, dieticians, social workers, case managers, and specialty or consultant physicians. Beyond the medical team, there exists the patient and his or her family. All of these individuals share a common goal: to provide the highest quality of medical care to a critically ill patient. Naturally, not all members of the team will agree on how to achieve this goal. It is thereby imperative for the team to have measures in place that promote collaboration and compromise, without sacrificing the advancement of medical care for the patient.

As in the PICU, teams working in the NICU encounter distinct clinical and ethical challenges because of their patient population. These teams serve infants at the extremes of life, children who are born prematurely, who if they survive the neonatal period, go on to have lifetime special needs. Given the volume of premature infants in most NICUs, often, the bedside nurse provides the primary communication between the medical team and parents, who may be recovering from childbirth, have other children who require care at home, or are so overwhelmed by the premature delivery and medical consequences that they may choose not to remain at the bedside. Although the attending physician is still ultimately responsible for the infant's care and the medical team will consist of many of the same practitioners as in the PICU, the characteristics of most NICUs shifts the roles in the medical team. Bedside nurses may assume a more significant role in direct communication with the family, but must also take care to remain impartial and consistent while at the same time empathetic to the patient and family's needs.

These examples highlight the need for a team structure that at once encourages all opinions to be heard and considered, but also permits clear and decisive patient management. In such a team, the attending physician assumes ultimate responsibility for the medical management of the patient, having taken into consideration the views of the team, but also using his or her experience, expertise, and judgment to provide directed care for the patient.

As the team leader, the attending physician must impart direction and cohesiveness to the team. This does not always imply complete agreement among team members; in fact, it is common for intensivists to make difficult decisions, particularly surrounding end-of-life discussions. What is imperative, however, is for the team leader to facilitate an atmosphere of open and candid communication.

The institution of family-centered care and family presence during medical rounds, resuscitation, and procedures in many pediatric intensive care units provides one such opportunity. *The direct participation of patients and their families can facilitate understanding, trust, and clarity within the medical team; however, it is not without its challenges.* Some team members may feel inhibited by the presence of families; for example, trainees may be reticent to ask questions that may suggest to families that they are not competent to care for their child. Additionally, when there is disagreement between the medical practitioners and the family about the plan of care, long-term outcomes, and disposition, it may be uncomfortable for such discussions to occur in front of parents.

The essential elements for successful team performance in neonatal or pediatric ICUs are fundamental to almost any discipline: strong communication, validation of individual team member's roles, and a team leader who provides direction and focus for the team. What is unique to ICU teams is the frequency with which they confront critical illness and the complex and emotional circumstances that the care of acutely ill children raises. For a pediatric clinical team to successfully navigate such issues, it must be prepared to incorporate families directly into its work, but also recognize the objective, yet nurturing role it must serve. Pediatric intensive care teams must also devise means for stress release and mutual support because their work is uniquely demanding and psychologically draining. If, however, all of these elements function well, pediatric intensive care teams are among the most skilled and proficient at caring for pediatric patients. Optimal team performance in the pediatric intensive care unit will be cohesive, yet facilitate a climate in which individual opinions regarding the child's care are readily expressed and valued; where there is a single clearly-identified team ultimately responsible for the child's care, despite collaboration with other medical specialists; and in which there is both regard and support for the emotional and professional stresses that uniquely accompany the care of such critically ill children.

Insight 2: A clearly-defined shared mental model of care is essential to goal achievement.

It is difficult for a pediatric clinical team to achieve its goals without a unified, structured plan of care, often termed a shared mental model. Without such a "roadmap," individual team members may independently be working toward goals of care without a defined endpoint or measures of success. Such behaviors place patients at greater risk because the propensity for task duplication and omission increases without a common goal. The value of shared mental modeling is particularly apparent within the ambulatory pediatric setting where the functional efficiency of the office depends on each team member fulfilling his or her role to completion; otherwise the "downstream" members of the team cannot work at maximum efficiency.

Ambulatory care settings are typically staffed by a multidisciplinary team. Each of these individuals plays an integral role in the care of the child, although unlike inpatient settings, there can be fewer opportunities for all team members to interact at once with the patient. Usually, the patient encounters each team member during different points of the care experience, thus what unifies the team is an unspoken understanding of their shared goal of efficient and quality care for the patient. Take for example a busy pediatric practice that sees both scheduled patients and walk-ins. If both patient types are not registered efficiently, they cannot be triaged appropriately by the nurse. The physician will not be able to evaluate patients in a timely fashion, and patient dissatisfaction will increase. Moreover, the nurses, therapists, or technicians who are waiting to execute the medical orders cannot maintain an efficient and well-balanced pace of work. What ensues is a chaotic, unhappy clinical environment for both patients and staff alike.

Pediatric ambulatory care team members must remember that even if unseen, their work is critical to the success of the patient encounter. Although the team members may seemingly work in parallel, rather than as one, communication is no less important. Frequent team debriefings and needs assessments will facilitate effective team performance in outpatient pediatric settings. *Thus for outpatient and hospital-based pediatric teams alike, situational monitoring and awareness, coupled with individual accountability and a shared mental model for patient care will deliver the highest success in patient care.*

Insight 3: Successful teams must strengthen both their adaptability and efficiency across clinical situations.

The pressures of time, resource and demand mismatch, and uncertainty pose unique challenges for the pediatric teams in the emergency department (ED). *Thus, high-functioning pediatric medical teams in this and other high-intensity zones of practice require a generalized team commitment to team efficiency and accuracy, the ability to rapidly mobilize resources, and the aptitude to perform consistently across a wide range of clinical diseases and patient types.*

Emergency department teams must be flexible, tolerant, and especially compassionate because their young patients are typically frightened and apprehensive when they present for care. In order to succeed, ED teams must further make a conscious effort to reach out to each other for support, pace themselves in their work, and strive for direct connections with their patients, even when their encounters may be brief. The performance of an ED team can affect an entire hospital, given that the decisions made by the emergency department affect hospital admissions, census, and revenue. Beyond that fact, the ED may be a family's first and only contact with the medical system, thus that initial interaction may color their future interactions with clinical teams, for better or for worse. At their best, clinical teams in pediatric EDs exemplify the best balance of protocol-driven and efficient models of care delivery coupled with the capacity to augment productivity and resources when faced with life-threatening situations.

Insight 4: Medical errors will occur: how teams deal with mistakes matters most.

Much has been made of medical errors that occur in the surgical environment, and specific initiatives designed to improve patient identification, to promote consistency in practice, and to prioritize patient safety are underway in many healthcare facilities. In addition to these strategies, team development, education and support must also be a priority. Children who undergo surgery bear special attention given that unlike many other pediatric environments, the sequestered nature of the operating room (OR) separates children and parents for a significant amount of time. Thus, there is a loss of ready patient advocacy and the additional mechanism of safety that parents at the bedside may add. Additionally, many ORs are shared between adults and children; therefore, special consideration must be given to the technical needs of the medical team as they work with children. From the anesthesiologist to the scrub nurses to the surgeon, all members of the operating room team must be deliberate and focused on their work to ensure safe practice and outcomes.

Despite the efforts to mitigate risk in such susceptible environments, errors do and will occur given that in the face of human subjectivity, no process can be entirely foolproof. When medical mistakes occur especially in children, several emotions—anger, remorse, disappointment, and mistrust—result among both the patient and clinical staff. Errors in care leave the medical team in a position of special vulnerability, and if not openly addressed, can essentially paralyze the subsequent therapeutic relationship with the patient and family. *Essential to the successful appraisal of medical mistakes are first, nonthreatening, secure forums in which providers can openly discuss potential deficiencies in clinical knowledge and understanding that may have contributed to the error; opportunities for experienced providers to discuss clinical alternatives to the choices made when appropriate; and methods of education and training to enhance staff competency and confidence.* Punition does not work, but rather serves to isolate team members and precipitate greater errors as a consequence of the atmosphere of fear, uncertainty, and disempowerment that such an approach breeds.

Insight 5: Practice may not make perfect, but makes better.

We cannot expect to improve medical outcomes, even in the face of scientific advancement without a true commitment to the improvement of the function and structure of pediatric medical teams. It is therefore valuable to consider the key elements of team development, education, and performance measurement.

Needs Assessment and Performance Measurement

Before developing strategies to optimize pediatric team performance, a needs assessment must first be performed. The goal of such an assessment is to define the existing role of the pediatric team in the given healthcare zone, to identify areas of strength and weakness in the team's performance, and to delineate objectives for the team's development and growth. The first step is to categorize the team's ongoing work in a framework of improvement. Doing so necessitates awareness of those events that may have led to the team's present vision and objectives; for example, a review of high risk events that have affected patient care or outcomes can provide insight into why the team functions as it does. An assessment tool such as a knowledge, attitudes, and practice survey is a useful means of prioritizing the medical teams' perceptions of and attitudes toward patient care. Other means of assessing team performance may include self-reporting mechanisms such as routine debriefings and audits, performance reviews, and external competency testing. All of these methods taken together serve the purpose of defining areas for potential improvement in team performance. The opinions of medical team members can significantly influence the direction and focus of the team's work—these individuals are among the true stakeholders, and their perceptions can inform the team transformation process.

Team Organization and Structure

As we have discussed, the integrated medical team structure in pediatrics incorporates patient, family, and medical personnel. These parties are united in their goal to provide high-quality medical care to the pediatric patient across a variety of zones of practice. Each environment will necessitate adaptations in team structure; however, fundamentally the team should maintain the same objectives for healthcare delivery. Key goals for pediatric team structure have been described in other settings with almost universal emphasis on providing a shared purpose, clear objectives, commitment to conflict management, principles of excellence and professionalism, and effective communication to the team.

In several organizations, a "change team" is charged with primary responsibility for initiating and directing team development. Before embarking on any successful implementation or practice change, it is important to establish a change team to ensure the change is introduced in a timely manner, as smoothly as possible and with maximal effectiveness. A typical change team consists of essential individuals from within the team who are particularly invested in performance improvement, have earned the credibility and respect of their colleagues through participation in other transitions, and are willing to invest the necessary time, creativity, and energy in the ongoing assessments and improvements. A change team offers experience, knowledge, and skills, which together can create substantially more energy around the initiative or project than any single individual may have the capacity to do. A change team also offers a broader base of relationships to handle issues on a personal level and an increased sense of purpose and importance about the change that will take place. Clear expectations must be relayed to potential change team members, including the anticipated time commitment, their roles and responsibilities as a change agent, and the length of time this commitment may require and operating guidelines. When used effectively, change teams can be invaluable in structuring a clinical team.

There are several models for team composition and structure that can be utilized in pediatric medical settings, but as we have emphasized, those models that enable patients, families, and medical personnel to function coordinately, rather than in parallel, are most likely to succeed. The ideal pediatric medical team model will incorporate the best elements of both "vertical" and "horizontal" team dynamics. In vertical teams, there is a defined leader who has primary responsibility for providing the direction, priorities, and goals for the team. The team may create a vision based on a shared mental model; however, the implementation of these goals is often dependent on the leader's initiative and commitment. The team leader is placed in a position of ultimate control for advancing the team's work. In contrast, horizontal-performing teams may also have a team leader; however, the entire team takes ownership for realization of the team's objectives. The team leader does not retain an isolated position of power, because hierarchy does not define horizontal teams. What such

a team resembles is one in which the needs of the pediatric patient are at the core of healthcare delivery; at various points during the care experience, team members may need to collaborate and compromise to advance the patient's care, but ultimately the medical team bears the responsibility for managing the child's medical needs. In such a system, all participants are invested in success, there is a means for ensuring accountability in the process, but the role of the medical providers does not overshadow the value of patient and family contributions to the medical care plan.

Team and Organizational Training

Given the attention that has been paid to clinical outcomes as a function of team performance, it is no wonder that team-training programs are growing in popularity. In recent years, many healthcare organizations have incorporated internal strategies to review and improve their team performance— simulated clinical scenarios, formal debriefings, and root cause analyses, as examples. Simultaneously, these same institutions have sought the expertise of consultants and educators to help promote a culture of safety, collaboration, and teamwork within the medical environment.

Successful characteristics of team and leadership development programs include broad applicability to all levels of the clinical team; use of real-life examples to characterize "what-if" situations; and a larger institutional commitment to their implementation. There is near universal emphasis on closed-loop communication, situational awareness, mutual respect, and positive, rather than negative reinforcement in the programs we have encountered. Additionally, processes such as patient hand-offs, escalation of clinical changes to appropriate staff, and mitigation of medical errors are targeted as key areas of risk for the pediatric patient, and thus are highlighted within such programs. We advocate the implementation of a structured, individualized team and leadership education program in all pediatric healthcare facilities.

CONCLUSION

We have demonstrated the unequivocal value of high-performing clinical teams across a spectrum of zones of pediatric practice and have provided guidelines for the establishment and sustainability of such well-functioning teams. A successful model of pediatric team performance will be based on a shared vision for safe, quality, and reliable clinical outcomes for the pediatric patient. The foundation of the clinical team will be mutual respect for the views of the patient, family, and medical team, with the knowledge that ultimately the medical team bears responsibility for achievement of the medical care plan.

Through a collaborative approach to team development and performance, pediatric medical providers can empower patients and their families. The value of teams to patients, families, and healthcare systems is significant and deserves prioritization across healthcare organizations. To that end, training physicians, nurses, and other team members should receive consistent and early education about their role in the team development process.

We have illustrated that the paramount goal of pediatric medicine—the delivery of safe, error-limited healthcare to children—cannot be achieved without first ensuring the availability of structured and resource-enabled clinical teams. We believe that with continued institutional, educational, and individual commitment to this goal, the medical care currently provided to children will only exceed our expectations.

SUGGESTED READINGS

Rosen, P., Stenger, E., Bochkoris, M., Hannon, M. J., & Kwoh, C. K. (2009). Family-centered multidisciplinary rounds enhance the team approach in pediatrics. *Pediatrics, 123*(4), e603–8.

Patel, D. R., Pratt, H. D., & Patel, N. D. (2008). Team processes and team care for children with developmental disabilities. *Pediatric Clinics of North America, 55*(6), 1375–90, ix.

Morison, S., Boohan, M., Moutray, M., & Jenkins, J. (2004). Developing pre-qualification interprofessional education for nursing and medical students: Sampling student attitudes to guide development. *Nurse Education in Practice, 4*(1), 20–9.

Ackerman, A., Graham, M., Schmidt, H., Stern, D. T., & Miller, S. Z. (2009). Critical events in the lives of interns. *Journal of General Internal Medicine, 24*(1), 27–32.

Devictor, D., & Floret, D. (2008). [Field 8. Safety practices in paediatric intensive care medicine. French-speaking Society of Intensive Care. French Society of Anesthesia and Resuscitation]. *Annals of French Anesthesia and Reanimation, 27*(10), e111–5.

Sands, S. A., Stanley, P., & Charon, R. (2008). Pediatric narrative oncology: Interprofessional training to promote empathy, build teams, and prevent burnout. *The Journal of Supportive Oncology, 6*(7), 307–12.

Krug, S. E. (2008). The art of communication: strategies to improve efficiency, quality of care and patient safety in the emergency department. *Pediatric Radiology, 38*(Suppl 4), S655–9.

Eppich, W. J., Brannen, M., & Hunt, E. A. (2008). Team training: Implications for emergency and critical care pediatrics. *Current Opinion in Pediatrics, 20*(3), 255–60.

Haller, G., Garnerin, P., Morales, M. A., et al. (2008). Effect of crew resource management training in a multidisciplinary obstetrical setting. *International Journal of Quality Health Care, 20*(4), 254–63.

Bognár, A., Barach, P., Johnson, J. K., et al. (2008). Errors and the burden of errors: attitudes, perceptions, and the culture of safety in pediatric cardiac surgical teams. *Annals of Thoracic Surgery, 85*(4), 1374–81.

White, C. T., Trnka, P., & Matsell, D. G. (2007). Selected primary care issues and comorbidities in children who are on maintenance dialysis: A review for the pediatric nephrologist. *Clinical Journal of the American Society of Nephrology, 2*(4), 847–57.

Catchpole, K. R., Giddings, A. E., Wilkinson, M., Hirst, G., Dale, T., & de Leval, M. R. (2007). Improving patient safety by identifying latent failures in successful operations. *Surgery, 142*(1), 102–10.

Zabari, M., Suresh, G., Tomlinson, M., et al. (2006). Implementation and case-study results of potentially better practices for collaboration between obstetrics and neonatology to achieve improved perinatal outcomes. *Pediatrics, 118*(Suppl 2), S153–8.

Brinkman, W. B, Geraghty, S. R., Lanphear, B. P., et al. (2006). Evaluation of resident communication skills and professionalism: a matter of perspective? *Pediatrics, 118*(4), 1371–9.

Thomas, E. J., Sexton, J. B., & Helmreich, R. L. (2004). Translating teamwork behaviours from aviation to healthcare: Development of behavioural markers for neonatal resuscitation. *Quality & Safety in Health Care, 13*(Suppl 1), i57–64.

Suresh, G., Horbar, J. D., Plsek, P., et al. (2004). Voluntary anonymous reporting of medical errors for neonatal intensive care. *Pediatrics, 113*(6), 1609–18.

Brown, M. S., Ohlinger, J., Rusk, C., Delmore, P., Ittmann, P., & CARE Group. (2003). Implementing potentially better practices for multidisciplinary team building: creating a neonatal intensive care unit culture of collaboration. *Pediatrics, 111*(4 Pt 2), e482–8.

Ohlinger, J., Brown, M. S., Laudert, S., Swanson, S., Fofah, O., & CARE Group. (2003). Development of potentially better practices for the neonatal intensive care unit as a culture of collaboration: communication, accountability, respect, and empowerment. *Pediatrics, 111*(4 Pt 2), e471–81.

Baker, G. R., King, H., MacDonald, J.L., & Horbar, J. D. (2003). Using organizational assessment surveys for improvement in neonatal intensive care. *Pediatrics, 111*(4 Pt 2), e419–25.

Margolis, P. A., Stevens, R., Bordley, W. C., et al. (2001). From concept to application: the impact of a community-wide intervention to improve the delivery of preventive services to children. *Pediatrics, 108*(3), E42.

Kohn LT, Corrigan JM, Donaldson MS (Eds). (1999). *To Err Is Human: Building a Safer Health System*. National Academy Press .

O'Connell, M. T. & Pascoe, J. M. (2004). Undergraduate medical education for the 21st century: Leadership and teamwork. *Family Medicine, 36*(Suppl)), S51–6.

American Academy of Pediatrics Policy Statement. (1998). Prevention of medication errors in the pediatric inpatient setting. *Pediatrics, 10*(2), 428–30.

Goldberg, R., Boss, R. W., Chan, L., et al. (1996). Burnout and its correlates in emergency physicians: Four years' experience with a wellness both. *Academic Emergency Medicine, 3*(12), 1156–64.

11

TRAUMA TEAMWORK AND PATIENT SAFETY

Kenneth Stahl, George D. Garcia, David J. Birnbach, and
Jeffrey Augenstein

INTRODUCTION

The risks our patients face, not from their injuries
or disease processes, but from the healthcare system itself, have many causes but limited solutions.
Although the exact magnitude of patient errors has
been debated, the fact that errors in patient care occur
and that some patients are seriously and sometimes
fatally harmed is no longer in dispute.[1] Trauma centers are beginning to investigate the nature of errors in
the management of injured patients, and these events
have become better understood. Preventable deaths
resulting from human and system errors account
for up to 10%[2-4] of fatalities in patients with otherwise survivable injuries cared for at Level I trauma
centers. These unintended deaths equate to as many
as 15,000 lost lives per year in the United States or
two lives lost per hour around the clock.[5] This rate of
death resulting from error in trauma patients is two
to four times higher than deaths resulting from errors
reported in the general hospital patient population.[6]

The scenarios that are most conducive to producing errors and lead to adverse patient outcomes are the
very environments in which trauma victims present;
unstable patients, fatigued operators, incomplete
histories, time-critical decisions, concurrent tasks,
involvement of many disciplines, complex teams,
transportation of unstable patients, and multiple
hand-offs of patient management. As such, trauma
care creates a "perfect storm for medical errors."[7]
Successful outcomes for trauma victims are characterized by the need to maintain mental acuity in the
face of fatigue or during quiet periods, make time-
critical decisions, and carry out intricate procedures
with life-or-death consequences. Successful care of
trauma patients also requires control of potentially
chaotic environments and rapid processing of complex and often incomplete information. These conditions not only define the circumstances under which
trauma care is delivered but also offers insight into
the worst-case scenarios from which adverse events
can result.[7] Successful management of trauma victims depends on maintaining order and providing
care in these environments, and teamwork and team
function is critical to accomplish this task.

High-risk and error-intolerant organizations,
known as high reliability organizations (HROs), have
pioneered and perfected methods to reduce errors
by avoiding many and when not possible to prevent
error to mitigate and trap small errors before they
can propagate through their systems, causing dis-
astrous outcomes. Among the most critical and successful methods that have been employed by HROs
to accomplish this task is crew resource management (CRM), which is a curriculum of material that
teaches principles of optimum teamwork and team

communication. There are elements of this body of knowledge that we can import into the management of trauma patients because the environment in which the trauma surgeon works closely mimics the cockpit environment that flight crews operate.

HIGH RELIABILITY ORGANIZATION SAFETY PRINCIPLES FOR ENHANCING PATIENT SAFETY IN TRAUMA

High reliability organizations are characterized as high-risk, error-intolerant systems that are capable of repetitively carrying out potentially dangerous tasks with low occurrence of adverse outcomes.[7] Commercial aviation serves as the primary example of the HRO safety model, as evidenced by a decade of annual Federal Aviation Authority statistics indicating that the risk of a major commercial carrier accident ranges from 0.00 to 0.218/1,000,000 flight hours.[8] An individual must fly 24 hours per day every day for 570 years before standing a 1% chance of being involved in a fatal commercial aviation accident. This safety record has been achieved and maintained based on a thorough comprehension of the mechanisms of errors gleaned from collecting incident and error reports. In aviation, as in other HROs, reporting and avoiding error has become a compulsion and a cultural norm.[7]

Detailed analysis of adverse events and near-miss case studies have generated a body of knowledge known as *high reliability theory* that defines a number of organizational features likely to reduce the risk of organizational accidents, human failures, and other hazards.[9] To adopt these organizational safety models for use in trauma patient safety, it is necessary to understand specific practices that can be abstracted from this body of information.[10] Designers of systems of care can increase safety by focusing on three tasks: designing a system to prevent errors; designing procedures to make errors visible when they do occur so they may be intercepted; and designing methods for minimizing the impact of adverse events when they are not detected and intercepted.[11] The hallmark of preventing adverse outcomes involves avoiding missteps in the first place as well as trapping small errors before they are allowed to become devastating mistakes.

Teams that exhibit behaviors and facilitate the characteristics and values held by the HRO may be defined as high reliability teams (HRT). Wilson and colleagues[12] have defined five guidelines for high reliability teams:

1. High reliability teams must use closed loop communication and other forms of information exchange to promote shared situational awareness regarding factors internal and external to the team.
2. High reliability teams must develop shared mental models that allow team members to monitor others' performance and offer back up assistance when needed.
3. High reliability teams must demonstrate a collective organization that allows members to be assertive, to take advantage of functional expertise, and to seek and value input from other team members.
4. High reliability teams must seek to recognize complexities of their task environment and accordingly develop plans that are adequate and promote flexibility.
5. High reliability teams must use semistructured feedback mechanisms such as team self-correction to manage, and quickly learn from errors.

TEAMWORK IS THE PRIMARY HIGH RELIABILITY ORGANIZATION SAFETY TOOL

Team skills are essential for successful trauma management. Team skills involve three core teamwork competencies: (1) A shared and common knowledge of team mission and objectives that is based on construction of the big picture by input from all team members; (2) skill competencies of mutual performance monitoring and adaptability of team members; and (3) attitude competencies of mutual trust and collective efficacy of the mission.[13] High reliability organizations further stress that teams are groups of people with similar objectives but differing levels of expertise and different skills; therefore, communication improvement strategies are best seen as the framework for supporting improved team function.[14] Medical teams generally and surgical teams specifically have been studied in depth by many authors.[15]

Failure to communicate critical information in the operating room occurs in approximately 30% of team exchanges.[16] Such failures lead to inefficiency, emotional tension, delay, workarounds, resource waste, patient inconvenience, and procedural error, all of which can portend poor patient outcomes.

Trauma teams are similarly composed of many individuals with different experience and skill levels and different responsibilities. High performing teams exhibit a sense of collective efficacy and recognize that they are dependent on each other and believe that, working together, they can solve complex problems. As defined in HRO safety models, effective teams are dynamic, they optimize their resources, engage in self-correction, compensate for each other by providing backup behaviors, and reallocate functions as necessary. Effective teams can respond efficiently in high-stress, time-restricted environments. Effective teams recognize potential problems or dangerous circumstances and adjust their strategies accordingly.[17] Good teamwork establishes and maintains group and individual situational awareness and provides mutual support. Key benefits of good teamwork include added knowledge and expertise available to confront situations, synergy of ideas and skills so that the combined expertise of the group is greater than any individual. This synthesis of ideas and skills make new options available. Good teams create the big picture of situational awareness together and share information, perceptions and ideas to keep everyone ahead of the evolving clinical condition. These principles are stressed in HROs and CRM used to train optimized teams.

In all aspects of healthcare, team care has been shown to be more effective than non–team care.[18,19] Bollomo et al.[19] have documented impressive reductions in mortality, morbidity, and length of stay in patients after major operations after institution of a formally trained emergency team. Their prospective cohort study shows a reduction in relative risk of 57.8% ($p < 0.0001$) for major complication, reduction in relative risk of postoperative death by 36.6% ($p < 0.0178$), and reduction of postoperative length of stay by four days ($p < 0.0092$). Observational studies in the operating room have consistently demonstrated that training clinicians in nontechnical and teamwork skills provides important safety nets.[20] Level II data support the conclusion that team training improves trauma and intensive care unit (ICU) team

performance and recognition of life-threatening injuries with reduction in death, adverse outcomes, and lengths of stay.[7]

TRAINING TRAUMA TEAMS

Among the most important skills that trauma surgeons learn during training years are how to form effective team units, how to be a good team member, and how to be a good team leader. The value of good teamwork, high-quality team communication, and accurate construction and exchange of the big picture of situational awareness have been documented in numerous organizations to increase safety and effectiveness. The same lessons hold true for medicine, and especially trauma and critical care management in our environment of complex patients, time compression, and task overload.

There are eight characteristics of effective trauma teams:

1. Establish an environment for open communication.
2. Hold preprocedure and postprocedure briefings that are thorough, interesting, and address team coordination and planning.
3. Make briefings open and inclusive of ancillary personnel and available to members of other teams.
4. Encourage a climate that is appropriate to the operational environment and patient criticality.
5. An attitude in which members are encouraged to and ask questions regarding team actions, plans and decisions
6. Promote an attitude in which members speak up and state their information in an appropriate, assertive, persistent, and timely manner.
7. Clearly state and acknowledge clinical decisions and priorities.
8. Coordinate activities to establish a proper balance between command authority and team participation.

The three major skill sets to build effective teams are communication skills, CRM, and effective leadership.

1. *Effective communication* is an essential skill in trauma management. High reliability organizations

view communication as the glue that holds teams together, understanding that team communication function is a central component of HROs and aviation safety. The Joint Commission (2003) (http://www.jcaho.org/accredited+organizations.htm) statistics have identified that 67% of the root cause of sentinel events are the result of errors in communication between team members.[21] Poor teamwork and communication lapses among members of healthcare teams have emerged as key factors in the occurrence of errors. In healthcare, understanding team dynamics and practicing functional team skills are important aspects of avoiding errors in the management of the trauma patient. Medical teams generally and surgical teams specifically have been studied in depth by many authors.[22] Failure to communicate critical information in the operating room occurs in approximately 30% of team exchanges.[23] Such failures lead to inefficiency, emotional tension, delay, workarounds, resource waste, patient inconvenience, and procedural error, all of which can portend poor patient outcomes. As an example, a potential source of increased risk would occur if the anesthesiologist and surgeon were not communicating well. It requires appropriate team training for them to learn how to effectively communicate with each other.

2. *Crew resource management (CRM)* is an educational program that has evolved over three decades of HRO safety studies. It has evolved from a program focused on individual attitude and awareness to a broad curriculum of behavioral skills and teamwork attitudes integrated with technical competencies. Crew resource management programs evolved steadily, in part because they were guided by data that validated the importance of human factors. Crew resource management encompasses skills such as clearly defining team roles and duties, managing distractions, prioritizing tasks, and avoiding task overload, all of which are integral components of a well-functioning trauma team. High reliability organization– and aviation-based CRM is defined as maximizing procedural effectiveness by using all available resources, including "hardware," "software," people, information, and environment. Crew resource management training results in positive reactions to teamwork concepts, increased knowledge of teamwork principles, and improved teamwork performance.[24] Crew resource management was rapidly adopted by airlines and is required not only for United States based carriers but also in the 185 countries operating under the United Nations' International Civil Aviation Organization (ICAO) mandate.

The byproducts of CRM skills are individual and team situational awareness, judgment, safety, resource preservation, and competitive advantage. This important set of skills has been emphasized in the medical literature also to optimize and manage workload and task assignments, clinical task planning, and review and critique strategies.[25] Skills such as pre-procedure briefs and "time-outs" and postprocedure debriefs are critical safety skills to plan procedures and capture just-lessons. Crew resource management skills are an indispensible element of communication and patient management in the operating room and Level II data support the conclusion that these skills enhance the performance of the operating team and patient outcomes.[26,27]

3. *Effective leadership and supervision* are crucial parts of team dynamics that have been repeatedly emphasized in HRO and aviation safety.[28] Trauma unit leaders perform three key functions; they provide strategic direction, monitor the performance of the team, and teach team members by providing instruction—all tasks that match those that researchers identified in the functional team leadership literature.[29] The characteristics of leadership in trauma teams has been studied by Yun et al. in a Level I trauma center.[30] They stress the importance of leadership adaptability because team leaders and their teams work in an uncertain and time-constrained environment. Trauma leaders cannot anticipate when critical patients will arrive or how many and what type of injuries they will face. They often do not know with accuracy such essential information as a patient's medical history and leadership adaptability becomes more important in uncertain and urgent situations. The ability to get the best performance from all team members and encourage each person on the team to share information and knowledge are traits of good leaders and supervisors that have been stressed in both the HRO literature as well as in reviews by The American College of Surgeons.[31]

TRAINING TRAUMA TEAMS

The Ryder Trauma Center at Jackson Memorial Hospital has the privilege of being home to the US

Army Trauma Training Center (ATTC) since its creation in late 2001. The ATTC is the only clinical, team-based training currently provided to US Army Forward Surgical Teams (FSTs), 20-person units whose role is to provide resuscitative surgery in an austere, far-forward location on the battlefield. Before deployment to a combat theater, every FST completes a 2-week training rotation at the ATTC. The primary goal of the ATTC rotation is to promote teamwork and thereby enhance the coordinated response to traumatic injury among team members that have rarely, and most often never, worked together in a clinical setting. The ATTC director (a trauma surgeon) and eight experienced ATTC instructors (physicians, nurses, and army medics) compose the primary training staff.

The ATTC curriculum is structured with an understanding of specific team knowledge, skills, and abilities that have been extracted from research on aviation teams. Medicine, especially trauma care, and aviation share a number of similarities, which include the need for decision making based on incomplete or conflicting information, the demand for coordination among professionals with varied skills and ranks, and the possibility of poor team performance leading to serious consequence or death (in this case of patients). There are few scenarios in medicine that fit this description more precisely than those faced by an army FST. US Army Trauma Training Center training recognizes that, as stated previously and stressed by HROs, each FST is a group of people with the same objective but widely variable levels of expertise and each with a unique skill set. Therefore, the primary emphasis of the training is to define each member's role on the team and begin functioning as a coordinated unit.

The initial phase of training consists of basic trauma management lectures given over the first 4 days of the rotation. In addition to lectures on clinical topics relevant to the FSTs, team members are given lectures on critical team concepts, trauma teamwork systems, and teamwork in the trauma resuscitation unit. These lectures, based on the TeamSTEPPS® model developed by the American Institutes for Research through a grant from the Agency for Healthcare Research and Quality (AHRQ) and the Department of Defense (DoD), introduce a set of core knowledge, team skills, and attitude competencies that are stressed throughout all phases of the

training rotation. The goal of the ATTC is not to give deploying FSTs a list of tasks to perform, but rather to train them in team and clinical competencies that will allow further growth and the adaptability to accomplish any task they face after deployment.

The first of these competencies is team leadership, and this is defined as the ability to direct and coordinate the activities of other team members, assess team performance, assign tasks, develop team knowledge, skills and abilities, motivate team members, plan and organize, and establish a positive atmosphere. Initially, the ATTC staff fills this role and clarifies each team member's role, provides performance expectations, and introduces acceptable interaction patterns. However, as the training progresses, members of the team emerge to assume this role. These leaders then synchronize and combine individual team member contributions to synergize efforts and coalesce the group into a highly functional team. A vital point that is emphasized is that this role is not limited to the FST commander or the surgeons; the team is encouraged to empower all members to act as leaders to facilitate team problem solving.

The second competency taught is mutual performance monitoring. This is defined as the ability to develop common understandings of the team environment and apply appropriate task strategies and priorities to accurately monitor teammate performance. Although initially seen as the role of the surgeons on the team, over the course of the training, even the team's most inexperienced members quickly gain confidence in their performance and begin develop the ability to monitor their teammates. This allows all team members to identify mistakes and lapses in other team members' actions so as to provide feedback that will eventually facilitate each team member's ability to self-correct and limit the number of mistakes made by the team as a whole.

Because each team member's role is described to the entire team, all members are able to anticipate each other's needs and shift workload during periods of high volume and/or pressure. This is the backup behavior competency and is relevant to army surgical teams, who face mass casualty incidents with far more frequency than their civilian counterparts. The redundancy that is built into the FSTs at this point closely parallels models of redundant skills in HRO safety models. Another vital competency for the FST members to master is the ability to adjust strategies and reallocate team resources (adaptability competency), both human and matériel, based on the rapidly changing conditions that are common on the modern battlefield. This allows all team members to potentially identify cues that a change has occurred, assign meaning to that change, and develop a new plan to deal with the changes. A common example would be an experienced medic left alone to monitor a critically injured patient while all the team's surgeons are occupied in the operating room. That soldier needs to not only identify a change in the patient's status, but also to understand what that change means and formulate a plan.

As these competencies are mastered, the shared mental model emerges. An army FST starts with the advantage of having a well-defined, single mission of which all members of the team are aware before attending the training offered at the ATTC. However, the shared mental model encompasses more than just being able to state the unit's mission. It allows team members to integrate how each team member will interact with the others within the scope of their mission and, therefore, function far more efficiently. They develop the ability to identify changes in their team, task, or teammates and implicitly adjust strategies as needed.

Effective communication, as outlined in the HRO team model, allows FST members to develop these other competencies. The importance of following up with team members to ensure a message was received and clarifying with the sender of the message that the message received is the same as intended is of paramount importance and is stressed through every simulation and all periods of clinical training. The simplest technique is the use of call outs and call backs. These basic techniques allow the sender of the message to confirm that it was not only received but acted on, and confirm that it was completed. The team's use of call outs and call backs is evaluated throughout the rotation.

SIMULATION AS A TOOL FOR TEAM TRAINING

Simulation has been recognized by HROs and team training of army FSTs as one of the critical safety tools to rehearse and train for error recognition and

recovery, as well as to enhance and practice safety skills. For decades, simulators have been used in the aviation industry and by the military and nuclear power plant operators for training and assessment of performance with excellent results. Similarly, simulation and role-playing allow trauma teams to replicate the task environments and stresses of patient resuscitation with no risk of adverse outcomes. Errors can be allowed to occur and their outcomes studied by replaying video recordings of the simulation, which are used so participants can see the consequences of their decisions. Presentations of uncommon but critical scenarios that require immediate recognition and attention can be programmed into the simulator and practiced for both pattern recognition and technical management skills.

Simulated training is conducted in several formats at the ATTC. The first is the use of the METIman (METI Medical Industries, Inc., Sarasota, FL), a physiologically responsive mannequin that allows the ATTC staff, and the team itself, to evaluate their ability to function as a team. On the second day of the rotation, treatment teams are presented with a patient scenario with little time to prepare. The exercise is repeated on the penultimate day of training to re-assess the team's ability to function together. Without fail, marked improvement is observed in all or nearly all of the competencies stressed throughout training.

The other major simulated training that is conducted is a mass casualty exercise. This exercise is undertaken on the last day of training before the beginning of the clinical rotation. The team is presented with multiple "patients" with simulated injury patterns of varying severity and complexity in a very short time coming very close to overwhelming the team's resources and available manpower. The exercise is conducted with IRB-approved live porcine models, so the sense of urgency in managing these "patients" is as realistic as possible. Both communication and adaptability are stressed during this exercise.

TEAM FUNCTION METRICS

Participants are surveyed before and after their experience at the ATTC regarding clinical and combat experience as well as knowledge of their purpose within the team. The ATTC has aggregated the survey data taken from 178 participants over 18 months to determine the typical profile of a participant in this rotation and evaluate the gains that are made in terms of team-building and clinical preparedness.

The pre-rotation profile of the participants highlights the necessity of didactic education and simulation in preparing participants for the challenge they will face in the field. Fifty-one percent have 0–6 months experience, and 27% have 6 months to 1 year. Only 22% have more than 1 year of experience in the field. Team building and role defining are essential components of this experience, because 49% of participants have worked together for less than 6 months. Fifty-six percent have had minimal involvement (<25% of their day) in patient care, reflecting the need for intense clinical education. Before the rotation, 74% of participants are unsure of how their team will function in the care of a trauma patient, and 30% are unfamiliar with their role within the team structure.

After the rotation and all training exercises have been completed, there is a significant improvement regarding participant perception of team performance as well as their role within the team. The awareness of subjects regarding the ability of their team to function in the care of a trauma patient improved from 26% to 84%, reflecting the overall course emphasis on teamwork and communication. Subject awareness concerning their role within the team improved from 71% to 95%, indicating that functioning as a team in the context of the MASCAL exercise along with clinical codes was beneficial. The clinical component of the rotation was considered by 47% to be the most valuable aspect of the training, with the MASCAL exercise receiving the second-most votes at 21%. These data support the value of team training and team management approach to trauma care and FST function.

FUTURE DIRECTIONS: SMART TECHNOLOGY

Acute management of surgical/trauma patients occur in a complex environment of admissions and constantly changing patient conditions on a 24-hour schedule that does not respect time of day or night. These patients do not always come with an accurate and detailed history of their prehospital care, which a unified hand-held device that is accessible by all clinicians can avoid. There are, in addition, multiple teams of caregivers who require this information and interact with differing schedules and responsibilities, which include primary clinical trauma and surgical services, consultants, nursing teams, and ICU teams. This no doubt contributes to the highest mortality in postinjury care.

The source of errors and adverse outcomes relates to a complex mix of human factors, teamwork, and system breakdowns that lead to communication mistakes and mishandling of critical patient information. Data from published studies in our institution confirm this finding and specifically document that 20.1% of critical patient care items were lost during a 24-hour observation period because of failures of communication among ICU team members.[32] Poor teamwork and communication lapses among members of healthcare teams have emerged as key factors in the occurrence of errors. In our study we documented that a structured checklist significantly reduces the incidence of lost information and communication lapses among trauma ICU team members at handoffs of care.

Our center has addressed these various causes of adverse outcomes in trauma care on multiple levels, which include understanding sources or errors, and training teams to avoid, catch, and mitigate errors. An understanding of these sources of error has led to the development of smart portable devices to aid clinicians and physicians-in-training in managing complex and chaotic environments. We have begun to beta test Mobile Care, a device based on pocket personal computer and smart phone technology. This electronic hand-held patient management and alerting system is designed to reduce the loss of patient critical data that contributes to error in the management of complex, injured patients. Further, this device will alert the carrier to incoming test and laboratory results, potentially dangerous trends in vital signs, and outstanding test results that need monitoring. This will enhance information management and link patients with their critical information wherever in the system or the world they are transported. This hand-held device also functions as a training aid to provide treatment guidance for unfamiliar clinical scenarios, provide live video links for telemedicine, and "tele-help" and audio checklists for procedures and patient care. In these ways the device will enhance communication regarding patient status and laboratory results. The device further has the capability to record direct dictation of procedures, progress, and clinical notes that can be stored electronically on the device and uploaded to central server storage and accessed via the Internet. Mobile Care is also being designed to include procedure prompting for complex, multistep tasks that are performed infrequently and an audio-guided checklist of all steps involved in the pre-procedure, procedure, and postprocedure debrief for more experienced clinicians.

This hand-held device is designed to deal with published data from our institution proving that patient critical data extinguishes over a 24-hour period.[5] This study demonstrates that a simple paper checklist that has become the template for our electronic patient management system, significantly reduced this error of lost data. Our trauma ICU study followed a total of 332 patient ICU days; 119 of those observation days were carried out during the control period and 213 during the study period. A total of 689 patient care items were tracked for a 24-hour period, 303 during the control period and 386 during the study period. Over this time, 75 discrete patient care items were lost (10.9%), 61 of 303 (20.1%) of observation patient care items were lost during the control period, and 14 of 386 (3.6%) of total patient care items were lost during the study period ($p < 0.0001$). Our electronic patient management system incorporates all the items on a paper checklist into one device that automatically uploads critical data, alerts the clinician, and disseminates this critical data eliminating communication errors.

CONCLUSION

Management of trauma patients is fraught with sources of errors that lead to bad outcomes. To manage this complex environment trauma must be considered a consummate "team sport." Trauma teams manage the changing conditions and immediacy of presentation of injured patients by sharing a common big picture, sharing and distributing workloads, and communicating patient critical information. Successful outcomes depend on successful team function.

REFERENCES

1. Weingart, S. N., Wison, R. M., Gibberd, R. W., & Harrison, B. (2000). Epidemiology of medical error. *British Medical Journal, 320,* 774–7.
2. Ivatury, R. R., Guilford, K., Malhotra, A. K., Duane, T., Aboutanos, M., & Martin, N. (2008). Patient safety in trauma: Maximal impact management errors at a level I trauma center. *Journal of Trauma,* 64, 265–72.
3. Gruen, R. L., Jurkovich, G. J., McIntyre, L. K., Foy, H. M., & Maier, R. V. (2006). Patterns of errors contributing to trauma mortality: Lessons learned from 2594 deaths. *Annals of Surgery,* 244(3), 371–80.
4. Teixeira, P. G., Inaba, K., Hadjizacharia, P., Brown, C., Salim, A., Rhee, P., et al. (2007). Preventable or potentially preventable mortality at a mature trauma center. *Journal of Trauma, 63,* 1338–47.
5. Miniño, A. M., Anderson, R. N., Fingerhut, L. A., Boudreault, M. A., & Warner, M. (2006). Calculation based on 161,269 resident deaths in the United States as the result of injuries. *National Vital Statistics Reports, 10,* 54.
6. Kohn, L. T., Corrigan, J. M., & Donaldson, M. S. (Eds.), *To err is human: Building a safer health system.* Washington, DC: National Academy Press.
7. Stahl, K. D., & Brien, S. (2009). Reducing patient errors in trauma care. In S. Cohn (Ed.), *Acute care surgery and trauma: Evidenced-based practice.* London: Informa.
8. Retrieved October 10, 2009 from: http://www.ntsb.gov/aviation/Stats.htm
9. Shojania, K.G., Duncan, B.W., McDonald, K.M., et al. (2001). (Eds.), *Making health care safer: a critical analysis of patient safety practices.* Rockville, MD: Agency for Healthcare Research and Quality.
10. Reason, J. (2000). Human error: models and management. *British Medical Journal, 320,* 768–70.
11. Nolan, T. W. (2000). System changes to improve patient safety. *British Medical Journal,* 320, 771–3.
12. Wilson, K. A., Burke, C. S., Priest, H. A., & Salas, E. (2005). Promoting health care safety through tracking high reliability teams. *Quality and Safety in Health Care, 14,* 303–9.
13. Morrison, G., Goldfarb, S., & Lanken, P. N. (2009). Team training of medical students in the 21st century: Would Flexner approve? *Academic Medicine, 85*(2), 254–9.

14. Hackman, J. R. (2003). Learning more by crossing levels; evidence from airplanes, hospitals and orchestras. *Journal of Organizational Behavior, 24*, 905–22.

15. Salas, E., Cannon-Bowers, J., & Weaver, J. (2002). Command and control teams: Principles for training and assessment. In R. Flin, & K. Arbuthnot (Eds.), *Incident command: Tales from the hot seat*. Aldershot, UK: Ashgate.

16 Awad SS, Fagan SP, Bellows C, et al. Bridging the communication gap in the operating room with medical team training. *Am J Surg, 190*, 770–4.

17. Baker, D. P., Salas, E., & Barach, P. (2003). *Medical teamwork and patient safety: The evidence-based relation. Final Report 2003*. Washington, DC: Center for Quality Improvement and Patient Safety and AHRQ and The Department of Defense.

18. Jeffcott, S. A., & MacKenzie, C. F. (2008). Measuring team performance in healthcare: Review of research and implications for patient safety. *Journal of Critical Care, 23*, 188–96.

19. Bellomo, R., Goldsmith, S., Uchino, J., Buckmaster, J., Hart, G., Opdam, H., et al. (2004). Prospective controlled trial of effect of medical emergency team on postoperative morbidity and mortality rates. *Critical Care Medicine, 32*(4), 916–21.

20. Healey, A. N., Undre, S., & Vincent, C. A. (2006). Defining the technical skills of teamwork in surgery. *Quality and Safety in Health Care, 15*, 231–4.

21. Retrieved August 17, 2009 from: http://www. jcaho.org/accredited+organizations.htm

22. Salas, E., Cannon-Bowers, J., & Weaver, J. (2002). Command and control teams: Principles for training and assessment. In R. Flin, & K. Arbuthnot (Eds.), *Incident command: Tales from the hot seat*. Aldershot, UK: Ashgate.

23. Awad, S. S., Fagan, S. P., Bellows, C., et al. (2005). Bridging the communication gap in the operating room with medical team training. *American Journal of Surgery, 190*(5), 770–74.

24. Salas, E., Burke, S. C., Bowers, C. A., & Wilson, K. A. (2001). Team training in the skies: Does crew resource management (CRM) training work? *Human Factors, 43*, 641–74.

25. Risser, D. T., Rice, M. M., Salisbury, M. L., Simon, R., Jay, G. D., & Berns, S. D. (1999). The potential for improved teamwork to reduce medical errors in the emergency department. The MedTeams Resarch Consortium. *Annals of Emergency Medicine, 34*, 373–83.

26. Awad, S. S., Fagan, S. P., Bellows, C., et al. (2005). Bridging the communication gap in the operating room with medical team training. *American Journal of Surgery, 190*(5), 770–4.

27. Lingard, L., Epsin, S., Whyte, S., et al. (2004). Communication failures in the operating room: An observational classification of recurrent types and effects. *Quality and Safety in Health Care, 13*, 330–4.

28. Day, D. V., & Halpin, S. M. (2001). *Leadership development: A review of industry best practices*. Technical Report 111. Alexandria, VA: US Army Research Institute for the Behavioral and Social Sciences.

29. Klein, K. J. (2006). *Teamwork in a shock trauma unit: New lessons in leadership*. Knowledge@ Wharton. Retrieved from: http://knowledge. wharton.upenn.edu/article.cfm?articleid=1048

30. Yun, S., Faraj, S., & Sims, H. P. (2005). Contingent leadership and effectiveness of trauma resuscitation teams. *Journal of Applied Psychology, 90*, 1288–96.

31. Healy, G. B., Barker, J., & Madonna, G. (2006). The surgeon as a leader. *Bulletin of the American College of Surgeons 91*, 26–9.

32. Stahl, K., Palileo, A., Schulman, C., Wilson, K., Augenstein, J., Kiffin, C., et al. (2009). Enhancing patient safety in the trauma/surgical intensive care unit. *Journal of Trauma, 67*, 430–5.

12

TEAMWORK AND SAFETY IN INTENSIVE CARE

Jill A. Marsteller, David A. Thompson,
Priyadarshini R. Pennathur, and Peter J. Pronovost

This chapter is dedicated to Christine A. Holzmueller, the consummate team member—always there when you need her.

INTRODUCTION

Intensive care units (ICUs) help many patients, but they also pose intrinsic risks because the environment is complex and the patients are vulnerable. Although many improvements in quality of care and patient safety have originated in ICUs, the opportunities for failure are multiplied by several aspects of care in this setting: the range in patient complexity and urgency of care needs; the requirements for both infrequent and routine procedures; the often large interdisciplinary team; the high specialization of care providers; the copious number of procedures; the use of advanced technology; and the abrupt changes in patient acuity in the ICU. Good teamwork is essential to help develop efficient treatment plans that encourage the patients' recovery while also keeping them safe. This chapter discusses the teamwork challenges that are aggravated by the ICU setting, the appropriate members of an ICU team, and the importance of effective communication for productive teamwork. It closes with a discussion of the norms on the unit that create the backdrop for

successful performance in team-based endeavors. Throughout the chapter, practical tips for improving teamwork are offered and a range of applicable tools from the Comprehensive Unit-based Safety Program (CUSP) are discussed (Table 12.1).[1]

THE INTENSIVE CARE UNIT AS A SETTING FOR TEAMWORK

Intensive or critical care is provided to hospital patients who are acutely ill or recovering from complex invasive surgeries. Between 10% and 15% of ICU patients die, compared with 5% of patients on less-acute inpatient floors.[2] Twenty-four–hour care and surveillance are required during a patient's ICU stay, and each patient is cared for by a complex array of providers. The typical length of stay in an ICU is 3 days, which is usually part of a longer hospital stay that often includes: (1) transition into the ICU from another unit; (2) transition out of the ICU to a step-down unit with less intensive care; and (3) hospital discharge, often to another healthcare facility such as a rehabilitation center.

Practical tip #1: Recognizing the effects of the work setting on how a team operates can help team members be watchful for potential problems. The ICU setting has unique challenges for providers endeavoring to work as an effective team. First, the work is highly complex because patient illnesses or injuries are severe and complicated by comorbidities, frailty, and interrelatedness of comorbidities. Patients rarely have a single problem. This complexity leads to a high degree of modularity, or breaking processes down into discrete chunks,[3] wherein staff specialize to handle a specific range of tasks, the summation of which establishes the entire process of care. Thus, there is minimal if any overlap of a given team member's expertise on the team.

Often, professionals from multiple disciplines care for the same patient. Although specialization generally means higher quality care from each provider, there is greater potential for poor communication and ineffective team functioning when the care process is broken up among multiple providers. Each healthcare provider is an expert in his or her discipline, but very few understand the daily responsibilities, needs, and communication and teamwork issues of other disciplines. Sometimes roles and responsibilities overlap or have ambiguous boundaries. For example, in different circumstances there may be a need for different team members, regardless of the typical hierarchy of disciplines, to act as the team leader, such as when nurses might be called on to teach resident physicians to operate new equipment. Communication is the thread that binds the various disciplines into an effective multidisciplinary team. When communication is ineffective, collaboration and teamwork fail, and patients are at increased risk of medical mistakes, sentinel events, or even death.[4]

Practical tip #2: Hierarchy on the team should vary by the urgency of the situation, and team members need to expect this kind of variation. The level of urgency of tasks varies across a wider range in ICUs than in other inpatient units. In the course of caring for a patient, there will be low urgency times when patients primarily need monitoring, and high urgency times when they require immediate attention. This variation in urgency both within and among patients creates a dynamic environment that requires constant surveillance and care coordination,

generating an interesting opportunity and challenge for teamwork. The amount of hierarchy on the team can and should vary by the level of urgency.[5] In quiet times, effective teams will tap the full potential of diverse staff, using a flat hierarchical structure that encourages free speech and open contribution and values individual participation. During urgent situations when action is needed, a command and control structure is usually warranted, with the team leader providing clear and decisive instructions and team members performing their assigned roles based on the team's shared understanding, often with little time for conversation or jockeying for leadership.[6] Thus, team leaders and team members must understand, accept, and use "situational" team interactive modes to be effective in the ICU setting.

Practical tip #3: Teams should strategically plan and train to handle novel or nonroutine tasks, as well as routine tasks. The variation in the novelty of tasks performed in ICUs present challenges for effective teamwork.[7] Many routine procedures are performed daily for which there are established rules, schedules, and protocols. However, staff also encounter a number of infrequent or rarely employed treatments or procedures to manage the complex or extremely fragile patient, the range of diagnoses among patients, and the high levels of technology used to maintain critical patients in the course of recovery or decline. Novel tasks require increased supervision, greater reliance on more experienced staff, customization of protocols or standard routines, and extreme mindfulness in administering care. As a result, interruptions, poor communication, and failure to support one another assume menacing seriousness when staff perform novel tasks. Opportunities to practice responding to novel circumstances have to be built into regular training so staff are better prepared for rare events.

Thus, complexity, modularity, urgency, and novelty of tasks performed in the ICU setting likely aggravate some of the typical challenges experienced by teams, accentuating the need for an organizational culture that supports teamwork, unimpeded communication, and tools to enhance multidisciplinary interaction. Teams must consider these influences on their work and plan appropriately in advance to be prepared for variations across these phenomena.

APPROPRIATE COMPOSITION OF THE TEAM

Patients in the ICU are usually cared for by their primary care physician, their specialist, or their surgeon, except where a hospitalist or intensivist is employed by the hospital. Nurses, pharmacists, respiratory therapists, nutritionists, social workers, and a variety of other consulting physicians are also engaged in the care process. This complex team is needed to provide high-quality care to critically ill patients, and usually works well, but the number of professionals involved and the sometimes unclear role boundaries pose risks for potentially harmful communication breakdowns.

Practical tip #4: Create opportunities to clarify roles and responsibilities on the team, because unclear roles in care often lead to communication problems. The primary caregivers in the ICU are the bedside nurse and the attending physician. Nurses provide continuous monitoring, participate in care plan development, and coordinate care decisions among physicians, deliver medications, manage wound care, provide preventive care, comfort, patient hygiene, patient and family education and support, and chart and document all care processes. They generally spend the most time with the patient and their family, and typically develop the closest relationship with them. Physicians lead the care team, evaluate and diagnose, select and order medications, perform procedures (e.g., central line insertion), develop care plans, monitor and interpret patient data, consult with specialists, document their medical interventions, and share care plans and progress with the patient and family. When overlaps in duties occur (e.g., developing the care plan, monitoring the patient, documenting activities, and communicating with the patient and family) opportunities for poor communication, disagreement, and conflict arise.

Practical tip #5: Use of intensivists can improve safety and quality of care in the ICU. Substantial evidence demonstrates improved patient outcomes when a critical care specialist, called an intensivist, is part of the critical care team. Two systematic reviews evaluating ICU staffing studies found reduced mortality and ICU length of stay associated with intensivist staffing.[8,9] In two other studies, the intensivist's timely management increased patient survival[10] and saved an estimated 162,000 adult patients in nonrural

ICUs in the United States.[11] Intensivist staffing is widely endorsed by prominent organizations, such as the American College of Critical Care Medicine,[12] the National Quality Forum (http://www.qualityforum.org/Home.aspx), and The Leapfrog Group. The Leapfrog Group developed the ICU physician staffing standard that many US hospitals have adopted (http://www.leapfroggroup.org/media/file/FactSheet_LeapfrogGroup.pdf).

Practical tip #6: Appropriate nurse staffing (one or two patients per nurse) improves safety and quality of care. Nurse staffing affects economic and clinical outcomes. Our team found that when nurses care for one or two patients versus three or four, length of stay in the ICU was reduced by approximately 50%, which is explained primarily by a reduction in pulmonary complications.[13] Other studies have found similar associations between nurse staffing and patient outcomes.[14] This should be expected because higher nurse workloads imply less time to provide preventive care that keeps patients from suffering complications. For example, nurses can help prevent pneumonia and re-intubations by ensuring patients ambulate, do breathing exercises, and cough regularly. Further, nurses who have sufficient time to observe their environments carefully likely catch many potential errors before they reach the patient.

Practical tip #7: Residents often identify inadequate training and supervision as a challenge of being a member of the ICU team. Hospitals should support physician training opportunities to improve quality and safety of care. Nurses are frequently offered in-service educational opportunities for new equipment, whereas physicians are rarely offered these continuing education opportunities. When computerized physician order entry was new, for example, user error stemming from insufficient training was commonly reported to the Intensive Care Unit Safety Reporting System multisite demonstration project.[15]

There is an undersupply of coverage needed to allow physicians to attend training that would benefit their clinical practice. Because most physicians are paid per unit of work, there is a strong economic disincentive for physicians to participate in training. Hospital leaders need to ensure that a mechanism is set up with sufficient resources to train and periodically evaluate the adequacy of training, which must include cross-coverage of patient care to ensure that physicians can allow adequate time to complete the training process.

Practical tip #8: Management support for out-of-hierarchy training roles, where required, should be made explicit. Nursing personnel and senior level physicians should supervise new members of the ICU team when they are operating new equipment or performing new procedures until they are proficient. Yet, such out-of-hierarchy roles (i.e., nurses supervising physicians) are difficult and pose risks to nurses. For example, even when seeking to ensure that physicians comply with an evidence-based checklist to reduce infections (that physicians and nurses unanimously agreed to use), nurses were reluctant to speak up and physicians were reluctant to be questioned.[16]

COMMUNICATION: THE KEY TO EFFECTIVE TEAMWORK

Errors in teamwork and communication are among the most common reasons patients suffer preventable harm. In The Joint Commission's database of sentinel events from 2004 to 2010, communication breakdown is high on the list of root causes every year for all event types (http://www.jointcommission.org/sentinel_Event.aspx). We have found that clinicians use teamwork tools more often when tools are perceived as evidence-based, modifiable, and effective mechanisms to reduce communication risks. Clinicians need both a forum and a framework for considering communication risks.

Practical tip #9: Teaching all unit staff a clear model of communication and strategies to deal with communication pitfalls can get everyone on the same page. To encourage the use of tools to enhance communication, we created a framework that builds on a communication model originally conceived by Shannon and Weaver[17] and adapted by Dayton (Fig. 12.1).[18] We detail five stages of team communication and the techniques to deal with communication barriers that arise in each stage and summarize them in Figure 12.2.

Deciding on a message: The first stage of communication is deciding what message to convey. In

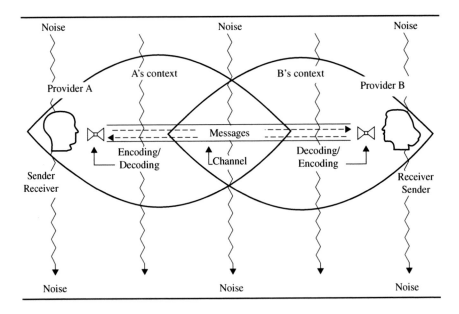

Figure 12.1
Some of the basic components and processes of communication, as derived from communication therapy and organizational studies, are shown.
Copyright Joint Commission Resources. Dayton, E., & Henriksen, K. (2007). Communication failure: Basic components, contributing factors, and the call for structure. *Joint Commission Journal on Quality and Patient Safety,* *33*(1), 34–47. Reprinted with permission.

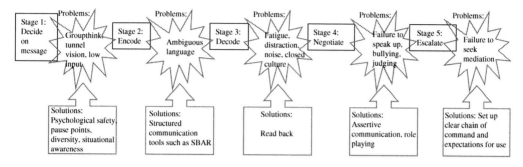

Figure 12.2
Stages of Communication, Common Problems and Solutions

---

team care, the leader should incorporate every member's input when making decisions about a patient's medical care because each will have different information based on their unique frame of reference that will help the leader make a wiser decision. Many problems can limit the effectiveness of team decisions and increase the risk of an error. Common problems include unclear information, failing to obtain broad and independent input, prohibiting members from contributing input, and following a path when available data refute the decision.[19] Another problem is groupthink, wherein teams limit the range of alternatives, or fail to question assumptions or engage in team dialogue.[20] Teams can improve their effectiveness through better situational awareness, wherein team members understand the system and their vulnerabilities in selecting actions, making a diverse team feel psychologically safe[21] enough to offer input, and building in "pause points" to allow divergent thinking (idea generation) and convergent thinking (selection of one course of action).

Encoding the message: In the second stage, the sender communicates the information, imparting deliberate and, often, unknown meaning to the message. Common problems can be nonverbal (e.g., emotional baggage; written symbols) and verbal (e.g., ambiguous language) content that leaves the receiver unclear about or misconstruing the intended message. Ambiguity is a major reason clinicians fail to comply with guidelines.[22] Communication tools can help clarify the message. For example, SBAR[23] (situation, background, assessment and recommendation) structures reporting between providers, and

operating room briefings establish situational awareness.[24] Paper tools such as lists or forms can also help deliver clear messages. Message senders should use unambiguous language, avoid indirect communication (e.g., hinting, winking), and ask the receiver to repeat their interpretation of the message to ensure the intended message has been relayed.

Decoding the message: In the third stage, the receiver translates (or decodes) the meaning of the message. In the ICU, the receiver is often distracted by competing tasks, noise, and fatigue, or intimidated by a culture that discourages questioning, all of which increase the risk for a decoding error. For instance, the physician may ask a resident to pull a chest tube, but perhaps the patient has two tubes and the resident translates this message to mean the right-sided one, without confirming this interpretation with the attending. Again, asking the receiver to repeat back the message aloud will allow the sender to confirm whether the message was decoded correctly. The daily goals checklist, for instance, uses repeat back and has improved communication among physicians and nursing during interdisciplinary rounds.[25]

Negotiation: If the receiver disagrees with the sender, together they must resolve any conflict and agree on an action plan (stage 4). Unfortunately, conflict resolution is often done poorly in healthcare. Unresolved conflicts among healthcare professionals can cause poor teamwork and morale,[26] stress, illness, missed work, and job turnover,[27] and may lead to preventable patient harm.[28] Moreover, conflict can lead to intimidation, not speaking up, judging others' intentions, and losing sight of what is best for the patient. Tools to rectify these problems include assertive communication techniques such as the two-attempt rule (trying twice to make oneself heard), and simulating conflict to prepare for difficult situations.

Escalation (going up the chain of command): If the conflict cannot be resolved, the persons involved should turn to a mediator to resolve the conflict (stage 5). In mediation, a neutral individual outside the team, usually with higher authority, helps resolve the issue. Common problems in this phase are an unclear chain of command, not engaging the chain of command in appropriate circumstances, and attacking the other person for seeking mediation. Importantly, this phase is not about attacking the other party or winning, it is about doing what is best for the patient.

Although we have outlined a model of various stages of communication, common errors and strategies to defend against those errors, communication is much more complicated than one can easily depict. Personal cognitive biases, team dynamics, and organizational culture influence every step of the communication process, affecting the way care is provided. In addition, information, especially in the ICU, is dynamic, influencing patient risk and the risks and benefits of decisions. It is essential to maintain situational awareness throughout the care process to keep track of ever-changing information. This can be accomplished by following standardized communication and teamwork practices during the care process. The next section presents several tools for standardization developed in the ICU.

COMPREHENSIVE UNIT-BASED SAFETY PROGRAM: TOOLS TO ENHANCE INTENSIVE CARE UNIT TEAMWORK

The CUSP program provides structured tools that enhance team interaction, improve communication, and help ICU staff learn from mistakes over time.[29]

This program was created with the knowledge that the local nursing unit is the microsystem in which work occurs[30] and safety climate is local.[31] Front-line staff are cognizant of the hazards in their workplace and, thus, should be empowered and provided resources to reduce these risks.

Practical tip #10: To reduce error, staff must be taught to look for the role of the system in producing error rather than seeking someone to blame. To begin CUSP, we educate participating ICU improvement teams (referred to as CUSP teams) on the science of safety and give them materials to educate other staff on the unit, including slides and access to a Web-based lecture (http://www.safercare.net/OTCSBSI/Staff_Training/Staff_Training.html). The training seeks to ensure that staff understand that safety is a property of a system and use the principles of safe design (standardize work, create independent checks with checklists, learn when things go wrong) to improve the system; recognize that they do both technical work and team work; and understand that teams make wiser decisions with diverse and independent input.

Practical tip #11: Front-line staff recognizes sources of error in their own environment and are often the best people to develop solutions to the problems. Another part of CUSP has ICU staff members identify actual and potential hazards in their unit. Sources that can be used to identify hazards include local error reporting systems, liability claims, sentinel events, and events discussed at morbidity and mortality conferences. Comprehensive Unit-based Safety Program teams also ask all ICU staff involved in patient care to suggest how the next patient might be harmed and what could be done to prevent that harm. A critical aspect of this exercise is the prospective identification of hazards before the patient is harmed.

After identifying hazards that should be addressed to prevent patient harm, CUSP teams learn from one defect (an actual or potential safety problem) per month[32] using a structured form that asks what happened, why it happened, what was done to reduce risk, and how the team knows the risk was reduced (e.g., staff report safety is improved, improved culture assessments). The use of this tool is described further in the section on learning from a defect (p. 161).

Practical tip #12: Meaningful partnership with a member of the hospital administration can help ICU staff resolve patient safety issues. Another feature of CUSP is that each team partners with a senior executive within their hospital. The senior leader's role is to round monthly with staff, review safety hazards, ensure the team has resources and political support to implement interventions that reduce safety risks, and hold the team accountable for mitigating hazards.[33] The more frequent the visits by an executive and the more risks they address, the greater the improvements in perceived safety climate.[34]

Practical tip #13: Teams can use or develop forms and tools to standardize specific processes, which improves communication and patient safety, and may shorten patient length of stay. Continuing with the CUSP example, teams should self-select teamwork tools that best address their communication needs given their local context and perceptions of safety climate.

Shadowing Another Provider was developed as a structured, user-friendly tool to help frontline ICU providers observe and understand the roles, responsibilities, and challenges of other clinical disciplines. To do this, the person shadowing must try to see things from the perspective of the person they are shadowing.[35]

To get started, the shadower (e.g., nurse) chooses a discipline he or she works with directly (e.g., physician attending) or indirectly (e.g., pharmacy technician). Next, the shadower explains the shadowing exercise to the individual he or she wants to shadow and arranges a block of at least 4 hours to follow them. During the exercise, the observer should use a structured set of questions to guide him or her in observing teamwork and communication issues among practice disciplines (e.g., physician, nurse, and pharmacist) that are important in the delivery of patient care. At the end of the session, the two individuals review the shadowing observation guide to address the issues raised and develop a plan to improve team effectiveness and communication. This is extremely important because physicians, nurses, and other healthcare professionals have divergent perceptions of teamwork and collaboration with other provider types.[36]

The issues exposed by using this tool include communication problems, such as not relaying information to a new provider during hand-offs, miscommunication during verbal orders, and incomplete written orders. Shadowers also identified personnel who were verbally abusive and failures to follow policies and procedures. Shadowing has been used effectively to orient individuals to a new unit as well.

A morning briefing is a way to improve situational awareness among all ICU team members and get staff on the same page with respect to what events (e.g., new admissions, transfers out) are planned on the unit for the day.[37] Two critical components of briefings are: (1) task-related interaction, and 2) relationship-related interaction. The task-related component requires the staff physician to review the technical details of expected unit-level flow and lead contingency planning. The relationship-related component is how the interaction unfolds and the tone of the communication. The discussion leader must open communication channels and allow team members to speak up, encouraging them to participate in the process. In general, briefings allow the exchange of information that can reveal threats to patient safety and help leaders build teamwork.

Observing patient rounds allows a member of the ICU team to scrutinize the rounding process. They can assess communication and interactions among providers, adequacy of case discussions and the development of patient care plans, existing mechanisms for transcription of orders, and the education of team members in an interdisciplinary environment. The observer later discusses his or her thoughts with the CUSP team and other unit staff regarding effective and ineffective components of rounds. This audit of interdisciplinary rounds should be conducted periodically. The same observer will often assess different teams of providers performing interdisciplinary rounds and note marked differences in interactions, and ultimately the impact of these interpersonal connections in achieving agreed-on patient care goals.

Learning from a defect (LFD) is a repeated exercise that investigates a selected defect (any undesirable event or circumstance) using a set of questions and a framework of potential system-based errors, from communication and team functioning to environmental properties.[32] The LFD process and tool teaches clinicians to identify the underlying systems-based problems and develop sound intervention plans. Clinicians are good at recovering from mistakes (e.g., find the missing supply), yet they rarely learn from mistakes (e.g., review inventory supply cabinet routinely to ensure it is stocked). The LFD tool is a practical method to help clinicians reduce risks that may harm future patients. Communication and team functioning are explicitly considered in all events investigated.

Intensive care units can improve communication, teamwork, and safety by using tools to standardize communication. Concentrating on these areas will help units develop norms and group traits that promote safety and collaboration and sustain healthy teamwork indefinitely.

ENCOURAGING NORMS FOR HEALTHY TEAMWORK

Practical tip #14: Sustaining good teamwork over time relies on developing widespread and enduring expectations or norms of team effectiveness among ICU staff. There are several traits that make teams effective in performing quality improvement, including team confidence in their own skills, autonomy, valuing individual contributions, goal agreement, cohesion, and felt support from the organization.[38] The usefulness of team effectiveness measures has been established in the literature.[39] Teams that self-assessed as more effective made more changes to improve quality of care that were expected to have stronger effects on patient outcomes.[38]

Team skill, reflecting the team's self-confidence in their abilities to make changes and successfully accomplish tasks, is an essential norm in the ICU because of the unusual range in urgency and novelty of tasks. For example, high levels of urgency force the team to fall into known and expected roles, in which each fulfills their role with minimal questions about the best approach to the situation. A team's strong assessment of its collective skills will smooth the path to coordinated action in which each team member knows his or her role and trusts others to do their part (situational awareness among all parties). In addition, in cases of novel procedures, a confident team will approach the task knowing that at least one member knows what to do and will take charge.

Autonomy empowers team members to self-govern their work and their decisions to change processes that improve safety. Autonomy is an essential part of daily clinical care, because leadership roles must be shared to manage complex patient needs that require modularity of care tasks and specialization. Moreover, there are times when the clinician taking charge is not a role-defined leader, but must lead and direct other staff. For instance, nurse staff may have recently been trained to use a new defibrillator when a patient codes. The ICU team responds and the nurse must lead, instead of the physician, when operating the defibrillator. Thus, autonomy is crucial to promote effective teamwork to do what is best for the patient.

Another norm that promotes high-quality patient care and good teamwork is valuing the contributions of each team member. This norm encourages individuals to share what they know to ensure that the team makes the wisest possible decision. This is especially important when modularity and complexity of care are high. When urgency is high, unique information has to be shared concisely, and at appropriate times, but is no less valuable.

To be effective, teams must also have a sense of unity (i.e., cohesion) and agree on goals. These unifying forces help teams move from idea generation to setting a plan, agree on common goals more quickly, and effectively manage emergency situations. In addition, as team leaders shift between the command and control mode (e.g., high urgency, extreme novelty) and group facilitator mode (e.g., low urgency, high complexity, high modularity/specialization), a sense of strong team unity will help members overcome feelings of alienation and appropriately adapt their behavior to respond to the demonstrated leadership mode.

Practical tip #15: Promote clinical leaders that foster good teamwork, not just those with high technical performance. Effective teams require organizational support in the way of resources and rewards that encourage their work. Executive leaders within the organization must share a norm for the importance of this support. Most norms are established by local unit leadership, however, which presents a difficulty when promoting norms for good teamwork. Expectations are primarily set and modeled by clinical opinion leaders and other managers within an organizational unit, in this case the ICU. Thus, local leaders must buy in to the need for these norms and actively promote them. In the past, individuals have been promoted to clinical leadership positions because of their technical expertise, regardless of their ability to promote or lead a healthy work environment. The healthcare field must start promoting leaders with good teamwork skills who also foster the team traits and norms described in this section. Many good team players are at the top of their fields technically, but the practice of selecting leaders without regard for their ability to manage, encourage, empower, and learn from others must become a thing

Table 12.1	Summary of Practical Tips
Section	**Tips**
The Intensive Care Unit as a Setting for Teamwork	1: Recognizing the effects of the work setting on how an ICU team operates can help team members be on the lookout for potential problems.
	2: Hierarchy on the team should vary by the urgency of the situation, and team members need to expect this kind of variation.
	3: Teams should strategically plan and train to handle novel or nonroutine tasks, as well as routine tasks.
Appropriate Composition of the Team	4: Create opportunities to clarify roles and responsibilities on the team, as unclear roles in care often lead to communication problems.
	5: Use of intensivists can improve safety and quality of care in the ICU.
	6: Appropriate nurse staffing (one or two patients per nurse) improves safety and quality of care.
	7: Residents often identify inadequate training and supervision as a challenge of being a member of the ICU team. Hospitals should support physician training opportunities to improve quality and safety of care.
	8: Management support for out-of-hierarchy training roles, where required, should be made explicit.
Communication: The Key to Effective Teamwork	9: Teaching all unit staff a clear model of communication and strategies to deal with communication pitfalls can get everyone on the same page.
Comprehensive Unit-Based Safety Program (CUSP): Tools that Enhance ICU Teamwork	10: To reduce error, staff must be taught to look for the role of the system in producing error rather than seeking someone to blame.
	11: Frontline staff recognize sources of error in their own environment and are often the best people to develop solutions to the problems.
	12: Meaningful partnership with a member of the hospital administration can help ICU staff resolve patient safety issues.
	13: Teams can use or develop forms and tools to standardize specific processes, which improves communication and patient safety, and may shorten patient length of stay.
Encouraging Norms for Healthy Teamwork	14: Sustaining good teamwork over time relies on developing widespread and enduring expectations or norms for team effectiveness among ICU staff.
	15: Promote clinical leaders that foster good teamwork, not just those with high technical performance.

of the past if we are to keep patients safe and promote healthy work environments for nurses, physicians, and their colleagues in other disciplines.

CONCLUSION

Intensive care units provide life-saving therapies. To do this, diverse team members collaborate to deliver complex therapies to critically ill patients. Too often, teamwork breaks down and patients suffer harm. This chapter presented a model for communicating in the ICU, discussed common errors in teamwork, and provided tools, advice, and practical tips to defend against errors and prevent harm (Table 12.1). If healthcare organizations focused on broadly improving teamwork and learning from mistakes, healthcare would be substantially safer, less costly, and more inspiring for those working to care for patients.

REFERENCES

1. Timmel, J., Kent, P. S., Holzmueller, C. G., Paine, L. A., Schulick, R. D., & Pronovost, P. J. (2010). Impact of the comprehensive unit-based safety program (CUSP) on safety culture in a surgical inpatient unit. *Joint Commission Journal on Quality and Patient Safety, 36*(6), 252–60.

2. Halpern, N. A., & Pastores, S. M. (2010). Critical care medicine in the United States 2000–2005: An analysis of bed numbers, occupancy rates, payer mix, and costs. *Critical Care Medicine, 38*(1), 65–71.

3. Ethiraj, S. K., & Levinthal, D. (2004). Modularity and innovation in complex systems. *Management Science, 50*(2), 159–73.

4. Greenberg, C. C., Regenbogen, S. E., Studdert, D. M., et al. (2007). Patterns of communication breakdowns resulting in injury to surgical patients. *Journal of the American College of Surgeons, 204*(4):533–40.

5. Pearce, C. L., & Sims, H. P. (2000). Shared leadership: Toward a multi-level theory of leadership. In: Beyerlein M, ed. *Advances in interdisciplinary studies of work teams.* Vol. 7. (pp. 115–39). Bingley, UK: Emerald Group Publishing.

6. Houghton, J. D., & Yoho, S. K. (2005). Toward a contingency model of leadership and psychological empowerment: When should self-leadership be encouraged? *Journal of Leadership & Organizational Studies, 11,* 65.

7. Hoeghl, M., Parboteeah, P. (2006). Autonomy and teamwork in innovative projects. *Human Resource Management, 45*(1), 67–79.

8. Pronovost, P. J., Angus, D. C., Dorman, T., Robinson, K. A., Dremsizov, T. T., & Young, T. L. (2002). Physician staffing patterns and clinical outcomes in critically ill patients: A systematic review. *Journal of the American Medical Association, 288*(17), 2151–62.

9. Young, M. P., & Birkmeyer, J. D. (2000). Potential reduction in mortality rates using an intensivist model to manage intensive care units. *Effective Clinical Practice, 3,* 284–9.

10. Durbin, C. G. Jr. (2006). Team model: Advocating for the optimal method of care delivery in the intensive care unit. *Critical Care Medicine, 34*(3 Suppl), S12–7.

11. Rollins, G. (2002). ICU care management by intensivists reduces mortality and length of stay. *Report on Medical Guidelines & Outcomes Research, 13*(24), 5–7.

12. Haupt, M. T., Bekes, C. E., Brilli, R. J., et al. (2003). Guidelines on critical care services and personnel: Recommendations based on a system of categorization of three levels of care. *Critical Care Medicine, 31*(11), 2677–83.

13. Pronovost, P. J., Dang, D., Dorman, T., et al. (2001). Intensive care unit nurse staffing and the risk for complications after abdominal aortic surgery. *Effective Clinical Practice, 4*(5), 199–206.

14. Kane, R. L., Shamliyan, T., Mueller, C., Duval, S., Wilt, T., & the Minnesota Evidence-based Practice Center. (2007). *Nurse staffing and quality of patient care.* Rockville, MD: Agency for Healthcare Research and Quality.

15. Pronovost, P. J., Thompson, D. A., Holzmueller, C. G., et al. (2006). Toward learning from patient safety reporting systems. *Journal of Critical Care, 21*(4), 305–15.

16. Pronovost, P. J. (2010). Learning accountability for patient outcomes. *Journal of the American Medical Association, 302*(2), 204–5.

17. Shannon, C. E., & Weaver W. (1969). *The mathematical theory of communication.* Urbana-Champaign, IL: University of Illinois Press.

18. Dayton, E., & Henriksen, K. (2007). Communication failure: Basic components, contributing factors, and the call for structure. *Joint Commission Journal on Quality and Patient Safety, 33*(1), 34–47.

19. Newman-Toker, D. E., & Pronovost, P. J. (2009). Diagnostic errors—the next frontier for patient safety. *Journal of the American Medical Association, 301*(10), 1060–2.

20. Kane, R. A. (2002). Avoiding the dark side of geriatric teamwork. In: M. D. Mezey, C. K. Cassel, M. M. Bottrell, K. Hyer, J. L. Howe, & T. T. Fulmer (Eds.), *Ethical patient care: A casebook for geriatric health care teams.* 1st ed. (pp. 187–207). Baltimore: The Johns Hopkins University Press.

21. Edmondson, A. C. (2003). Managing the risk of learning: Psychological safety in work teams. In: M. West, D. Tjosvold, & K. Smith (Eds.), *International handbook of organizational teamwork and cooperative working.* Hoboken, NJ: Wiley.

22. Gurses, A. P., Seidl, K. L., Vaidya, V., et al. (2008). Systems ambiguity and guideline

compliance: A qualitative study of how intensive care units follow evidence-based guidelines to reduce healthcare-associated infections. *Quality and Safety in Health Care, 17*(5), 351–9.

23. Haig, K. M., Sutton, S., & Whittington, J. (2006). SBAR: A shared mental model for improving communication between clinicians. *Joint Commission Journal on Quality and Patient Safety, 32*(3), 167–75.

24. Makary, M. A., Holzmueller, C. G., Thompson, D. A., et al. (2006). Operating room briefings: Working on the same page. *Joint Commission Journal on Quality and Safety, 32*(6), 351–5.

25. Pronovost, P., Berenholtz, S., Dorman, T., Lipsett, P. A., Simmonds, T., & Haraden, C. (2003). Improving communication in the ICU using daily goals. *Journal of Critical Care, 18*(2), 71–5.

26. Makary, M. A., Sexton, J. B., Freischlag, J. A., Holzmueller, C. G., Millman, E. A., & Pronovost, P. J. (2006). Teamwork in the operating room: Teamwork in the eye of the beholder. *American College of Surgeons, 202*(5), 746–52.

27. Saxton, R., Hines, T., & Enriquez, M. (2009). The negative impact of nurse-physician disruptive behavior on patient safety: A review of the literature. *Journal of Patient Safety, 5*(3), 180–3.

28. Rosenstein, A. H., & O'Daniel, M. (2008). A survey of the impact of disruptive behaviors and communication defects on patient safety. *Joint Commission Journal on Quality and Patient Safety, 34*(8), 464–71.

29. Sexton, J. B., Berenholtz, S. M., Goeschel, C. A., et al. (2011). Assessing and improving safety climate in a large cohort of intensive care units. *Critical Care Medicine, 39*(5), 934–9.

30. Sexton, J. B., Thomas, E., & Pronovost, P. J. (2005). The context of care and the patient care team: The safety attitudes questionnaire. In P.P. Reid, W. D. Compton, J. H. Grossman, G. Fanjiant (Eds.), *Building a better delivery system. a new engineering health care partnership.* (pp. 119–23). Washington, DC: National Academies Press.

31. Huang, D. T., Clermont, G., Sexton, J. B., et al. (2007). Perceptions of safety culture vary across the intensive care units of a single institution. *Critical Care Medicine, 35*(1), 165–76.

32. Pronovost, P. J., Holzmueller, C. G., Martinez, E., et al. (2006). A practical tool to learn from defects in patient care. *Joint Commission Journal on Quality and Patient Safety, 32*(2), 102–8.

33. Pronovost, P. J., Weast, B., Bishop, K., et al. (2004). Senior executive adopt-a-work unit: A model for safety improvement. *Joint Commission Journal on Quality and Safety, 30*(2), 59–68.

34. Frankel, A., Grillo, S. P., Pittman, M., et al. (2008). Revealing and resolving patient safety defects: The impact of leadership walkarounds on frontline caregivers assessments of patient safety. *Health Services Research, 43*(6), 2050–66.

35. Thompson, D. A., Holzmueller, C. G., Lubomski, L., Pronovost, P. J. (2008). View the world through a different lens: Shadowing another provider. *Joint Commission Journal on Quality and Patient Safety, 34*(10), 614–8.

36. Makary, M. A., Sexton, J. B., Freischlag, J. A., et al. (2006). Operating room teamwork among physicians and nurses: Teamwork in the eye of the beholder. *Journal of the American College of Surgeons, 202*(5), 746–52.

37. Thompson, D. A., Holzmueller, C. G., Cafeo, C. L., Sexton, J. B., & Pronovost, P. J. A morning briefing: Setting the stage for a clinically and operationally good day. *Joint Commission Journal on Quality and Safety, 31*(8), 476–9.

38. Shortell, S. M., Marsteller, J. A., Lin, M., et al. (2004). The role of perceived team effectiveness in improving chronic illness care. *Medical Care, 42*(11), 1040–48.

39. Strasser, D. C., Smits, S. J., Falconer, J. A., Herrin, J. S., & Bowen, S. E. (2002). The influence of hospital culture on rehabilitation team functioning in VA hospitals. *Journal of Rehabilitation Research and Development, 39*(1), 115–25.

13

RAPID RESPONSE TEAMS

Celeste M. Mayer, Tina M. Schade Willis, Renae E. Stafford, and Sara E. Massie

In the hours preceding a cardiac arrest, warning signs of physical or psychological deterioration are present.[1-4] Intervention at the earliest sign of deterioration can save lives.[5,6] A hospital-based rapid response team[7] (RRT)* provides a safety net for patients who show signs of deterioration and require immediate medical attention when the level of care needed is not readily available. An RRT is considered a contingency team—a time-limited team that may be composed of members from various teams that is formed for emergent or specific events.[8] The members of an RRT have unique roles and abilities and must work together, in conjunction with the primary team, to ensure that patients receive coordinated care. In larger systems, these contingency teams may have never worked together and must come together and function as a cohesive team in an emergency.

Given that the RRT may be composed of healthcare providers who do not know each other and must collaborate with others who may have limited teamwork skills, how is it possible for such a team to exemplify teamwork? In this chapter, we provide insights on implementing an RRT with optimized teamwork skills. In addition, we describe strategies for addressing barriers to teamwork, based on our experience at University of North Carolina (UNC) Hospitals. We start by reviewing a case study that illustrates the consequences of poor teamwork in an RRT activation.

---

*RRTs are part of a larger rapid response system. This system includes four arms: an efferent arm, i.e., the RRT, for medical response and intervention, an afferent arm for case detection and response triggering, and evaluative or process improvement arm, and a governance or administrate arm to provide structure and oversight.[7]

Case Study 1: Poor Teamwork in a Pediatric RRT Event

On the pediatric surgical ward, a 2-year-old Hispanic boy with a history of a complicated liver transplant and prolonged hospitalization experiences sudden onset of fever to 105°F, respiratory rate of 60 breaths/minute, heart rate of 180 beats/minute, and blood pressure 70/30 mmHg. The patient's mother, who does not speak English, is at the bedside with the new surgical resident. The resident orders blood cultures, a fluid bolus, and antibiotics. As the initial fluid bolus is infusing and antibiotics are primed for infusion, the patient's heart rate increases to 220; he appears flushed, agitated, and has some faint wheezing. His mother appears more concerned and begins to cry. The bedside nurse asks the resident whether they should activate the pediatric RRT for assistance. He responds that he wants her to wait for the fluid bolus to finish and then call his senior resident before calling the RRT. As the fluid bolus is completed, the patient becomes lethargic and develops worsening pulmonary status, with continued tachycardia at a heart rate of 210 beats/minute.

The ward charge nurse arrives to assist the patient's nurse with orders and immediately becomes concerned about the patient's appearance and vital signs. She states that the pediatric RRT should be called, and the surgical resident repeats that he needs to discuss it with his senior resident first. The charge nurse replies that she is going to call anyway and activates the RRT. The resident becomes angry and leaves to page his team. The pediatric RRT arrives and recognizes the patient and his mother from his lengthy stay in the pediatric intensive care unit. The RRT assesses the patient and begins treatment without getting the details of the situation. The team obtains additional intravenous access, begins rapid fluid administration, and places the child on oxygen. The ward charge nurse begins to complain to the RRT nurse about the surgical resident and his inability to respond to their concerns, stating that they "had been calling all morning" and the only response from the surgical team was to send a first year resident to see the patient. As the surgical resident returns to the room, he overhears her stating that they were "lucky the kid didn't code."

The rest of the primary surgical team physicians arrive and criticize the junior surgical resident for not calling them sooner. The noise in the room escalates and multiple individual conversations occur while the patient's work of breathing continues to worsen and his blood pressure starts to fall. At this time, he also develops worsening hives and decreased peripheral pulses. The RRT physician thinks the child may be having a reaction to something and asks if the patient had been receiving a medication when the event started. The patient is given antihistamines, albuterol, and an additional fluid bolus and shows some improvement in his vital signs and work of breathing.

Meanwhile, the surgical team reviews his medication list with the bedside nurse, and they discover that the patient did not receive his ordered premedication regimen for a medication administered before his deterioration. Several punitive comments are made to the nurse causing her to start crying while the child's mother looks on. The RRT physician suggests that the patient be moved to the intensive care unit (ICU) for further treatment and monitoring, and the surgical team agrees. The RRT physician asks the ward charge nurse to call for an interpreter to tell the mother about her son's status and to where they are moving him. The RRT transports the patient to the ICU before an interpreter arrives to communicate with the mother.

The situation leaves the junior surgical resident and patient's nurse feeling helpless and crestfallen. The RRT physician returns to the ICU and complains about the surgical ward stating to her colleagues, "they can't take care of anyone up there." The patient's mother remains at the bedside for the next 48 hours without sleep, despite his improvement, and expresses concern with return to the surgical ward area. She is given reassurances from the transferring team, but this does nothing to ease her concern.

Although the individual clinicians in this case study were highly skilled and dedicated, a lack of teamwork prevented them from providing the best care. The RRT encountered many challenges and barriers. First, the RRT, the primary team, and the patient's family at the bedside did not communicate effectively about the patient's status early in the RRT's assessment. This resulted in delayed diagnosis of an adverse medication reaction that contributed to delayed treatment. Second, the patient's nurse did not feel empowered to call the RRT when the physician told her not to do so. Rather than coming together to assess and treat the patient, the nurses and physicians demonstrated an "us-versus-them" attitude, creating barriers to effective communication. Third, a "silo culture" between the ICU and surgical ward teams was apparent throughout the response, instead of both services coming together for the patient in one team structure. Fourth, none of the team members provided information or support for the patient's mother, and the mother observed the tension between individuals and lost confidence in their future ability to care for her child. Finally, an error occurred with the missed premedication order, but this was not addressed in a constructive manner to prevent recurrence. Instead, the patient's nurse was solely blamed for the error, and possible system issues were not discussed.

The RRT's experiences in this case study are, unfortunately, not unusual in healthcare. Our experience at UNC Hospitals changed for the better when our RRT began routinely practicing good teamwork skills. The following insights represent our new understanding of the importance of teamwork and how to achieve short- and long-term success.

Insight 1. *Good teamwork and encouraging patients and/or family members present to be part of the medical team is vital during the first five minutes of an RRT event.*

Good teamwork during the first 5 minutes of an RRT event is critical to an RRT's performance. It is during the first 5 minutes that the RRT members can set the tone for quiet, controlled, and orderly communication using standardized language and tools. The RRT leader can establish the leadership role and, in this role, encourage active participation from the primary team members. In addition, during this time, the patient and family members should share any information they think would be useful to the RRT. This is important because they can provide information that others in the room do not have. Family members can often recognize changes in their loved ones before any of the medical team members do. This is especially true for very young patients and those with chronic medical conditions or developmental delay.

Insight 2. *Excluding the primary team or giving negative feedback to callers, the primary team, or even patients leads to alienation and poor communication and teamwork in the future.*

Experiences of poor teamwork between bedside nurses and medical teams may lead to stressful day-to-day interactions because of the unresolved conflict. In addition, it is likely that individuals involved in or witnessing a poor teamwork event (or those they tell the story to later during break) will recall the unpleasant experience and be hesitant to call the RRT in the future for fear of a similar experience. We have found that repeated positive experiences, shared stories, and education have led to increased use of the RRT, with calls coming from a variety of professionals (nurses, physicians, and respiratory therapists).

Following RRT activations, we distribute satisfaction surveys to evaluate the primary team members' experience during the event. Questions assess level of comfort with calling the RRT and satisfaction with the overall experience. The survey also includes space for open-ended comments. These comments help us to monitor the perception and experience of teamwork.

Insight 3. *Good teamwork affects the patient/family experience.*

Chaotic, unorganized responses are noisy and frightening for patients and family members. Although they may not recognize outstanding clinical skills, they can recognize good teamwork as controlled, organized, and calm. Most patients and their families perceive all they experience as "the organization" and do not see the organizational divisions that can be barriers to good communication and teamwork. In the first case study, the child's distraught mother did not recognize one group as intensive care providers and another as the surgery team. The language barrier increased her confusion. At our institution, families interviewed after RRT activations do not detect separate services working together. Instead, they see the medical care in the institution as one system without the "silo culture" that staff members see.

Insight 4. *Holding a debriefing after RRT events provides time for immediate performance improvement and promotes long-term culture change.*

One of the most important things any team can do to strengthen its performance is to conduct team debriefings following an event. A debriefing should be done routinely after all RRT events. In a debriefing, the RRT leader spends 5 minutes with the team members who reflect on and share observations of what went well, what did not go well, and what could be done differently next time. The leader sets the tone that the debriefing is not to point out individual failings, but to reinforce the team's positive performance and identify ways to improve teamwork and system-related issues in the future.

Debriefings have led to many improvements at our institution. For example, in the case of a patient who had a plugged tracheostomy tube, a debriefing revealed that one clinical area rarely dealt with patients who had a tracheostomy tube, and the nurses in this area did not feel comfortable with the tubes and troubleshooting. This was identified as a systems issue, and a multidisciplinary team was formed and created an algorithm for patients with tracheostomy tubes, which our institution now uses as a training tool for residents, respiratory therapists, and nurses.

If the individuals participating in a debriefing have some exposure to teamwork skills, knowledge of when and how to use the skills and a positive attitude about the value of teamwork, then the debriefing can be used as the one teamwork tool that facilitates day-to-day feedback and reinforcement. During a debriefing, however, teams may encounter unanticipated behavior. For example, a participant in a debriefing may feel personally responsible for not identifying signs of patient deterioration before the RRT event and, as a result, may be emotional. Other participants may exhibit anger and hostility or refuse to participate in the debriefing. Box 13.1 provides suggestions for handling such behavior.

Box 13.1   How to Handle a Difficult Debriefing

Assisting an Emotional Team Member

Participants in a debriefing can be emotional. In some cases, an individual will be fearful of a potentially punitive experience. The debriefing leader should reassure participants that debriefings are standard practice after all RRT activations. At the end of the RRT event, the following script can be used to set the tone and expectations. "OK, thanks for activating the team. Now that we have completed the RRT call, we always complete a debriefing to identify what went well, any issues or questions to address, and changes that are recommended based on the call. If you are able to wait here for the 5-minute debriefing, I will make sure we get through the debriefing efficiently."

Managing Anger and Hostility

It is not unusual for the primary nurse and physician to disagree regarding notification of the RRT and a nurse will often say to the responding RRT, "I have been calling them about this all day, and they didn't want to call you." In these cases, it is sometimes useful to do a group debriefing

(Continued)

Box 13.1   (Continued)

after separate debriefings for RRT physician with primary physician and RRT nurse with primary nurse. After reassurances in separate debriefings, a more constructive group debriefing can occur, focusing on communication tools and earlier activation of the team. It is not always feasible to have an efficient and effective group debriefing if anger or hostility is not diffused easily. If not diffused easily, a follow up review should be completed. Disruptive or inappropriate behavior should not be tolerated. Structured debriefings can be a tool to identify repeat behaviors that should be addressed at an administrative level.

Addressing Accusations
At times, punitive comments are made in a debriefing that do not allow collective learning and identification of safety issues. In a debriefing, a member of the primary team may be accused of harming the patient, which prevents collective review of the system including human, computer, and communication errors. The leader of the debriefing should handle this with redirection such as, "Errors like this can happen through any number of scenarios, and we are not providing the best care for this patient and others if we are not able to openly discuss medication errors in a non-punitive manner." If the accusations continue, the debriefing should be completed without further discussion of the error, and a separate review should occur with assistance from the unit's leaders. Further exposure of the staff to punitive statements in a debriefing can lead to future avoidance in activating the Rapid Response System, significant employee dissatisfaction, and failure to promote a culture of safety.

Dealing with Team Members Who Fail to Participate
A debriefing may sound time consuming and unfamiliar to some team members who decide to "opt out" when approached for the debriefing. At our hospital, we have found it most useful to use an introductory statement, such as, "It is our policy that we conduct a debriefing to make sure we identify any systems issues that can be improved in the future. It should only take five minutes of your time, and we can do it now." In fact, the debriefing has been written into hospital policy for our Rapid Response System, which provides a structure for the statement and lends to a culture where communication and systems thinking are a part of daily operations. If individuals continue to refuse to participate in an event debriefing, conduct the debriefing without them.

Insight 5. *When a high-functioning RRT interacts with a primary team with poor teamwork skills, leadership, mutual support, situation monitoring, and communication can improve the experience for all and the outcome for the patient.*

The teamwork skills of leadership, mutual support, situation monitoring, and standardized communication make it possible for individuals unfamiliar with each other to work as an efficient team during routine and emergent situations. These skills that are valuable in all types of teams and in all types of events are considered *transportable teamwork skills.*[9] Leadership skills include clear role identification, delegation, and role modeling of teamwork. Communication skills include open sharing of information with all present. Paying attention to this open sharing while monitoring the patient's condition and other team members' performance is called *situation monitoring*. Situation monitoring contributes to a shared mental model, and situation monitoring skills are honed in teamwork trained RRT members. Mutual support skills involve providing assistance when any team member is observed to need or requests help. This can balance the workload and potentially decrease the risk of adverse events.

An RRT exemplifying teamwork skills and strategies can effectively and efficiently assess and intervene in a given patient care situation. We have found that an optimally functioning RRT can effectively provide patient care and primary team support even when the primary team does not have the same teamwork skills training or is not exhibiting the expected teamwork skills. One RRT activation at our institution required the pediatric RRT to respond to a chronically ill 17-year-old patient in an area of the hospital that cares primarily for adult patients. The patient was awake and alert but experienced sudden onset of severe respiratory distress, in the presence of several of his family members, including his mother. The pediatric RRT was unfamiliar with the ward, including its resources and staff. Multiple staff members and physicians who were not part of the patient's team gathered in the immediate area, creating noise and confusion. In response, the RRT leader, nurse, and respiratory therapist, who were the only members present with formal team training, fell into a routine they had practiced multiple times.

The team leader assigned roles, controlled the crowd, and removed unnecessary personnel. Participating staff who had not undergone team training fell into the routine as well, responding to the calm, controlled tone, callouts, and reassurances to the patient and family. Prior to intubation, the team leader held a briefing to detail role assignments, provide reassurance, describe the events to the patient and family, and discuss how to appropriately collect and prepare intubation and monitoring equipment. After the successful intubation, a debriefing occurred with all present during the event. At the end of the debriefing, the patient's care was handed off to the adult ICU team members with a clear history and plan of care. This example illustrates how leading with the intention to promote and maintain teamwork can be effective.

RRT Teamwork Training

Organizations planning to begin RRT teamwork training might benefit from consideration of the following insights gained from our experience.

Insight 6. *Whether beginning a new RRT or working with an established team, the introduction of training and performance expectations should follow guidelines for successful change management.*

Training plans should include identifying teamwork champions from multiple disciplines who are either recognized or respected formal or informal leaders. A leadership team should be established to share the responsibility of oversight and provide the training. The team should identify an aim with a set of purposeful actions and measures for success. Finally, to sustain change, timely feedback and reinforcement are necessary.[10] The action planning steps included in the TeamSTEPPS® Instructors Guide[8] incorporate principles for successful change management.

Insight 7. *Teams that work together should train together.*

RRT teamwork training should be provided to interdisciplinary groups rather than professional group silos, to facilitate removal of the barriers of hierarchy and excessive professional courtesy, which can undo the best of team training. The primary reason professional groups are trained separately is the difficulty of matching schedules and the limits of time. Training should use a blended learning approach,[11] which addresses the needs of adult learners by integrating face-to-face and online learning. In addition, this approach minimizes scheduled time commitment challenges. The commitment to overcome schedule conflicts for interdisciplinary training is one best made in the early planning stages by the leaders and teamwork champions.

We have been successful using the TeamSTEPPS® system for implementation planning and modified TeamSTEPPS® material for training.[8] Our teamwork training consists of two parts:

1. An independent learning session that includes relevant readings and a 50-minute video covering all training topics, and
2. A 1-hour interdisciplinary group session that combines didactic and interactive learning through a slide presentation with embedded videos.

The coleaders of the group session typically come from different professional backgrounds (e.g., a physician and respiratory therapist) and have extensive training in teaching and providing unit-based, in-the-moment coaching of teamwork behavior. We believe that even during training the facilitators can model teamwork, and we often point out when mutual support is provided to one another. The session includes many examples from the learners' environment and a relevant role-play exercise to promote shared language and expectations of consistent teamwork performance. Although many announce that they "hate role-play," the exercise always turns out to be fun for participants, with the secondary benefit of additional team building. Our posttraining evaluations show that participants highly rate the value of the role-play, relevant examples from the work environment, and the use of video.

Potential Barriers to Effective Teamwork

RRTs may encounter barriers to effective teamwork during teamwork training or an RRT activation.

Insight 8. *It is important to address and monitor barriers and challenges before initial implementation of RRT teamwork training.*
    Many of the barriers to effective teamwork can make already tense situations more difficult. RRT events can become chaotic and unorganized, leading to poor care, missed diagnoses, and delayed treatment. A successful RRT must have not only the necessary knowledge and skills to assess and intervene with critically ill patients, but also teamwork skills that allow for efficiency and effectiveness in working with unfamiliar personnel in unfamiliar areas. Box 13.2 describes five common barriers to effective teamwork in RRTs: refusal to participate in training, lack of teamwork skills, unfamiliarity among team members, conflict at the bedside, and lack of crowd management.
    At the beginning of this chapter, we presented a pediatric RRT case with multiple breakdowns in teamwork. We now re-present that case study, illustrating many of the teamwork elements we have described as essential for optimum RRT outcomes.

Box 13.2   How to Handle Barriers to Effective Teamwork in RRTs

Refusal to Participate in Training
Change can be perceived as threatening, and we have found that introducing teamwork training can heighten feelings of threat to the status quo and professional integrity. The nonparticipation of a single individual is unfortunate and the outcome is uncertain: the individual may engage later after trust has developed, may attempt to sabotage change, or may ultimately choose to find other work. If only one professional group is motivated to participate in training, the teamwork champion and/or leadership team should use change management approaches to gain support from the leaders of the nonparticipating groups. This can be done by appealing to what is most important to those individual groups and emphasizing the purpose and plan for measurement of success and regular feedback.

(Continued)

Box 13.2   (Continued)

Lack of Teamwork Skills
RRTs must often interact with an individual or individuals who do not have the same teamwork skills. To overcome this, the RRT can provide role modeling, continued focus on teamwork during the event, and good leadership. RRT teamwork skills can be promoted with interteam reinforcement, often provided by the leader (e.g., saying, "Good callout, thanks.").

Unfamiliarity among Team Members
If the RRT is composed of team members that are dispersed throughout the organization until needed, team functioning can be maximized by having a check-in briefing with each change of team members. This short in-person meeting or conference call can include introductions, role clarifications, and reports of any primary responsibilities that may result in a mid-shift replacement and who that replacement will be. A dedicated (nondispersed) RRT can also use the check-in briefing to share self-assessments such as fatigue, stress, or illness that help other team members provide mutual support, if needed, during a team event later in the day.

Conflict at the Bedside
RRT leaders need to practice the skills to temporarily diffuse conflict during the RRT intervention and follow up for teambuilding after the event. It is common to encounter role conflict that is expressed by primary team members through challenging the need and presence of the RRT at the bedside, or challenging decisions made by the RRT leader. Scripts should be practiced such as, "We can talk about that later. How can we work together now to help the patient?" or "Thank you for bringing your concern to my attention. Let's get more information and make our decisions together to help the patient."

Lack of Crowd Management
One of the biggest threats to a high-functioning team's performance is lack of crowd control or "onlooker management." At our institution, the RRT activation system includes a pager message to individual RRT members and an overhead page throughout the hospital. The overhead page alerts the primary team that an event is unfolding with one of their patients, and many people arrive at the event to "help and learn." The crowd interferes with team member recognition and communication and often upsets the patient and family. Managing the crowd through role identification and obtaining support from hospital police are strategies that can be used.

Delay in Calling the Rapid Response Team
Although RRTs are intended to intervene before an emergency unfolds, at times, the rapid deterioration of the patient is minutes away. Often, antecedents or signs of impending patient deterioration are not recognized early enough or acted on when first noticed. This reluctance or delay in calling the RRT is, in part, due to teamwork deficiencies throughout healthcare, which have a negative effect on the afferent arm of the Rapid Response System. The barriers of hierarchy and excessive professional courtesy, as well as more overt behaviors related to personal confrontation and challenge, all contribute to under-triaging patients who could be helped by early intervention with the RRT. RRT members should be aware that their teamwork behavior can not only partly compensate for delays secondary to organizational and cultural barriers that can potentially diminish the effectiveness of the RRT intervention, but can pave the way for organizational improvement and future earlier activation of the RRT for the good of the patient.

Case Study 2: Good Teamwork in a Pediatric RRT Event

On the pediatric surgical ward, a 2-year-old Hispanic male with a history of a complicated liver transplant and prolonged hospitalization experiences sudden onset of fever to 105°F, respiratory rate of 60 breaths/minute, heart rate of 180 beats/minute, and blood pressure 70/30 mmHg. The patient's mother, who does not speak English, is at the bedside with the nurse and a new surgical resident. The surgical resident orders blood cultures, a fluid bolus, and antibiotics. As an initial fluid bolus is infusing and the antibiotics are primed for infusion, the patient's heart rate increases to 220 beats/minute; he appears flushed, agitated, and has some faint wheezing. His mother appears more concerned and begins to cry. The bedside nurse tells the resident that she is going to activate the pediatric RRT for assistance, and he responds that he wants her to wait for the fluid bolus to finish and call his senior resident before an RRT call. She states that she is concerned about the patient's sudden change and uncomfortable with managing care without more nursing assistance, as well as the patient's safety and her inability to see her other patients.[†] For that reason, she needs to call the pediatric RRT to help her while he pages his senior resident. Although the surgical resident appears displeased with the decision, the nurse activates the RRT and asks her charge nurse to assist her until their arrival.

The pediatric RRT members arrive, announce their names and roles, and recognize the patient and his mother from his lengthy stay in the pediatric ICU. A Spanish interpreter arrives to assist with communication, and the primary nurse and resident report the reason for the call to the responders in SBAR[‡] format. The surgical resident appears tense and apologizes to his senior resident as the additional surgical team members arrive. The patient's mother, through the interpreter, relays that the patient had a similar appearance when he had a "bad reaction" to one of his IV medications, and she believes that he received the medication today.

The RRT assists with obtaining additional IV access and rapid fluid administration, placing the child on oxygen, and administering medications for possible anaphylactic reaction. The primary surgical team and RRT discuss the patient's status and make a joint decision to transfer the patient to the ICU. A multidisciplinary debriefing occurs with the responding and primary teams. The nurse who activated the team is thanked for the call, and the members identify that good communication was used during the activation, with little noise and disruption. The team identifies that the patient did not receive his ordered premedication regimen prior to a medication administered before his deterioration, and this error is reported as a system medication error. During the debriefing, the RRT leader reassures the new surgical resident who was unfamiliar with the RRT that the team is called only to assist the primary team, and patients often stay on the ward after the response is completed. He and the other primary surgical physicians are later copied on an e-mail thank you to the activating nurse from the president of the hospital.

Prior to the patient's transfer to the ICU, the RRT physician and interpreter update his mother in detail about the likely medication reaction and what will be done to assure that it does not happen again. She is encouraged to ask questions regarding medications in the future and is told about the pediatric Rapid Response System and how non–English-speaking family members can call it. The patient's vital signs and clinical status improve over the next 12 hours, and the patient returns to the wards with a new medication regimen and additional pretreatment for his transplant medications.

[†]Structuring critical language using the words "concerned, uncomfortable and safety" is a non-threatening way to get other team members' attention while advocating for the patient. In TeamSTEPPS training, this tool is known as "CUS."[8,12]

[‡]SBAR is an abbreviation for Situation, Background, Assessment, and Recommendations. It is a communication tool for structuring communication in a logical, concise format.

Box 13.3   Insights into Teamwork in Rapid Response Teams

1. Good teamwork and encouraging patients and/or family members present to be part of the medical team is vital during the first 5 minutes of an RRT event.
2. Excluding the primary team or giving negative feedback to callers, the primary team, or even patients leads to alienation and poor communication and teamwork in the future.
3. Good teamwork also affects the patient/family experience.
4. Holding a debriefing after RRT events provides time for immediate performance improvement and promotes long-term culture change.
5. When a high-functioning RRT interacts with a primary team with poor teamwork skills, leadership, mutual support, situation monitoring, and communication can improve the experience for all and the outcome for the patient.
6. Whether beginning a new RRT or working with an established team, introduction of any training and performance expectations should follow guidelines for successful change management.
7. Teams that work together should train together.
8. It is important to have a plan for addressing and monitoring barriers and challenges before initial implementation of RRT teamwork training.

SUMMARY

Teamwork is vital to an RRT. A high functioning RRT can enhance the contribution of the primary team during patient assessment and intervention, and ultimately, save patients' lives. Typical barriers to effective teamwork training can be minimized by training in teams and taking advantage of blended learning. Teamwork training can be part of the original RRT implementation plan or added later with established teams. Our experience providing teamwork training for RRT members and observing the impact of good teamwork has led to the insights summarized in Box 13.3. These insights can help guide other organizations as they pursue improved teamwork in their rapid response systems.

REFERENCES

1. Hillman, K. M., Bristow P. J., Chey, T., Daffurn, K., Jacques, T., Norman, S. L., et al. (2002). Duration of life threatening antecedents prior to intensive care admission. *Intensive Care Medicine, 28*(11), 1629–34.
2. Hodgetts, T. J., Kenward, G., Vlachonikolis, I. G., Payne, S., & Castle, N. (2002). The identification of risk factors for cardiac arrest and formulation of activation criteria to alert a medical emergency team. *Resuscitation, 54*(2), 125–31.
3. Fieselmann, J. F., Hendryx, M. S., Helms, C. M., & Wakefield, D. S. (1993). Respiratory rate predicts cardiopulmonary arrest for internal medicine inpatients. *Journal of General Internal Medicine, 8*(7), 354–60.
4. Schein, R. M. H., Hazday, N., Pena, M., Ruben, B. H., & Sprung, C. L. (1990). Clinical antecedents to in-hospital cardiopulmonary arrest. *Chest, 98*(6), 1388–92.
5. Jones, D., Bellomo, R., & DeVita, M. A. (2009). Effectiveness of the medical emergency team: The importance of dose. *Critical Care, 13*(5), 313. Retrieved April 4, 2012 from: http://ccforum.com/content/13/5/313.
6. Sharek, P. J., Parast, L. M, Leong, K., Coombs, J., Earnest, K., Sullivan, J., et al. (2007). Effect of a rapid response team on hospital-wide mortality and code rates outside the ICU in a children's hospital. *Journal of the American Medical Association, 298*(19), 2267–8.
7. DeVita, M. A., Bellomo, R., Hillman, K., Kellum, J., Rotondi, A., Dan Teres, et al. (2006). Findings of the First Consensus Conference on Medical Emergency Teams. *Critical Care Medicine, 34*(9), 2463–78.
8. Agency for Healthcare Research and Quality. (2006). *TeamSTEPPS™ Guide to Action: Creating a Safety Net for Your Healthcare Organization.* AHRQ Publication No. 06–0020–4.

9. Cannon-Bowers, J. A., and Salas, E.. (1997). Teamwork competencies: The interaction of team member knowledge, skills, and attitudes. In: H. F. O'Neil, Jr. (Eds.), *Work Force Readiness: Competencies and Assessment.* (pp. 151–74). Mahwah, NJ: LEA.

10. Institute for Healthcare Improvement (2008). *Improvement Methods.* Retrieved November 17, 2009 from: http://www.ihi.org/IHI/Topics/Improvement/ImprovementMethods/.

11. Garrison, D. R., & Vaughan, N. D. (2008). *Blended learning in higher education: framework, principles, and guidelines.* San Francisco: John Wiley & Sons.

12. Leonard, M., Graham, S., & Bonacum, D. (2004). The human factor: the critical importance of effective teamwork and communication in providing safe care. *Quality and Safety in Health Care, 13*(Suppl 1), i85–90.

14

IMPLEMENTATION

Mary L. Salisbury

ON PAPER, IMPLEMENTATION is the ability to effectively execute planned change. In practice, organizations recognized for their excellence in leadership and ability to advance their agendas, invest heavily in the resources required to ensure projects are effectively implemented and managed over time. Established as a critical dimension of improvement science and discussed on a continuum over time, implementation is described specific to a implementing a team initiative over, industry-standard, phases: (1) readiness to engage; (2) training, kickoff, and early implementation; (3) evaluating, coaching to improve, and integration to sustain over time. Issues identified are addressed at both the macro- and micro-system levels and where helpful, case-based scenarios and lessons-learned tips illustrate and provide experience as evidence to the various points.

In a nutshell, to be successful at implementation is to be: (1) knowledgeable; (2) disciplined; and (3) diligent to the detail. After that, it should go pretty well.

M. L. Salisbury

Someone must just pay attention! Healthcare organizations are ever-changing in matters that are increasingly complex and vital to their survival. Change to an organization is as blood to the living organism; it is its very life and future.[1] Therefore, if planned change is important, it is unfathomable that the actions critical to such change be left to chance. Yet regularly, large-scale, million dollar initiatives approved in the board rooms are promptly placed in the hands of front-line leaders who, although well intentioned, may not be well skilled and capable of implementing, project managing, and sustaining as large an initiative as teamwork. Wished well and expected to manage, all hope for the best as front-line managers press yet another new task into the priorities of their day.

> Case scenario. *A recent assessment in a department newly implementing their team initiative provided the opportunity to observe a shift charge nurse managing her own patient load, as well as maintaining mastery over the newly implemented teamwork initiative. The nurse collaborated and coordinated the department flow and function while prioritizing and balancing patient care requirements with the available staff resources. She recruited staff to cover holes in the yet-to-be-published schedule, covered sick calls and meal breaks, which she used as a captive opportunity to provide performance feedback, hand out and gather in a focused survey, as well as teach and credential staff on the new intravenous pump while managing parallel operations—working to find beds and missing teeth, sending the supply aid for missing respiratory equipment, tagging and sending a monitor for repair, mourning with a grieving loved one, calling the priest and social services, comforting a crying child with an ice pop, and resolving a widespread interdepartmental, interdisciplinary, interpersonal care delivery and customer conflict, complicated by the unnerving elements of consultant and family member fury.*

In the midst of these multiple challenges it is clear that without a sound strategy and stratified team approach to shepherd and attend the detail of their planned team change, the initiative left to the care of this one individual, predictably, is doomed to fail. More is needed.

Tip: Powerful organizations focus on powerful teams. Implementation requires a system that structures the staff to recognize and mitigate all hazards to the process. It is a matter of using simple practical steps to reduce the complexity and manage the variability of what would otherwise overwhelm. Someone has to own the initiative. Someone has to pay attention.

Planned change is implemented typically in a three-phase approach: (1) assessment, planning and readiness preparation; (2) training, kickoff, and implementation of the intervention; and (3) sustaining and integrating behaviors into practice and operations over time. Each phase possesses steps that have the potential to impede implementation and thwart the overall impact of the initiative unless successfully completed.

IMPLEMENTATION PHASE I.
SETTING THE STAGE: PREPARING YOURSELF, PREPARING OTHERS

Units change within the context of the whole. Before an organization undertakes planned change it must understand the complexities of the program under consideration and match-up or skill-up its people to take on, to literally become and role

model, the vision of team-driven safety while in parallel providing the necessary steps to project manage and bring about change. Leaders, managers, and staff must be provided clear roles and responsibilities with the built-in accountabilities to perform. Effective leaders and implementers of change must demonstrate a working knowledge of the relevant: (1) theories of change; (2) standards and health regulatory agency policies or guidelines governing planned team change; (3) organizational factors that may facilitate, block, or impede success; (4) program as well as the requisite strategies and resources; (5) organizational history when implementing other similar change initiatives; and (6) the use of evaluation to drive implementation. Any discussion on implementation would be incomplete without some consideration of each.

#1. Know the theories. "*There's nothing as practical as a good theory.*" (Kurt Lewin) Leaders of excellent change and implementation methodologies use theory to guide practice. Leaders of planned change benefit with a working knowledge of several theories: system theory; theory on measurement and evaluation concepts specific to medical quality and process improvement; theories governing leadership and culture; learning and evaluation theory; the theory, methods, and application of team performance assessment; and the theory of behavioral change. Broadly speaking, these theories pivot on the element of behavior and to that end, the seminal work of Lewin provides a basic framework upon which the

works of many modern theorists now build,[2] and that all embarking on implementing team-driven change should consider.

Tip: By accounting for the many elements of change, theory brings practice into focus and gives meaning to evaluation. Theory allows for prediction and what can be predicted can be planned for and avoided or advanced.[3]

#2. Know the standards, guidelines, health policy, and law. Executive leaders, project managers, department leaders, and change team members cannot design or execute an implementation plan without a thorough knowledge of all applicable standards, as well as labor and regulatory guidelines. The Institute of Medicine recommends the education of healthcare professionals to deliver evidence-based patient-centered care as a member of an interdisciplinary, high-quality, high-tech improvement team.[4] Quality and regulatory organizations extend advisories and safe practice guidelines, whereas professional organizations and credentialing bodies move safety into interprofessional education, licensing, and performance evaluation.

Tip: Leverage all applicable guidelines, recommendations, and standards to define performance, drive evaluation and engage patients to properly frame the full vision of safe, compliant care.

#3. Know the relevant organizational factors. Although many venues report the positive impact teams have on healthcare, the same reports have wide variation in the implementation strategies and processes used to achieve such impacts. Research concludes 20% of variation found in team performance attributable to training quality, with the remaining 80% resulting from organizational factors.[5] These data provide critical insights regarding the allocation of time and resources:

- Training accounts for a very small portion of learning, yet is where the majority of organizations focus

- Organizational factors account for a large portion of learning and impact and yet are barely considered at all

Seven organizational factors were found to be critical to consider if learning is to successfully transfer into practice: (1) align training objectives and safety aims with the goals of the organization; (2) provide organizational support; (3) ensure the involvement of front-line leaders; (4) establish the climate and prepare the environment for the initiative; (5) determine and secure the necessary resources; (6) facilitate the use of skills; and (7) use evaluation to drive implementation.[5]

Tip: To ensure effective implementation, organizations must develop strategies and embed into operations positive solutions for each of these factors.

#4. Know the program, manage the program, and leverage the lessons learned. Whether working at the macro- or micro-system level, it is critical to be educated on the program to be implemented; exactly what the program is and what it can do for the organization; how to monitor, manage, evaluate, and properly resource so as to include the roles and responsibilities each has in the implementation process. Leaders, change team, and staff must know the course and the factors affecting its effective implementation and work to develop strategies capable of ensuring its success. All decisions must be made from the perspective of "Where is the patient in the middle of this decision? Is he or she more or less safe?" In this manner, consensus is gained when change is needed. When it comes to progressing patient safety there are no sacred cows.

Tip: Everyone has a role and responsibility to facilitate successful program implementation. From that perspective, each must closely observe the process itself and provide feedback to ensure the early identification and mitigation of all risks to the plan. This shared environment of learning and responsibility to improve yields the shared understandings necessary for cross-organizational goal alignment toward the shared mental model of safety.

Case scenario. *Following his training, the executive officer of a mid-size organization used one of his employee FORUM sessions to create a shared understanding of the upcoming team initiative by providing an overview of TEAMS to all staff. With a town-meeting methodology, he talked of the hospital's vision for team-driven, patient-engaged, safe, high-quality care. Trainers*

(Continued)

(Continued)

provided high-level content and a video demonstration of caregivers at work using team skills, tools, and strategies to plan, problem solve, and improve outcomes. The chief executive officer (CEO) projected his commitment to provide the resources necessary to optimize performance stating his commitment to: (1) integrate into walking rounds the action of asking staff and their patients the plan for their stay or care; (2) release department leaders from standing meetings for the first 3 months post team kickoff with the expectation they attend team briefs and debriefs, perform real-time observations, and provide formative feedback to encourage new behaviors into performance; (3) require front-line coaches to provide the ongoing formative feedback that facilitates long-term team outcomes; (4) provide staff with the opportunity, time, and place to effectively plan, problem solve, and debrief so that performance would be improved and team strategies strengthened over time; and (5) "walk, watch, learn and look to help."

#5. Know the history. A critical element of implementation readiness and the ability to execute is to analyze organizational past experience when executing large-scale projects. What went well? What did not? And, most important in either case, why? The likely cause of implementations that stutter or fail is that steps critical to readiness, training, implementing, and sustaining were missed or one or more of the organizational factors left underattended.

Tip: Understanding past implementation successes provides the insight vital to an implementation effort and the experience-based adjustments required to ensure planned and improved outcomes.

#6. Know the data. **You get what you stroke.** When employees are not achieving, leadership may not be either.[6] Team performance does not just happen; however, what you pay attention to does happen. High leadership visibility, close monitoring, interactive debriefing, feedback, and problem-solving sessions are all opportunities to get and give feedback on the implementation process. Executive and front-line leaders and change team members need to leverage opportunities to observe or hear the information to ensure project and process risk identification so as to understand, problem solve, and co-create corrective solutions as well as event-based reward and recognition. Supported and cared-for teams flourish and the project succeeds. In turn, successful teams take every occasion to care for and enrich the patient experience. This is the business for which no one can be too busy. This is the business in which everyone has a role.

Case scenario. *The CEO of a large medical center ran a full-to-the-brim calendar. To integrate performance evaluation into his already overloaded role, he walked to and from his car through a different department every day. He stopped and asked staff how "this team thing" was going—what was going well, what needed more attention, what had they tried, and what they might need him to do. He viewed every conversation as an opportunity to obtain information critical to his ability to support the teams. He obtained information both about staff performance as well as his leadership team and their ability to be clear on the priorities, provide necessary resources, and prepare the climate and environment in which teams thrive. Contrary to the expectation of department leaders, teams rarely took him up on the offer to intervene. Why? He speculated that his query "What had they tried?" expressed confidence in the team's ability to address and resolve their issues. However, when interviewed, his staff stated, "He expects us to make this thing work." They said they "never knew when or which unit he would 'visit' next." They also said that they "welcomed his visit." "He pays attention." "He cares." He had to go to and from his car anyway, so the evaluation cost nothing, although the yield was great.*

Tip: Data are critical to determining a successful implementation process. These data can be gathered in both formal and informal ways. High visibility of leaders to gather feedback from those working the process provides valuable program data while sending the strong message that "This initiative is important. We share the responsibility of making it happen."

IMPLEMENTATION PHASE II. TRAINING AND KICKOFF

A solid implementation plan ensures that organizations standardize and replicate an implementation process designed to ensure team success across units or facilities as well as within or across a system over time.

Where organizations have experience and success using a specific implementation or change model, they should stick with what they know.

Without a model, the work of John Kotter provides a stepped approach successful in healthcare and non-healthcare industries alike. The steps are: (1) setting the stage and creating a sense of urgency; (2) building the guiding team; (3) developing a change vision and strategy; (4) creating understanding and buy in; (5) empowering others; (6) developing short-term wins; (7) never letting up; and (8) creating a new culture.[6] When all the elements are present, implementation is facilitated and change occurs. When any one is missing, something different from the expected may result.

Tip: The complexities of change are managed with a good plan against which all actions of concern can be monitored.[6]

Step #1: Setting the stage and creating a sense of urgency uses inquiry to answer for staff and leaders questions of "Why teams?" "Why now?" and "What's in it for me?" When communication degrades to unexplained chaos, trust erodes.

Case scenario. A "setting the stage" exemplar is illustrated by the CEO (discussed earlier) who used one of his employee FORUM sessions to provide an overview of TEAMS to all hospital staff, to talk of the hospital's safety journey and the vision for teams to drive the organization from good to excellent in all categories of safety.

Case scenario. A "creating a sense of urgency" exemplar is illustrated when the sponsoring vice president opens the training session for the emergency medicine change team by telling the story of a child who entered their organization for treatment and things went very, very wrong. The vice president ends with the vision for teams to safeguard the journey for other and all children so that "this sad thing might never happen again." Strikingly stated, the vision was clear—for teams to safeguard the care journey for all patients by equipping all healthcare givers working within their system with the team tools and strategies to be safe.

Tip: Trust is a byproduct of open transparent communication in which staff engage in a safe zone team debrief of all events of care, expressing all celebrations or concerns, and in which those concerns are heard and a formal response is provided.

Step #2: Pulling together a guiding team provides a core team to undertake the mission to resource, monitor, and manage team implementation and the actions that safeguard five of the seven

organizational success factors. The guiding team ensures the involvement of front-line leaders who are responsible to establish the climate and prepare the environment to receive the initiative. The team determines and secures the necessary resources, plans and designs skill facilitation (e.g., regularly scheduled case review and analysis sessions), and provides opportunities for event-based simulation experience.

Case scenario. *In response to the queries "Are all staff represented?" and "Do we have the resources we need?" the change team added to their membership a medical resident, Post-Graduate Year 4. Over time, when provider-raised issues involve personnel who are not serving on the change team, the team assembles small subcommittees to consult on the matter of interest. In this manner, the size of the change team remains small enough to work well and achieve intended outcomes, yet is capable of flexing up and adding members for the focused but time-limited work of emerging needs or new initiative demands.*

Tip: Kickoff and short-term performance may occur without the multidisciplinary, multi–skill mix of executive sponsors, directorate, and front-line formal and informal positive, influential leaders (the change team), but long-term implementation to sustain and integrate into daily operations will not.

Step #3: Senior leaders are responsible to develop and cast the vision and guide the strategies necessary to ensure values translate into expected behaviors. This step ensures that the intervention objectives and safety aims align with the goals of the organization that in turn dictates the resources necessary to implement and sustain.

Case scenario. *Intent on ensuring involvement, the CEO of a mid-sized community hospital attended all preparation and learning sessions. Together, leader and team created their "elevator speech" as a three-sentence story expressing the future of their organization using enquiry to engage staff to answer "What is teaming and why are we doing it?" "Why now?" and "What's in it for me?" Once completed, the executive worked to guide the team in discovering and developing a strategy capable of achieving that vision. Although directly involved, he took no action other than using enquiry and high-level facilitation skills to guide the team's work. The team expected answers. He simply asked more questions. The team, frustrated over what they at the time perceived as a lack of direction, were surprised to see that they had gained skill at the task and actually completed their work ahead of all other hospitals in the session.*

Tip: Although it may be easy to understand why a well-cast and communicated vision facilitates change, deciding specifically what, when, and why to change is not. There are a few principles to consider. The change must (1) solve a problem about something that matters; (2) answer the question, "What's in it for me;" and (3) have clear roles and responsibilities for staff to successfully engage.

Step #4: Communicating for buy-in is to seize every staff interaction as an opportunity to connect the vision of teaming back to the power of teams to create safer cultures of care by improving performance and solving the everyday problems experienced by caregivers and their patients and, in turn, add meaning to work. Be very certain to speak to all staff one-on-one. Provide the opportunity to ask questions or state concerns up front.

Change theorists predict resistance at this stage; therefore, be prepared. Expect and be willing to hear the confrontation of resisters because it may contain valuable information to safeguard patients, caregivers, or the initiative itself. However, all resistance is not equal. Therefore, it is important to distinguish between the resistance exerted by good-willed professionals who need additional or clarifying information and the cognitive distortion experienced by chronic resisters. (A second type of cognitive distortion resistance exists that is rooted in true pathology, comprises less than 1% of staff, and exceeds a team's skill level to resolve. The additional skills of Human Resource specialists are required to assist the individual in adjusting and committing to the role of supporting the patient's right to experience high-quality, safe, nondisruptive care.)

Case scenario. *The physician and nurse project leaders of a large academic medical center designed their "communicating-for-buy-in" plan with the goal of speaking to every staff member individually. They used a staff meeting to announce the purpose of these one-on-one interviews and that they would speak with all members over the next 2 weeks. They requested that each member gather their thoughts or concerns in preparation for the discussion. They agreed to keep the conversation to about 5 minutes and used their elevator speech as the opener for each session. Both had a spreadsheet prepopulated with their half of the staff member names next to columns and spaces for logging staff questions, concerns, and suggestions or solutions for the change team to consider. After the opener, they asked the team member, "What will teaming do for you?" "What do we need to consider to ensure teaming supports all staff and patients?" "What haven't we thought of or considered yet?" All questions were answered, concerns logged, and handed over to the change team to resolve or respond to and names checked off the list in front of staff, providing visible evidence of their claim to speak with all.*

Tip: Resistance to change is normal and is the most common obstacle to implementation. Knowledge and skill are required to support the resistor. Although information resolves some resistance, using the patient's perspective to reframe and guide simple thinking distortions may resolve others. Patience, engagement, and clear accountabilities are essential for all.

Step #5: Removing obstacles and empowering others to act. Opportunities to practice and facilitate behaviors are planned into implementation with staff gaining skill just by exercising the processes (e.g., performing team briefs, huddles, and debriefs) or in the planned team practice of event-based simulation experiences.

Up to this point in implementation, much time has been spent involving staff in understanding the purpose and power of teams to drive safety. In response, most staff will be eager to engage. However, despite good will and the intention to act, anticipated and unanticipated obstacles to implementation and performance will arise. To facilitate the uninterrupted use of skills, all barriers must be identified and resolved immediately.

Obstacles rooted in the *nature of the system* must be quickly identified and addressed. Obstacles rooted in the *nature of humans* must be identified and acted on immediately as well. Although resistance is normal, resisting nonperformers must have immediate feedback and support to manage their career toward excellence; nonengagement is not an option. Change team members, coaches, and staff must be hypervigilant to performance goals and team successes or events of nonperformance and intervene quickly and frequently with verbal rewards or formative feedback.

Case scenario. The system as an obstacle. *At their in-class training session, the executive sponsor, department physician, and nurse leader, change team leaders, and staff came to understand the burden the team initiative was about to place on front-line managers and staff. In addition to implementing the Joint Commission's medication reconciliation guidelines, the department was also absorbing increased patient volume arising from the recent closing of a local hospital. The decision was unanimous to stage the initiatives, train-up the teams first, use the teams as a method to drive and safely care for patients while under the stress of the increased volume, and then provide the team with the templates and scripts necessary to ensure all elements of medication reconciliation, embedding key actions into all events of care.*

(Continued)

(Continued)

Case scenario. Human nature as an obstacle. *With all staff trained and performance expectations clear, a senior nurse on the night shift does not attend team briefs, does not huddle, and does not task assist but openly declares, "You know what, you all just do your thing and I will do mine. I just come here to do my work and then go home, that's it." When asked by teammates why she was not attending team briefs, the nurse blew up, retorting, "Hey, you all knock yourselves out if you want to. I don't need this team thing. Nobody asked me anyhow." The team leader was quick to respond, "You are correct, you were not involved. You were out on leave when we began teaming. But, here is what I know to be true, teaming is not about you or me personally, it's about us professionally and what we can do for the patients. They need you to represent their plan at the team brief where the team can review for risk and structure for success. By hearing the plans, we catch and interrupt errors so they never occur. It's really about patient advocacy."*

Teammates in this scenario experienced human nature as an obstacle and appeared to have expected the responses they received. Perhaps they even rehearsed how to support this evidence- or information-based resisting by an otherwise good-willed individual and do so with information and an appeal to the concept of patient expectations and professional deportment. Regardless of the trigger, the action worked.

Tip: Strengthening team skills and facilitating the legitimate behaviors of communication, workload management and care flow is an effective method by which to address the day-to-day conflicts to the normal delivery of care.

Step #6: Rewards, recognition, and positive feedback are critical reinforcers of a team's hard work. Using data as the standard to reward and recognize performance successes encourages staff, fosters good morale, helps build performance momentum, and builds in the organizational factor—using evaluation to drive implementation. Given the opportunity, staff will define meaningful, budget neutral, means of recognition.

Case scenario. *With the charge to develop a budget-neutral reward and recognition system, change team members of a large sprawling multi-acre medical center, randomly interviewed staff members from all roles regarding their opinion on a meaningful but no-cost reward system. Overwhelmingly, the number one request was a parking space in the front lot for a week. At no cost to the organization, the executive sponsor worked with building and grounds personnel to carve out and post signage reserving a space within the front lot as a reward for the "Team Member of Excellence."*

Tip: Embed the mutually agreed-on vision of team-driven safety into the bedrock of operations—new person orientation, policy and procedure, performance evaluation, credentialing, and the extension of privileges, rewards, and recognition and career management.

Step #7: It is easy to say never let up, but difficult to do. When eager or conflicted leaders or teams are pressed for results or time, it is easier to claim victory than to hold fast to the fact that implementing planned change is a process over time. Therefore, it is critical to post the team's implementation timeline and planned event markers as an objective method to ensure that organizational and front-line leaders and staff do not lose sight of where they are in the implementation process and where they have yet to go. It is important for the change team to periodically update the timeline through huddles with front-line leaders and team members specific to the pace of implementation. Staff are masters at their work and are to be trusted when progressing their growth.

Case scenario. Give teams control of their growth. *To optimize success, the decision was made to complete the physician order entry roll-out that was already in progress before starting the team training initiative. This delay pushed team roll-out into the summer, a busy summer with increased volume and staffing patterns stressed by vacations, unexpected long term leaves-of-absence, and unplanned resignations. The first team behaviors to roll out—early shift team briefs—required staff to: (1) provide a 5-minute heads-up to whiteboard rounds; (2) assemble to present all patient plans of care in SBAR format; (3) openly dialogue to review all plans for risk; and (4) develop contingencies capable of structuring the plan (and therefore the patient) for success when risks exist. Running well, the teams were using their communication bundle— structured communication—SBAR, call-outs, check-backs, and hand-offs of care. During the interview, team members provided stories in which the team briefs resulted in good catches. Executive leaders openly broadcast the "team victories" and encouraged the teams to push on. Despite the accolades and early successes, the teams did not believe they could advance the performance expectations as defined in the roll-out plan. They were exhibiting signs of increased stress with common descriptors, "Our plates are full," "People are struggling just to keep up with care," "What's the big deal? We apparently already work pretty well as a team," and "How much do they expect a team to do?" The change team and executive sponsor met and agreed that pressure was high and action was required. A staff meeting was called. The executive sponsor attended, but the change team conducted the meeting to: (1) acknowledge executive acclaims and as well verbally reward the great work the teams were doing; (2) recognize that the teams were not yet where they wanted to be; while also (3) recognize and agree with the staff's request to "hold on the plan for the summer." The change team told team members that even in this early stage of teaming, they were performing the skills more safely than before teaming. They stated that the decision to stand down the timeline made good sense. They requested that each team member commit to maintaining all current actions of whiteboard rounding and the use of their communication bundle. The change team established weekly staff meetings to regularly take the team's "pulse." In turn, they would keep the executive leader apprised of the team health. They established 4 weeks hence as a time to re-gather formally, determine the climate of the department. They agreed that without further reasons for delay they would re-start implementation in 6 weeks. Reports came back that "the staff feel heard" and "the staff are energized."*

Case scenario. Never let up. *In a mid-sized community hospital, the sponsoring vice president and project manager work to achieve the vision of team-driven safety. Before any training, leaders at the macro- and micro-level were educated about the purpose of teaming and their role in the initiative. Staff were educated in overview sessions specific to the mission of teaming to achieve the vision of high-quality, safe, care that they would be performing on behalf of the organization to enhance safety and that they would be supported with the resources necessary to do so. Whole hospital implementation would be achieved staging implementation over one year. Units would be bundled in partners when feasible or trained alone when size or specialty dictated. In parallel, master trainers were created and charged along with the Quality and Education Department to embed teaming agreements and performance expectations into*

(Continued)

(Continued)

all elements of employee orientation, ongoing learning, credentialing, and performance expectations. Based on early successes, a template for whole hospital roll-out was developed for use throughout their five-hospital system. The executive team instilled teaming into the organizational pillars of excellence. Coaches attend monthly debrief learning and performance improvement strategy sessions. At 6 months after kickoff, unit change teams formally convert into collaborative practice teams, in which physicians, nurses, and leaders work to address patient- and provider-raised issues of care, developing solutions that improve process and outcomes over time. Interested staff are regularly rotated onto the team with the expectation that one-third of the membership will turn over annually.

Tip: Understand the environment in which implementation is occurring. Never create a safety issue to solve one. When pressure from the top and the need to claim victory is high, resist. Short of full implementation, the initiative is at risk to be nonsustaining. When pressure from the front-line is high, partner with staff to manage or modify the implementation timeline while ensuring that good gains remain. The arbiter of safety success is the patient, not the pressure.

Step #8: Creating a new culture looking back to move forward. It requires reframing the questions of preimplementation where inquiry transitions to reflection. "Why are we doing this team thing?" transitions to "Why did we do this?" "What's in it for me?" becomes "How have the new skills, tools, and strategies helped you improve your work and better care for your patients?" And "What will the new culture look like?" becomes "What do you see?"

Tip: If you want to know from whence you came, engage the past. If you want to know where you have yet to go, engage the patient. Patients will tell you how far you have to go before you reach a true culture of safe high-quality care.

IMPLEMENTATION PHASE III. STRUCTURING SUSTAINMENT

Implementation is a process that begins with the end in mind. Initiatives are more likely to obtain and proceed into sustainment in organizations that prepare leaders, staff, and the environment to monitor, manage, and receive a team initiative, secure the organizational success factors, and embed new behaviors into everyday operations.[5] Someone must own it. Someone must pay attention. Departments of simulation provide vibrant event-based learning environments for on- and off-site safe experiences in which to practice and improve performance over time. Although simulation does not have to be costly, it does have to be well designed.

CONCLUSION

Today's healthcare mission is to deliver safe, high-quality, team-driven care in time-compressed circumstances amidst shifting and ever-changing priorities. A solid implementation methodology provides the structured approach by which teams and all improvement initiatives of planned change come into being. Without the ability to change, the life of the organization as well as the lives of the patients are at risk.

REFERENCES

1. Schein, E. H. (1999). *The Corporate Culture: Survival Guide*. San Francisco: Jossey-Bass.
2. Schein, E.H. (1995). Kurt Lewin's Change Theory in the Field and in the Classroom: Notes Toward a Model of Managed Learning.Invited paper for a special issue of Systems Practice edited by Susan Wheelan.Section I, 7, Personal and Relational Refreezing.
3. Schein, E. H. (1999). *The corporate culture: Survival guide*. San Francisco: Jossey-Bass.

4. Institute of Medicine Committee on Quality of Health Care in America. (2001). *Crossing the quality chasm: A new health system for the 21st century.* Washington, DC: National Academy Press.

5. Salas, E., Almeida, S., Salisbury, M., et al. (2009). What are the critical success factors for implementing team training in health care? *Joint Commission Journal on Quality & Patient Safety, 35*(8), 398–405.

6. Kotter, J. P. (1996). *Leading change.* Boston: Harvard Business School Press.

15

SUSTAINMENT OF TEAMWORK

Heidi B. King and Stephen W. Harden

SUSTAINABILITY AND ORGANIZATIONAL CULTURE: LESSONS LEARNED FROM HIGH RELIABILITY ORGANIZATIONS

Somewhere in the world, right now as you read this, a US Navy aircraft carrier is plowing through wind-swept seas as the crew prepares to launch jet aircraft from its flight deck. This dangerous and nerve-racking task is accomplished for the most part by young men and women with an average age of 22 or 23. They are part of the 4,600 sailors and pilots aboard this giant floating steel city that is as long as the Empire State Building is tall. Surrounding the carrier are another 12 to 15 vessels and submarines providing security and protection for this billion-dollar asset of the US government.

The entire formation of ships, called a carrier task force, is capable of fending off any unexpected or potential attacks by enemies. Despite its size, a carrier is surprisingly agile and speedy, able to zig and zag when needed, except when it is launching or recovering aircraft. Then it is vulnerable to attack because its path through the water is steady and predictable. To launch aircraft, it must turn into the wind and hold a fixed course, making it a sitting duck for anyone wanting to attack.

Consequently, the process of launching aircraft must be executed like clockwork, with no delays

because of slipshod performance. Every second the carrier holds a steady course to fling its jets into the sky is another second it is at most risk of attack. To minimize delays and therefore risk, launching aircraft is a carefully scripted and choreographed procedure. Each movement and action is planned, scrutinized, and rehearsed.

As the supersonic fighter jets prepare for flight in the choreographed chaos of the flight deck, they are directed to launch point by young men in yellow jerseys. Navy pilots trust these "yellow shirts" with their lives, depending on their sure directions and instincts to guide them to the takeoff position without incident. Once in place, each jet is hooked up to a catapult and final preparations made for launch. Powerful machines embedded in the flight deck hurl the 25-ton aircraft from zero to 150 miles per hour in about 2.5 seconds. At these sudden speeds and G forces, there is absolutely no room for error. Mistakes have deadly consequences.

One of the last things to happen just before the launch of each airplane is the final check. An aircraft mechanic, sometimes a startlingly young sailor, crawls underneath the airplane, and despite the danger from the jet's powerful and deadly engines, checks it out from nose to tail. He ensures that everything is ready for the pilot's rocket ride down the catapult rails. If he finds anything amiss—flaps not set, equipment loose on the wing, open inspection panels, leaking hydraulic fluid—he signals the catapult officer to suspend the launch until the discrepancy is investigated and corrected.

In the ultimate example of a "stop the line" behavior, this 20-something-year-old sailor, who may be only a few years out of high school, causes the entire carrier task force to take a brief and perilous pause in its steady drum beat of launching aircraft. During this break, young men and women scramble underneath the jet to assess and fix the problem. Despite the risk to the carrier, nothing more happens to launch this airplane until its problem is fixed. Senior officers, including admirals, as anxious as they may be to proceed, respond to this event instigated by one of the most junior sailors on the team as if it were a normal occurrence. This young well-trained but inexperienced mechanic has the power to affect what happens to 15 ships and thousands of sailors. No one yells at him or berates him for making this decision to stop the line. It is his job. It is expected. It is the way things are done. It is part of the culture.

Surprisingly there is no variation in this scene on any of the Navy's aircraft carriers. On every ship there is a final check. In every case when something is amiss, the line is stopped. Every time it is stopped there is a flurry of activity, but the response is measured and routine. Although risky and unwanted, stopping the line is part of normal naval operations everywhere and is expected. It is part of the culture on every carrier. And this has been normal operations for generations of sailors.

The Navy has a well-practiced capability to turn a 20-year-old, fresh out of high school, into a member of the team capable of such confident, life-saving behavior during impossible mission stress and demanding environmental conditions. The Navy is able to do this because of its exceptional training program producing sustainable results. Earlier chapters of this book have described the elements of effective training. Navy training is an exemplary case of the exceptional use of those concepts and methodologies.

SUSTAINABILITY DEPENDS ON ORGANIZATIONAL CULTURE

How does the Navy sustain the effect of its training programs to get this sort of stop the line behavior every day, on every ship, for generation after generation of sailors? The lesson learned from the success of the Navy is that *sustainability of teamwork training depends on embedding the teamwork behaviors into the culture of the organization.* Teamwork must become the way things are done in the daily work flow.

What is true for the Navy is also true for healthcare organizations. If there is one thing we have learned in 11 years of helping healthcare facilities thoughtfully adopt the best training practices of high reliability organizations such as commercial aviation, aircraft carriers, and nuclear power—it is this: Hospitals and other healthcare facilities wishing to sustain the improvements in behavior and performance resulting from their teamwork training programs must do two things well:

1. Provide multiple opportunities for staff members to practice the use of those teamwork behaviors, and
2. Take the necessary actions to embed those teamwork behaviors into the organization's daily work culture.

HOW TO EMBED TEAMWORK INTO THE CULTURE OF DAILY WORK

How do you embed teamwork behaviors into the culture of the organization? Here's the formula used successfully in the navy, commercial aviation, and healthcare organizations that have sustained teamwork training performance improvements:

Thoughts + Actions + Habits + Character = Culture

This formula means that to change culture you must first change the character of the people within the organization. To change character, change individual habits. To change habits, change actions. To change actions, change how people think at the moment of truth in each process.

Here's an example. Observe a surgical team conducting the Joint Commission Universal Protocol. The first moment of truth occurs in this process when the Time Out is announced. Does everyone stop what they are doing and tune in to the process, giving it their undivided attention? If not, it is because of their thoughts about the importance of the Time Out and the role they individually play in it. To get a different thought process, and therefore a different action, training—as described in previous chapters—is needed to inform and motivate the surgical team.

If the training is effective, the thought processes will be different and will lead to a different action—mindfulness, focus, and participation during the accomplishment of the Time Out. Once that action is seen, make it become a habit by ensuring the action is repeated until it becomes second nature. The actions seen during the Time Out should be done the way airplanes are launched from aircraft carriers—with habitual participation, focus, and mindfulness, because that is "just the way things get done." To help make those actions become habits, successful healthcare institutions hardwire the desired actions by implementing system tools such as checklists, communication scripting, or standard operating procedures. For example, the surgical team might use a preprocedure checklist incorporating the requirements of the Universal Protocol (e.g., the WHO Surgical Safety Checklist). Use of the checklist makes it easy for the surgical team to do the right thing—focus and participate—and hard to do the wrong thing—ignore the accomplishment of the Time Out.

Once the habit is formed, to ensure it stays a habit and that the character of the individual is changed permanently, hospital administration and managers must continue to lead the transformation by taking very specific actions and making targeted structural changes to the organization. These leadership actions will support and nurture the habits that form the work character of the individuals in the organization.

To summarize:

- To affect *Thought Processes* and *Actions*—conduct effective training;
- To hardwire *Actions* and make them become *Habits*—implement safety tools like checklists, scripting, protocols, etc.;
- To nurture and sustain *Habits* that form and change *Character*—perform Leadership actions;
- Change *Thoughts*, get *Actions*, and create *Habits* and you will change *Culture* and sustain training performance improvements.

Here are 13 specific tips for sustaining performance improvements and supporting the performance change resulting from your investment in teamwork training. The tips are grouped in the three areas for creating a supportive culture: training, hardwiring behavior, and leadership actions.

EFFECTIVE TRAINING

Sustainability Tip #1. Teamwork and Communication Skills Training Must Be Provided to All Clinicians and Staff Involved in Providing Care.

Sustainability begins with effective training. To effectively change thought processes and therefore behaviors, training must include all of the concepts previously covered in this book, such as simulation-based training and medical debriefs. In our experience, the most important of these for sustainability are:

- Interdisciplinary. Actual patient care is provided by an interdisciplinary team; therefore, teamwork training *must* be provided to the entire team. The "teams" working together in your classroom educational activities should closely mirror the teams providing care in your organization, with each team having physician, nurse, and staff representation. Training nurses without physicians, or vice versa, is ineffective and sometimes counterproductive.
- Skills-based. "Telling" is not "training." Teamwork training must be experiential, with opportunities for practice and feedback. Knowledge-based training is insufficient to teach behavioral skills.[1] Knowledge-based learning is perishable and is not sustainable. Although knowledge is important to learning new skills, it is not sufficient to sustainably change behavior. Effective skills-based training gives your staff the ability "to do"—actually to use specific behaviors in their daily work activities.
- Attended by leadership: Make sure your leaders learn and practice the skills as well. To get the maximum buy-in from the staff, it is extremely important that your leaders support these behaviors by modeling them for the entire organization.[2]

Sustainability Tip #2: Conduct Periodic Refresher Training on Teamwork Skills.

The skills used in teamwork-based patient safety programs are just like technical skills and knowledge. If not used and refreshed, they decay over time.[3] Use it or lose it. A single didactic exposure is not enough to sustain long-term change.[4]

Organizations must identify which teamwork skills are decaying most rapidly through data collection and analysis. Direct observational studies, error and near miss reporting systems, sentinel event root cause analysis, and quality data can be mined to highlight which skills need focus and attention through refresher training.

Sustainability Tip #3: Conduct New-Hire Training.

Healthcare employee turnover in most states averages 15.6% yearly. For every 100 staff members involved in your team training initiative, about 16 will be replaced in the coming year. Each one of those new employees will need teamwork training to equip them with the same skill sets the rest of the team now has, and align them with the corporate focus on teamwork and safety. Alignment between the values of the organization and the teamwork competencies of the employee is a key indicator of motivation and satisfaction. If an employee's values and abilities are close to those defined as "core" by the hospital, they are more likely to be productive, motivated, satisfied, and well rewarded—four critical elements to long-term sustainment of your training initiative.[5]

HARDWIRE TEAMWORK BEHAVIOR

Sustainability Tip #4: Customized, Site-Specific Safety Tools (e.g., Checklists, Communications Scripting, Standard Operation Procedures) Thoughtfully Adapted from High Reliability Organizations, Must Be Created and Implemented.

Effective, experiential, interdisciplinary classroom or simulator training is only the first step in sustainability and in most cases does not permanently change behavior[6] or create culture changing habits. Safety tools, such as checklists, standard operating procedures, and standard communication protocols are needed to ensure the behaviors learned in the training are actually used on a daily basis. Successful tools have these important characteristics:

- Safety tools are created by the people who actually do the work. Tools "borrowed" from other organizations and not locally customized are rarely effective because they do not account for local and site-specific workflows. These sorts of off-the-shelf tools have no personal investment and support from the people who actually use them. Even the designers of the WHO Surgical Safety Checklist recommend their product be customized locally.
- Safety tools are updated and refined frequently. Tools are rarely perfect the first time they are used and should be treated as living documents, to be revised and updated as needed by the people doing the daily work.
- Every written tool (e.g. checklist, briefing guide, etc.) must have the tool owner's name, version number, and date clearly visible. This allows the team to know who is responsible for the updating and revision process and that they are using the most current version of the tool. This also reinforces the thought process that this is a living document to be refined as needed.
- All safety tools must be formally embedded into the organization's policy and procedure manual or other official unit documents describing how work is accomplished in the department. For example, if you create a patient handoff script, ensure the requirement to use the script during patient transfers is written in to the policy and procedure manual.

Safety tools that hardwire behavior are the "engine" producing real and measurable change and the key ingredient of sustainability. Long after the effects of classroom training have worn off, safety tools will ensure permanent behavior change.

LEADERSHIP ACTION AND ORGANIZATIONAL STRUCTURE

Sustainability Tip #5: Managers and Administrators Must "Round" on Departments That Have Implemented Teamwork Training and Safety Tools.

Rounding is a version of "management by walking around." Rounding means that managers get up, leave their office, and daily and personally visit departments conducting teamwork training and implementing safety tools. Leaders touch base with physicians and staff to find out what is working with the training initiative and what improvements can be made. This is the key leadership action that helps ensure sustainability. In our experience, every organization that has failed to sustain their performance improvements over time has also failed to Round. An effective leadership Rounding program:

- Is conducted according to a written schedule with people, places, and times specifically designated. Without a specific schedule, Rounding will not happen.
- Is emphasized in the first month after the first safety tool is implemented in the department.
- Includes key executive leadership such as the chief operating officer, chief medical officer, and chief nursing officer, as well as departmental leadership such as the chief of service and departmental directors and managers. Leaders must be present in the unit and demonstrate support of the team training initiative by providing positive messages about the initiative and positively reinforcing observed teamwork behaviors,[8]
- Collects key information on the success of the initiative by having managers ask these questions:

  – What is working in our initiative?
  – What needs to be fixed?
  – Who should I thank for doing a good job?
  – Do you have everything you need to make this successful?

- Analyze and act on the information collected during Rounding. Leaders should make sure there is a formal feedback program for the

information obtained during these Rounds. Managers must fix what needs to be corrected and ensure their efforts and improvement results are publicized to their personnel.

- Reward positive behavior that is helpful to your teamwork training initiative. Be especially alert for significant examples of supportive behavior from champions and difference makers. When discovered during Rounding, send personalized "thank you" notes, write letters of appreciation for personnel files, and recognize individuals during departmental meetings.

Staff members want to know the effort they are expending on this initiative is important. The presence and interest of their managers and leaders signifies its importance. Additionally, they want to know that what they are doing has an impact and makes a difference to their patients. Rounding enables leaders to collect the anecdotal success stories for publication and dissemination.

Sustainability Tip #6: Leadership Must Embrace and Conduct Coaching to Improve Performance, Including Imposing Consequences for Poor Performance.

Research shows that in the typical healthcare organization 34% improve performance after training and stay at their new level, 58% improve and stay there if their performance is reinforced, and 8% do not improve.[8] Everyone must be held accountable as professionals for their behavior and impact on the organization. Leaders as coaches notice and praise high team performers and are obligated to coach low performers to change. If performance doesn't improve over time, consequences through termination are recommended. By hanging on to the low performer, leaders sabotage the sustainability of their team training initiative.

What you permit, you promote. Toxic colleagues who are allowed to persist with low performance cause 48% of your staff to decrease the quality of their work and 78% decrease the level of their commitment to the initiative.[9] Failing to impose consequences on low performers causes those who support your training initiative to be pulled backward, and your champions become frustrated. Dealing with low performers is one of the most critical leadership actions required for sustainability of training.

Sustainability Tip #7: Ensure Safety and Teamwork Become Part of the Corporate Mission or Annual Goals.

Behavioral change begins and is sustained when organizational leadership communicates its vision for the role of teamwork in achieving safe and quality care. Sustained individual behavior change is more likely to occur when the strategic priorities and mission are clearly communicated. Written corporate mission statements, yearly goals, and other organizational commitments must include an emphasis on teamwork and its role safety and quality. Institutions have little chance of convincing their medical staff and employees of their serious commitment to teamwork and safety without the willingness to put that commitment in writing.

Here are a few examples of mission or vision statements from hospitals that have successfully sustained their teamwork training improvements over time:

General Hospital provides care that is safe, efficient, patient-centered, timely, effective, and equitable. To do this, we will excel technically, be experts in teamwork, and follow our policies, procedures, and protocols to provide the highest standard of care.

Memorial Hospital provides safe, efficient, and compassionate care of the highest standard through teamwork, technical proficiency, and adhering to guidelines, policies, and procedures.

Notice that both examples include the concept of "teamwork." Teamwork must become part of mission statements, yearly goals, and other written commitments because executive performance assessment and compensation tend to follow those corporate goals (as discussed in Sustainability Tip #9). The more closely aligned the written corporate goals are with your training initiative, the more executive assessment systems will be aligned

with your teamwork training program, and the more focus and attention your leaders will give the effort.

Sustainability Tip #8: Safety and Quality Metrics Must Be Part of the Dashboard Used to Measure Performance.

Many hospitals today use a dashboard system of metrics to gauge their financial and clinical health. Dashboards must also include metrics that include teamwork-based safety and quality issues. Measurement and transparency drive accountability and allow leaders and staff to adjust their actions to get the results they want. Data collection and analysis also allows the organization to objectively hold individuals accountable for results. Last, including teamwork-based safety measures in the corporate or unit dashboard allows alignment of daily behaviors to the goals of your initiative. If teamwork-based safety performance is not measured, organizations will not get the behaviors they need to make the initiative a success. As results improve, passion is ignited in the organization for the initiative, and sustainability becomes easier.

Here is an example of how the failure to include safety and quality issues in the corporate dashboard affected organizational performance. As we began our work with one large hospital in the south, not one dashboard metric covered safety or quality issues. Every single metric focused on efficiency, throughput, or profitability. It came as no surprise when we discovered the hospital had one patient-harming event in surgery every 60 days. The staff was clearly rushing and focusing on throughput, trying to respond to what was important to leadership. Leaders wanted more throughput to compensate for the reduction in reimbursement rates. By driving the staff to see more cases, the hospital generated more revenue on the front end, but they were losing much of that revenue on the back end in errors and claims. Realizing this, the leadership changed their dashboard to include safety and quality metrics.

A typical example of a dashboard for a successful teamwork-based patient safety initiative is shown in Table 15.1.

Table 15.1 Example of Data Collection and Analysis Plan	
Goal/Outcome	**Measure**
A. Safety/Quality Outcomes	1. Reduce surgical error.
	2. Eliminate operating room sentinel events.
	3. Eliminate wrong surgeries.
	4. Reduce post op infections.
	5. Increase compliance with pre-op antibiotics.
B. Teamwork and Communication	1. Improvement in Employee Satisfaction Scores.
	2. Improved physician satisfaction.
	3. Decreased turnover among staff.
	4. Improved patient satisfaction.
	5. Decreased vacancy rate.
C. Efficiency	1. Operating room turnaround times.
	2. Improved first procedure start times
	3. Decreased instances of required equipment not there or not operable.
D. Reliability/Standardization	1. 100% compliance and use of Hardwired Safety Tools.
	2. Decreased specimen errors.
	3. Decrease in returns to surgery.

Sustainability Tip #9: Executive Assessment and Reward Systems Must Be Aligned with Teamwork-Based Safety Initiatives.

Teamwork training initiatives must have continual management attention and focus to be sustained over time. Therefore, executives and managers must be held accountable, and rewarded, for meeting the goals of the initiative. Without alignment between your organizational teamwork training goals and individual performance assessment and reward, management attention will drift and become devoted to what is assessed and rewarded. Managers will pay attention to the projects that affect their personal performance evaluations.

An organization might want to see a 20% improvement in compliance with the Universal Protocol, but if a manager's evaluation is not tied to this metric, the increase is merely a nice idea—not a "must do" for that manager. If, however, the manager's assessment system is revised to reflect that increased compliance in the department becomes 10% of her evaluation, the initiative will get constant leadership attention. There is a simple principle at play here—behavior

that gets rewarded gets repeated. Sustained organizational change requires the ongoing support of leadership.[2]

Sustainability Tip #10: Physicians Must Be Actively Recruited as "Partners" in Support of the Teamwork-Based Safety and Quality Program.

Physicians play a critical role in the sustainment of teamwork-based training initiatives. They are clinical workplace leaders, set the example of teamwork, and influence the standards of conduct for the organization. Without their active support and partnership, few facilities are able to sustain their training improvements. The physician who treats his or her patient with care, cooperation, and effective communication when working with that patient, but otherwise displays a complete lack of teamwork and collaboration with the staff will undermine the clinical team's ability to sustain the teamwork training initiative.

Leaders of the training program cannot allow physicians to sit on the sidelines and wait for the training program to bear fruit. They must convince physicians of the need for their commitment from the very beginning of the initiative, and that their influence, example, and leadership are critical to sustained success. In our experience, following a strategy of "Let's train everyone else and hope the physicians come onboard later" is not a winning game plan. Sustainable training initiatives follow these steps in creating and supporting physician partners:

- Provide the "evidence" for teamwork—the data and literature that support teamwork training as a method to improve processes and clinical outcomes.
- Insist on physician involvement in experiential, skills-based teamwork training. Prescriptive training conducted with the rest of the clinical team is critical for performance improvement.
- Provide feedback on performance data collected and analyzed to measure progress of the training initiative. Ensure that your physicians can see the results of their efforts in a systematic and comparative way.
- Recruit physician champions to the cause and equip them with the "scripting" and data to conduct one-on-one conversations with their peers. The support of respected physicians for the team training program is crucial in the informal process of convincing physician colleagues to make practice pattern changes.
- Ensure physicians are crystal clear about your organization's behavioral expectations resulting from your teamwork training program. "Over communicate" your revised Mission, Values, and behavioral standards. Where needed, revise Med Exec By-Laws to include verbiage supporting your teamwork behaviors and ensure these are well communicated to all physicians.
- Create patient demand for teamwork by making your patients aware of the collaborative role you expect them to play. Patient expectations for teamwork can have a tremendous influence on physician behavior.
- Reward and recognize supportive physician behavior discovered during Rounding and observations.

Sustainability Tip #11: Revise the Policy and Procedures Manual and Other Unit Documents to Include Teamwork and Behavioral Guidelines.

If the hospital desires specific teamwork and communication behaviors from its physicians and staff it must put those expectations in writing. Policy and procedure manuals and other written documents governing how work gets done should contain behavioral guidelines for teamwork, communication, coordination, decision making, and performance feedback. These written policies drive procedures and practices on a daily basis. Including these performance guidelines creates alignment among the organization's philosophy, as expressed in their mission statement, their written policies, and the daily practices of the staff. Employees are keen to discern any disconnects among the mission, value, policies, and actual daily work practices. If the organization is unwilling to create policies supporting the new teamwork-based safety initiatives, there is great risk that the effort will fail. Changing the policies is a way for leadership to commit publicly, in writing, to the necessary changes.

It is difficult to implement any sense of the standards of teamwork behavior until the standards are clearly articulated. By revising the documents that govern how work is done, the organization is simply saying, "This is how we do things here." Including behavioral guidelines for teamwork and collaboration helps create a system in which teamwork is not dependent on which team or which department chooses to use them, but rather all teams in all departments all of the time will have the same behavioral standards.

Here are examples of policy statements a hospital inserted into its policy and procedures manual to support training sustainment:

> *All members of the surgical services team at General Hospital will be trained in teamwork skills and are expected to use these teamwork skills in their daily work and in their professional communication with other members of the General Hospital healthcare organization.*

It is the personal responsibility of each member of the team to cross-check other members of the team.

Any Red Flags, or potentially unsafe or nonstandard situations shall be brought to the attention of the team and team leader in a respectful but assertive manner.

Sustainability Tip #12: Employed Physicians, Nursing, and Staff Member Evaluation Systems Must Include Teamwork and Communication Behavior Metrics.

Most of the assessment systems in use in healthcare organizations have a heavy emphasis on clinical performance and procedure. Few assessment systems evaluate communication and teamwork behaviors. True change in support for teamwork training programs in aviation organizations did not occur until flight crews were assessed on their teamwork skills, and the same is true for healthcare personnel. What is assessed becomes important to those being evaluated. The evaluation system becomes the linking bridge between the employee and the organization's goals. Changing the evaluation system changes the employee.

Additionally, the assessment program can feed valuable data back to the training program so that future teamwork training targets areas of need as indicated by data analysis.

Sustainability Tip #13: Institute a System to Capture Teamwork–Based Safety Program Successes and Publicize Those to the Organization.

The culture of silence is so pervasive in many healthcare organizations that most departments have no idea of their actual safety record. For instance, many of the surgical departments with which we have worked are shocked to find out that their department has had a record of wrong surgeries. That culture of silence also prevents many institutions from documenting and publicizing those instances in which a staff member did assertively speak up and prevent an impending adverse outcome.

Without transparency of unit performance or awareness of the unit track record, many staff members will see no reason to do anything differently. As well, if the staff never sees the results of the effort they have invested in the new safety initiatives, they see no reason to continue that effort. In short, success breeds success. The institution must absolutely capture, document, and publicize data documenting improvements in safety and quality to sustain their teamwork training program.

CONCLUSION

Sustaining the gains in performance resulting from teamwork training programs is best accomplished by creating an organizational culture supporting the teamwork, communication, and collaboration behaviors provided by the training initiative. Table 15.2 summarizes the steps to improve sustainability.

Culture change begins with providing effective, skills-based, and interdisciplinary team training to the organization. Effective teamwork training programs also include periodic refresher training to prevent atrophy of skills, and new-hire training to equip new employees with the same skills possessed by incumbent staff.

Sustainability is also dependent on the ability of the organization to hardwire teamwork behaviors into daily work life. Successful training initiatives equip physicians and staff with the skills to create and employ customized, site-specific safety tools such as checklists, communication scripts, and standard operating procedures to make it easy to do the right thing, and hard to use the wrong behavior. Hardwiring behavior is an iterative process, and hardwiring tools must be constantly refined by those who use them.

Finally, and most importantly, sustainability is primarily a function of specific leadership actions and the changes made to the organizational structure by those leaders. Only leadership can blast through the many sources of organizational inertia. Only leadership can motivate the actions needed to alter behavior in any significant way. Only leadership can get change to stick, by anchoring it in the very culture of the organization. Key leadership actions to change the culture are Rounding, coaching low performers, terminating hard-core resistors when needed, recruiting physician champions, and collecting, analyzing, and publishing performance data documenting the effect of the training initiative.

Table 15.2   Steps to Improve Sustainability

1. Provide teamwork and communication skills training to all clinicians and staff (including physicians) involved in providing care.
2. Conduct periodic refresher training on teamwork skills.
3. Conduct new-hire training.
4. Create and implement customized, site-specific safety tools thoughtfully adapted from high reliability organizations (e.g. checklists, communications scripting, standard operation procedures).
5. Ensure managers and administrators "round" on departments that have implemented teamwork training and safety tools.
6. Embrace and conduct coaching to improve performance, including imposing consequences for poor performance.
7. Ensure safety and teamwork become part of the corporate mission or annual goals.
8. Include safety and quality metrics on the dashboard used to measure organizational performance.
9. Align executive assessment and reward systems with teamwork-based safety initiatives.
10. Actively recruit physicians as "partners" in support of the teamwork-based safety and quality program.
11. Revise the policy and procedures manual and other unit documents to include teamwork and behavioral guidelines.
12. Include teamwork and communication behavior metrics on performance evaluation systems for employed physicians, nurses, and other staff members.
13. Institute a system to capture teamwork-based safety program successes and publicize those to the organization.

In summary, sustainability is not the result of any single strategy, but the combinative effect of proven steps to create a culture that supports and rewards the use of teamwork behaviors.

REFERENCES

1. Beukelman, D. (1990). Information alone does not change behavior. *Michigan Consortium on Assistive Device Delivery Systems: Resource Directory.* 2nd ed. (pp. 79–82). Lansing, MI: PAM Assistance Centre.
2. Kotter, J., & Cohen, D.S. (2002). *The heart of change: Real life stories of how people change their organization.* Boston: Harvard Business School Press.
3. Helmreich, R., Merritt, A., & Wilhelm, J. (1999). The evolution of crew resource management training in commercial aviation. *The International Journal of Aviation Psychology, 9*(1), 19–32.
4. Beeson, S. (2006). *Practicing excellence.* Gulf Breeze, FL: Fire Starter Publishing.
5. Jones, K. D. (2001). The impending crisis in healthcare. *The Internet Journal of Healthcare Administration,* 1(2). Available at: http://www.ispub.com:80/journal/the-internet-journal-of-healthcare-administration/volume-1-number-2/the-impending-crisis-in-healthcare.html
6. Sarafino, E. P. (2001). *Behavior modification* (2nd ed.) Boston: McGraw-Hill.
7. Tannebaum, S. I., & Yukl, G. (1992). Training and development in work organizations. *Annual Review of Psychology, 43,* 399–441.
8. Studer, Q. (2008). *Results that last.* Hoboken, NJ: John Wiley & Sons.
9. Porath, C., & Pearson, C. (2009). *How toxic colleagues corrode performance.* Cambridge, MA: Harvard Business Review.

PART FOUR

THE SCIENCE OF TEAM TRAINING

16

DOES TEAM TRAINING WORK? WHERE IS THE EVIDENCE?

Tripp Driskell, Elizabeth H. Lazzara, Eduardo Salas, Heidi B. King, and James B. Battles

On the mountains of truth you can never climb in vain: either you will reach a point higher up today, or you will be training your powers so that you will be able to climb higher tomorrow.

—Friedrich Nietzsche

INTRODUCTION

Over the past couple of decades, an increasing amount of attention has been focused on teams and teamwork.[1-4] Increasingly, organizations have come to rely on teams to achieve desired organizational goals. In fact, organizations that do not rely on teams have become exceedingly rare. Because of the dependence on teams within organizations, teams have a direct role in determining performance and organizational outcomes. Thus, it is essential that the teams that fulfill vital roles within organizations perform effectively and efficiently.

There are various approaches to improving team effectiveness including selection, training, and design.[4-6] By almost any standards, team training has had a considerable record of successful application. It has been illustrated to be effective in many different areas, including military operations, aviation, and business. From early efforts of Briggs and Naylor[7] to more recent efforts of Cannon-Bowers and Salas[8], much has been learned about team performance and team training. In addition, there is evidence to suggest team training has a significant, positive impact on key measures of aviation performance[9,10] and business performance.[11,12] We know a great deal more about team training and its effectiveness than we did a decade ago. However, although extensive amounts of literature exist on the effectiveness of team training in different arenas, the effectiveness of team training—specific to healthcare—is relatively limited.

The importance placed on team training in healthcare has been well documented throughout this book. With healthcare organizations facing an increase in competition and collaboration; a need exists to engage a mixed workforce; a need to embrace developments in information technology; and a need to increase patient and employee safety.[13,14] The demand to foster these changes is essential in a healthcare organization where negative outcomes have the potential to cost human lives.

In comparison with aviation and the military, medicine has notably "arrived late" in adopting a team level perspective on performance effectiveness.[15,16] Perhaps as a consequence of the high status that the primary care physician has held in our culture, people have tended to view healthcare as an individual level phenomenon. In other words, traditionally, when we think of healthcare, we tend to think of the actions of a single person, perhaps aided by others. However, as this book attests, this view has changed, and the healthcare community has adopted the team level perspective on enhancing performance effectiveness wholeheartedly. Moreover, healthcare is unique in that it has great potential for catastrophic outcomes. To this end, patient and employee safety is directly impacted by teamwork and team performance. Moreover, the relationship between teamwork and patient outcomes is illustrated by a recent RAND report.[17] This report reviewed 16 empirical studies and support for the link between teamwork behaviors (e.g., coordination, shared goals, debriefing, etc.) and clinical patient outcomes (e.g., risk-adjusted mortality, adverse events, complications, etc.). As the understanding of this link has developed, so to has the importance of optimizing teamwork in healthcare organizations. Team training has been adopted as the strategy of choice for optimizing teamwork. Moreover, it has become a focused effort, especially with the release of the TeamSTEPPS program by the Department of Defense and the Agency for Healthcare Research and Quality. However, healthcare is an evidence-based field; therefore, evidence that team training works is vital to its acceptance. This evidence is required to increase the buy-in from the healthcare community.

Despite existing evidence that demonstrates the effectiveness of team training, we would not expect healthcare professionals to simply accept these innovations with open arms. This concern harkens back to the problems identified in innovation adoption by the US Department of Agriculture in the 1950s. They found that when introducing a new hybrid seed, the users (i.e., farmers) were not just passive recipients of information but actively evaluated and made decisions regarding these new technologies. This led to the demise of the "better mousetrap" theory; that if you built a better mousetrap, the world would beat a path to your door. Instead, they concluded that without a concerted effort to engage the users in innovation acceptance, potentially useful innovations could easily fall by the wayside. The point is that user acceptance of a new innovation should not be assumed. Users from farmers to healthcare providers are actively involved in determining whether a potential innovation is of value to meet their needs. Therefore, chapters such as this one are tools that can be used to make this case—to demonstrate the value of team training for healthcare.

The purpose of this chapter is to document what is known about the evidence-based effectiveness of team training. The following sections of this chapter are organized as follows. We first present the evidence for the overall effectiveness of team training, reviewing two relevant metaanalyses on team training effectiveness. Second, we review one industry in which team training has been successfully implemented—the application of crew resource management (CRM) in aviation—and discuss the relevance of lessons learned in this industry to healthcare. Third, we will present the evidence for the effectiveness of team training, specific to healthcare. We examine the evidence in terms of Kirkpatrick's four levels of evaluation: (1) reactions, (2) learning, (3) behavior, and (4) results.[18]

In brief, this chapter will attempt to answer the following questions: Does team training work? Does team training impact patient safety? Does team training improve the work environment?

DOES TEAM TRAINING WORK?

The fundamental assumption of team training interventions is straightforward: Teams perform better when they participate in a training intervention directed toward the team as a whole. This assumption has been generally accepted, even with a noticeable lack of empirical evidence to support this statement. Team Training interventions have classically been delivered using one or more of the following instructional methods: information, demonstration, and practice. A brief description of each instructional method is provided below in Figure 16.1.

It was not until recently that researchers sought to provide a comprehensive empirical evaluation of team training interventions. Several recent

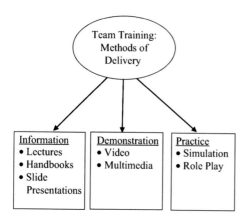

Figure 16.1
Team Training: Methods of Delivery

metaanalytic reviews have provided ample evidence of the benefits of several team training interventions developed to increase team effectiveness and team performance.[19,20] This section will review these metaanalyses of team training interventions and present the evidence that was found.

In a recent effort to summarize the relative contributions of several team training interventions, Salas et al. conducted a metaanalysis on this topic.[19] Specifically, they investigated the efficacy of three team training strategies: namely, cross training, coordination and adaptation training, and guided team self-correction training. The researchers found evidence suggesting that for the overall database, team training lead to a significant improvement in team performance. This overall finding was not moderated by the type of measurement (i.e., objective versus subjective). When the researchers examined each type of measurement separately, there remained a significant trend for team training to improve team performance.

This overall effect supports the ideology that team training improves team performance. However, the researchers were interested in more than an overall effect. They were interested in the extent to which the specific strategies of team training (i.e., cross training, coordination and adaptation training, and guided team self-correction training) had an effect on team training. *Cross-training* refers to a team training intervention where team members are trained on each others jobs in order to develop an understanding of the knowledge, skills and attitudes (KSAs) required to successfully perform the tasks of other team members.[21] The aim of cross-training is to provide team members with a general understanding of the team's task and how each individual's role is important to it. *Team coordination and adaptation training* refers to a team training intervention developed to train teams to adapt to demands by shifting from explicit to implicit modes of coordination, in addition to selecting appropriate strategies during high stress (e.g., acute and sustained) and high workload conditions.[22] Team coordination and adaptation training is proposed to modify a team's coordination strategy, while reducing the degree of communication required to successful perform tasks. Finally, guided *team self-correction training* refers to a team training intervention in which team members learn to identify and diagnose the complications and to develop effective solutions through event review, error identification, feedback, and planning.[23] Guided team self-correction training is proposed to promote correct expectations (i.e., shared mental models) among team members, subsequently enhancing team performance and team behaviors. Focusing on these three specific training strategies, Salas and colleagues found that both guided team self-correction and team coordination and adaptation training significantly improved team performance, whereas cross-training did not. The researchers noted in their findings that the relative contributions of these team training strategies may be unclear because of covariance among the specific strategies. Taking this concern into account, the researchers applied statistical techniques in an effort to more accurately gauge the independent contributions of the three team training strategies. Results bore this out. Cross-training and guided team self-correction training did not make an independent contribution to the effectiveness of team training. However, team coordination and adaptation training was shown to make a significant independent contribution to the effectiveness of team training. See Table 16.1 for results.

Summary

These results suggest that having team members to rotate positions during (i.e., cross-training) may not be the ideal team training intervention, especially for healthcare where individual roles can be very

Table 16.1   Team Training Metaanalysis

Outcome Type	Team Training Component			Overall	Overall Summary of Findings		
	Cross Training	Team Coordination and Adaptation Training	Guided Team Self-correction Training		Small	Moderate	Strong
Performance (r)	−0.09	0.45	0.61	0.29	☑	☑	
Objective Performance (r)	–	–	–	0.28	☑	☑	
Subjective Performance (r)	–	–	–	0.34		☑	

Source: Salas, E., Nichols, D. R., & Driskell, J. E. (2007). Testing three team training strategies in intact teams: A meta-analysis. Small Group Research, 38, 471–88.

specialized. Moreover, having team members identify and diagnose team complications, and develop and implement effective strategies (i.e., guided team self-correction training) may result in an improvement in team performance, but may not be the optimal team training intervention. However, the results suggest that an optimal team training intervention seems to involve team members being trained to modify their coordination strategy, subsequently reducing the amount of required communication during team performance (cf. Burke et al. for a review[24]). Team coordination and adaptation training is proposed to assist team members learning about teamwork skills, as well as how to optimize periods of low demand by predicting and discussing potential problems. The evidence from the metaanalysis on team training interventions indicates that team coordination and adaptation training is the most effective team training intervention.

In a metaanalysis aimed at building upon and expanding these findings, Salas et al. reviewed a database consisting of a total of 93 correlations from 45 primary studies.[20] The overall results supported the notion that team training does work. Specifically, for the combined set of independent outcomes, team training demonstrated a moderate, positive effect on team functioning. This metaanalytic integration was contructed on 52 effect sizes representing 1,563 teams. The results of the analyses revealed team training to have a positive effect on all four outcomes under examination: team-level cognitive outcomes, affective outcomes, process outcomes, and performance outcomes (Table 16.2).

The content of training interventions was examined as a potential moderating variable (i.e., taskwork, teamwork focus, mixed). Team training targeting taskwork seeks to develop the task related proficiencies of team members.[25] In comparison, team training targeting teamwork focus on improving how team members successfully work together as a team. Mixed training interventions utilize a mix of taskwork and teamwork content. Overall, although each team training intervention was shown to be useful (Table 16.3), however, there was insufficient evidence to conclude that mixed content interventions were superior to taskwork or teamwork interventions in isolation. Moreover, taskwork, teamwork, or mixed training content interventions showed little variability in respects to improvements in performance. However, for process outcomes (e.g., improved team behaviors), taskwork training was shown to be inferior to teamwork or mixed content training. Similarly, teamwork focused training was shown to result in enhanced affective outcomes (e.g., attitudes and assessed worth of training) in comparison with taskwork training respectively. Caution should be taken by the reader in the interpretation made on the estimated correlation for taskwork content on affective outcomes, because it is was based on one point estimate and did not take into account the calculated error range for their results.

In addition, Salas and colleagues looked at the effects of team stability (i.e., intact versus ad hoc) on team training effectiveness. There was no clear evidence that the effectiveness of team training was limited to one type of team in comparison to the other.

Table 16.2   Analysis of Effectiveness of Team Training Based on Outcome Type

Outcome Type	Number of Teams	Mean Observed Correlation(r)	Summary of Findings		
			Small	Moderate	Strong
Cognitive	554	0.38		☑	
Affective	465	0.32		☑	
Process	607	0.39		☑	
Performance	1,024	0.33		☑	
All outcomes	1,563	0.34		☑	

Source: Salas, E., DiazGranados, D., Klein, C., Burke, S., Stagl, K. C., Goodwin, G. F., Halpin, S. M. (2008). Does team training improve performance? A meta-analysis. *Human Factors, 50*, 903–33.

Table 16.3   Analysis of the Effectiveness of Team Training Based on Training Content

Training Content	Outcome Type	Number of Teams	Mean Observed Correlation(r)	Summary of Findings		
				Small	Moderate	Strong
Taskwork	Cognitive	242	0.28	☑	☑	
	Affective	90	0.10	☑		
	Process	145	0.27	☑	☑	
	Performance	240	0.35		☑	
Teamwork	Cognitive	86	0.52			☑
	Affective	326	0.37		☑	
	Process	236	0.40		☑	
	Performance	374	0.35		☑	
Mix	Cognitive	226	0.45		☑	
	Affective	49	0.36		☑	
	Process	226	0.47		☑	
	Performance	410	0.30		☑	

Source: Salas, E., DiazGranados, D., Klein, C., Burke, S., Stagl, K. C., Goodwin, G. F., Halpin, S. M. (2008). Does team training improve performance? A meta-analysis. *Human Factors, 50*, 903–33.

For performance outcomes, team training appeared to work as effectively for intact teams as for ad hoc teams. The results for process outcomes were similar for intact and ad hoc teams.

The studies included in the metaanalysis were also divided into three categories as a result of the average size of the teams under investigation (small, medium, and large). This was done in order to determine the potential moderating effect of team size on team training effectiveness. The results suggest that team size was a significant moderator. Team training, for instance, was shown to impact cognitive outcomes to a larger extent in medium sized teams. Alternatively, compared to medium and large teams, small teams benefited the most in terms of improvements in affective and process outcomes.

SUMMARY

The findings from the above metaanalysis provide insight into the extent to which team training interventions relate to team outcomes. Specifically, team training efforts were successful across a wide variety of settings, tasks, and team types. The findings suggest that team training works, and that team training interventions are a sensible approach for organizations to adopt in order to improve team outcomes. These results suggest that team training interventions are useful for improving cognitive outcomes, affective outcomes, teamwork processes, and performance outcomes. The metaanalysis showed that team training accounted for 12% to 19% of the variance in the outcomes under investigation. The authors note that this percentage is likely an underestimate of the theoretical and practical significance of the relationships between the variables investigated in the metaanalysis.[26]

APPLICATIONS: AVIATION/CREW RESOURCE MANAGEMENT

Similar to healthcare organizations, within the aviation environment, deficits in teamwork are both unwelcome and frequently highly publicized, and can lead to dire consequences. The aviation industry introduced Crew Resource Management (CRM) training in an attempt to mitigate some of the consequences of failed teamwork, in addition to the subsequent safety concerns.[27,28] The aim of CRM training was to train aircrews to use all resources available to them (e.g., equipment, people, information) through effective team communication and coordination. Currently, CRM enjoys over 30 years of active application, and has necessarily undergone numerous evolutions coinciding with advancements in science and technology.[29-31] The aviation industry represents an example of an industry that has adopted a team training perspective with a positive response from users and proven effectiveness. Moreover, the aviation industry acts as an excellent source of lessons learned for the application of team training to healthcare.

The aviation community has invested a considerable amount of resources into developing and implementing CRM training. As with any investment, it is important to be aware of the return on investment. For the aviation industry, that return should provide evidence that CRM has improved, or has failed to improve, team performance. As reported by Salas et al., the data supporting the effectiveness of CRM are encouraging.[6] Not without its critics,[32-34] reviews by Salas and colleagues[9,35] conclude that evidence supporting the benefits of CRM training exists. Specifically, evidence suggests that CRM training is an effective intervention at certain levels of evaluation (e.g., attitudes), although the evidence is not as clear as it should be after 30 years. The dearth of research illustrating cause and effect is a significant limitation. Even so, given that CRM training is an essential factor that may affect the practice and effectiveness of team behaviors, the data supporting CRM training effectiveness are encouraging. Specifically, CRM training has generally resulted in positive reactions from trainees, improved learning, and has encouraged desired behavioral changes.[35]

RELEVANCE TO HEALTHCARE

As previously mentioned, healthcare is unique in that failure to perform effectively as a team (or individual) has the potential for catastrophic outcomes. Teams in healthcare (e.g., rapid response teams, intensive care units, etc.) work in an environment that is dynamic, stressful, and where increased importance is placed on making correct decisions. Healthcare is a prime example of a high-reliability organization. High-reliability organizations are those organizations that are required to function in

dangerous, dynamic, fast-paced, and complex systems, at or near, error-free for an extended length of time.[36] In addition to healthcare, aviation and military operations also constitute this type of environment. The medical community could appreciably improve medical team training by applying lessons learned from aviation and CRM. In addition, the medical community can look to other fields where team training interventions have been implemented and have proven to be successful. Moreover, the healthcare community can apply research that has examined individual and team performance under stress.[37,38] Of particular interest to healthcare, the Tactical Decision-Making Under Stress (TADMUS) program is a good example of a line of research that can positively impact medical team training programs. TADMUS made great strides in elucidating the mechanisms in which individuals and teams make decisions during periods of stress.[8] Researchers have noted the similarities between the conditions studied under the TADMUS program and the conditions emergency management workers encounter.[39] Numerous medical team training programs have adopted CRM training principles as well as other team training principles into the design of team training programs. The following section will present the existing evidence for the effectiveness of team training interventions in healthcare.

DOES TEAM TRAINING WORK IN HEALTHCARE?

A vital question for healthcare organizations adopting a team training approach is whether or not these types of interventions produce desired outcomes. Historically, there has been much debate regarding the general impact of team training interventions.[23,40-44] However, numerous research reports and publications have championed the need to improve performance and safety in healthcare, identifying team training as a key component in achieving this goal.[45-49] In a review aimed at summarizing the present state of practice for healthcare team training, Weaver et al. conducted a qualitative review of 40 peer-reviewed empirical articles describing the evaluations of healthcare team training interventions.[50] Of the 40 reviewed articles, 27 (68%) reported evaluations at more than one level (i.e., reactions, learning, behavior, and organizational impact). Specifically, from these 40 articles, 24 (60%) collected reactionary data, four (10%) collected changes in learning, 25 (63%) evaluated behavior change, and 11 (28%) reported changes in trainee affective measures such as safety attitude surveys. The researchers question the validity of the methods used to evaluate behavior, noting that evaluation methods ranged from self-report measures to observations of team behavior. Lastly, 12 (30%) studies made an effort to evaluate organizational outcomes. A consolidated list of these articles by level of evaluation is presented in Table 16.4. Overall, the results demonstrated that healthcare programs clearly benefit from training interventions when they are predicated on the science of team training, learning theories, and theories of human performance. The qualitative review by Weaver et al. helps convey the message that to determine the effectiveness of team training programs for

healthcare, the first step is adopt a comprehensive approach to evaluating training effectiveness.[50]

By and large, the most commonly used framework for evaluating training is Kirkpatrick's typology.[18] Kirkpatrick presented a multilevel approach to evaluating training evaluation at four levels: (1) reactions, (2) learning, (3) behavior (i.e., extent of performance change), and (4) results (i.e., organizational impact). Within recent years, this typology has been expanded by several researchers.[92,92] For purposes of this chapter, we will use Kirkpatrick's typology for training evaluation, because it is the most well-known and widely accepted model for measuring the effectiveness of training programs.[18] Specifically, the following sections are organized by the type of training evaluation. (i.e., reaction, learning, behavior, and organizational impact).

As a result of the patient safety crisis identified by the Institute of Medicine, a proliferation of medical team training programs (MTT) have been developed

Table 16.4	Levels of Evaluation
Reactions	Blum et al. (2005), Cole and Cambell (1986), Dunn et al. (2007), Flanagan et al. (2004), Flin et al. (2007), France et al. (2005), Gaba et al. (1998), Grogan et al. (2004), Haller et al. (2008), Haycock-Stuart and Houston (2005), Le Blanc et al. (2007), Moorthy et al. (2006), Morey et al. (2002), O'Donnell et al. (1998), Østergaard et al. (2004), Paige et al. (2009), Reznek et al. (2003), Robertson et al. (2009), Sehgal et al. (2008), Shapiro et al. (2004), Sica et al. (1999), Stroller et al. (2004), Wallin et al. (2007), Weaver et al. (2010b), Youngblood et al. (2008)
Learning	Ammentorp et al. (2007), Blum et al. (2005), France et al. (2005), Gibson (2001), Grogan et al. (2004), Haller et al. (2008), Haycock-Stuart and Houston (2005), Morey et al. (2002), Østergaard et al. (2004), Paige et al. (2009), Pratt et al. (2007), Robertson et al. (2009), Sax et al. (2009), Stroller et al. (2004), Wallin et al. (2007), Weaver et al. (2010b), Youngblood et al. (2008)
Behavior	Awad et al. (2005), Berkenstadt et al. (2008), Blum et al. (2005), Cashman et al. (2004), Cooley (1994), DeVita et al. (2005), Dunn et al. (2007), Gaba et al. (1998), Gibson (2001), i Gardi et al. (2001), Jacobsen et al. (2001), Moorthy et al. (2006), Morey et al. (2002), Murray et al. (2006), Nielsen et al. (2007), Østergaard et al. (2004), Paull et al. (2009), Robertson et al. (2009), Sax et al. (2009), Shapiro et al. (2004), Sica et al. (1999), Stroller et al. (2004), Taylor et al. (2007), Wallin et al. (2007), Weaver et al. (2010b), Youngblood et al. (2008)
Organizational	Dunn et al. (2007), Jacobsen et al. (2001), Le Blanc et al. (2007), Marshall and Manus (2007), Moorthy et al. (2006), Morey et al. (2002), Nielsen et al. (2007), Pratt et al. (2007), Sax et al. (2009), Taylor et al. (2007), Weaver et al. (2010b)

Source: Adapted from Weaver SJ, Lyons R, DiazGranados D, et al. (2010a). The anatomy of health care team training and the state of practice: A critical review. Academic Medicine, 85(11), 1746–60.

and implemented within healthcare organizations.[15] The MTT programs have been implemented in both military and civilian medicine and range from specialty-specific programs (e.g., anesthesia, obstetrics) to more general programs (e.g., medical emergency team). The bulk of MTT programs fall within two specific categories: simulator-based programs and traditional instructor classroom-based programs. We identify three major MTT simulator-based programs: Anesthesia Crisis Resource Management (ACRM), Team-oriented Medical Simulation (TOMS), and Multidisciplinary Obstetric Simulated Emergency Scenarios (MOSES). These programs employ patient simulators to train both individual and teamwork skills in a controlled safe environment. We identify six MTT classroom-based programs: TeamSTEPPS, MedTeamsTM, Medical Team Management (MTM), Dynamic Outcomes Management© (DOM, renamed LifewingsTM), Managing Obstetric Risk Efficiently OB (MORE OB), and Geriatric Interdisciplinary Team Training (GITT). These programs employ traditional instructional methods (e.g., lectures, PowerPoint, manuals, etc.). Despite the difference between the two categories of MTT programs, all are influenced to a large degree by CRM. Moreover, they share the common goal of mitigating medical errors through training teamwork-skills. Unfortunately, there has only been a relatively few number of studies that have evaluated the effectiveness of simulator or classroom based MTT programs. However, the studies that evaluate the effectiveness of these programs will be discussed in the following sections.

EVIDENCE ON TRAINING REACTIONS: DO HEALTHCARE PROFESSIONALS LIKE TEAM TRAINING?

The first level of Kirkpatrick's typology[18] is reaction evidence and reflects trainee's feelings and reactions in regards to a training intervention. Reaction data are measured after training and examine trainee's perceptions of training. Typically reaction data aims to examine if training is viewed as relevant, interesting, and valuable, amongst other perceptions.

On the basis of the available literature, findings revealed that, overall, healthcare professionals reacted positively to MTT programs. For example,

of the thousands of trainees who were exposed to ACRM training, the majority evaluated it positively.[94] Moreover, trainees reacted positively to ACRM's "death scenario," which is designed to evaluate how trainees manage a dying patient. Overall, trainees believed that ACRM training is an important factor in increasing safe practice of anesthesiology. Additionally, these beliefs were shown to last for up to 6 months after training.[94] Comparable participant reactions have been reported for TOMS. Similar to the simulator-based MTT, classroom-based MTT programs have yielded positive trainee reactions. In a study evaluating the effectiveness of the MedTeams project, Morey et al. found a significant increase in emergency department staff reactions toward teamwork, and staff assessments of institutional support significantly increased.[63] Furthermore, the general reaction to the content of TeamSTEPPS has been viewed favorably. Trainees reacted positively to the training in terms of both organization and practicality. For example, 81% had more confidence in their ability to work as an effective team member after training.[74] In addition, staff members have commented on the usefulness of the specific teamwork behaviors and skills being trained.[95] Research on the effectiveness of DOM has indicated that trainees attitudes toward the importance of teamwork in the operating room (OR) increased, as well as their view on the worth of DOM training.[96] In case study analyses of MedTeams, MTM, and DOM conducted by Baker et al., results suggested that participants had positive reactions to each of the three training programs.[97]

Summary

The above studies that evaluated trainee reactions to MTT programs lend considerable support to the conclusion that these programs generate positive reactions in healthcare organizations. In general, healthcare professionals have a positive response to training and view MTT as a valuable and suitable tool. While reaction data represents the simplest method of evaluation, it reflects the viewpoint of individuals, which is indispensible to a training programs successful adoption. Moreover, reaction data can drive higher-level evaluations of training and importantly, enhance a trainees motivation to learn.[9]

EVIDENCE ON LEARNING: DO HEATH CARE PROFESSIONALS LEARN DURING TEAM TRAINING?

Kirkpatrick's second level of evaluation, evaluation of learning, refers to "the principles, facts, and skills which were understood and absorbed by participants" (p. 11).[18] It is worth noting that this level of evaluation does not include displays of learned behaviors. Instead, evaluation of learning reflects the amount of learning that occurred during the training. Also measured in the evaluation of learning is the degree to which training leads to attitude change (e.g., positive attitudes towards MTT programs). Both changes in learning and attitude change are measured within this level of evaluation because each process mediates performance, and thusly, ought to be assessed together. The evaluation of learning provides direct evidence that the training program was or was not impacting targeted KSAs, in addition to developing relevant feedback and identifying areas that need of improvement.

Once we move away from reaction-type evidence and delve deeper into the levels of training evaluation, less literature is available that presents empirical evidence supporting or denying the efficacy of team training. In that learning evidence includes the degree to which training leads to attitude changes, a considerable amount of information exists regarding attitudinal changes in the healthcare literature. As mentioned in the previous section, overall reactions toward MTT programs are positive. Intuitively, if MTT programs are viewed positively by the trainees, there should also be an increase in desired attitudinal changes. Overall, research supports this claim. Grogan et al. demonstrated that an 8-hour didactic CRM course on teamwork improved operating room staff attitudes toward teamwork.[58] Specifically, Grogan et al. found that of 489 trainees, 95% of the respondents believed that CRM training would help mitigate errors in their practice. Moreover, responses to the Human Factors Attitude Survey developed by the researchers illustrated that training had a positive impact on managing fatigue, team building, communication, identifying adverse events, team decision-making, and performance feedback. In the research conducted to evaluate the MedTeams Project, Morey et al. found an improvement in staff attitudes toward team training.[63] Moreover, when MedTeams program principles were adopted by the Beth Israel Deaconess Medical Center (BIDMC) Labor and Delivery

unit, the L&D staff showed more positive attitudes about the unit's safety than the rest of the hospital.[78] Although plentiful evidence exists regarding attitude chances, few evaluations of MTT programs have measured improvements in learning. However, in one such evaluation of Team STEPPS, the researchers found that the training program participants did in fact achieve desired learning benchmarks.[74]

Summary

Although more data are needed to get a fuller understanding of the effectiveness of MTT on learning outcomes, the general trend is that MTT has a positive effect on this type of outcome. Sufficient evidence exists to support the notion that desired attitudinal changes are directly impacted by team training programs. Although initial results indicate that training interventions have a positive effect on knowledge and learning, more research is needed to make more generalizable and concrete conclusions.

EVIDENCE ON BEHAVIORAL CHANGE: DO HEALTHCARE PROFESSIONALS APPLY THE LEARNED TEAM TRAINING BEHAVIORS?

Evaluation of behavior represents the third level of Kirkpatrick's typology.[18] This level of evaluation provides an assessment of whether or not the learned KSAs transfer to observable changes in behavior. This level of training evaluation is important in that it provides: (1) an indication of the extent to which trainees learned how to perform the KSAs taught during training, in addition to when and where to apply the KSAs, and (2) a measure of trainee readiness and overall program effectiveness.[98]

The evidence for the effectiveness of MTT at the behavioral level has been well documented. Because of the suggestion by Cannon-Bowers et al.[98] that this level of evaluation indicates overall program effectiveness, and the reality that organizational outcomes are difficult to accurately measure, researchers have generally used behavioral outcomes as a final measure of training effectiveness. In the evaluation of MedTeams conducted by Morey et al., they found that the training program resulted in significant improvement in the quality of team behaviors.[54] Regarding team behavior of ACRM and TOMS, researchers evaluated a selection of important team skills through behavioral observation using skilled raters. Results indicated that both MTT programs effectively improved overall behavioral outcomes.[99,57] Furthermore, recent research illustrates that trainees' self-efficacy increases and self-reported anxiety decreases in ACRM training.[100] Awad and colleagues offered a training session involving didactic instruction, interactive participation, role-play, training films, and clinical vignettes to a surgical service by the Veterans Affairs National Center for Patient Safety exercising CRM principles.[80] The researchers developed a Likert scale survey to measure the effectiveness of communication between nurses, anesthesiologist, and surgeons. Results indicated that anesthesiologist and surgeon communication increased after the MTT program. The researchers concluded that MTT using CRM principles can improve communication in the operating room. Moreover, this increase in communication can lead to a safer environment, which can help mitigate errors. In the evaluation of Team STEPPS, Weaver et al. found an increased degree to which quality teamwork occurred in the OR suite.[74]

Summary

The findings from the aforementioned studies provide encouraging evidence that MTT programs positively impacts behavioral outcomes. Moreover, previous research on team training suggests that evidence offered at this level of evaluation is likely to positively impact overall program effectiveness.[98] Nevertheless, caution should still be taken when extrapolating from these results. There remains a need for more research to be conducted at this level of evaluation and beyond. At this point, the weight of available evidence lies in favor of MTT programs improving behavioral outcomes in healthcare.

EVIDENCE ON ORGANIZATIONAL IMPACT: IS HEALTHCARE SAFER BECAUSE OF TEAM TRAINING?

The final level of evaluation in Kirkpatrick's typology is organizational impact (e.g., increased safety, reduction in errors, monetary savings, etc.).[18]

Although this type of evidence is a terminal outcome of team training programs, few evaluations are conducted at the organizational level due to the difficult nature of evaluation.

Of the training programs that have been evaluated at this level, many have offered positive evidence of training effectiveness on organizational outcomes. In the evaluation of DOM training at the Methodist University Hospital, researchers found a 50% reduction in the number of surgical count errors.[96] However, the researchers identify several limitations to this evaluation. First, the researchers note that the small sample size affects external validity. Second, lack of a control group impacts internal validity. In other words, it is not possible to rule out other explanations for the founded results. When evaluating the MedTeams training, Morey et al. found a significant decrease in clinical error rate, from 30.9 % to 4.4%, concluding that the CRM based training is a fundamental factor in error reduction.[63] In addition, MedTeams research has demonstrated improved patient safety and satisfaction, in addition to a potential savings of $4 per patient visit. However, the findings should be interpreted with caution because the research was unable to apply random assigned to experimental and control groups, and the raters were not blind to experimental conditions. Shapiro et al. studied how the addition of simulation training to CRM training affected training outcomes in emergency department settings.[70] In this study, the experimental group with additional simulation education showed an increased error aversion by 67% and decreased observable errors by 58% as compared to the control group. Regarding Team STEPPS, the researchers noted that the training program demonstrated positive changes in patient safety culture.[74] An additional simulator-based training program, Advanced Cardiac Life Support (ACLS) training, found that after training, simulated survival (based on a predetermined criteria for death) increased from 0% to 89%. Moreover, results indicated that initial team task completion rate was 10% to 45% and appreciably increased to 80% to 95% throughout the third training session.[84] Most recently, Neily et al. evaluated the effects that a Veterans Health Administration's (VHA) national team training program had on patient outcomes.[101] Specifically, the researchers examined the relationship between the MTT program and the rate of change in the mortality rate. Specifically, these researchers examined mortality rate 1 year after the MTT program was implemented and compared this with the year prior to the MTT program. These researchers also investigate mortality rates at nontraining sites. Results from this study indicated that the 74 facilities that enrolled in the MTT program showed an 18% decrease in annual mortality compared with a 7% decrease amongst the 34 facilities that had not enrolled in training. Although this represents a veritable change, the risk-adjusted mortality rates at baseline were 17 per 1,000 procedures per year for the facilities enrolled in training and 15 per 1,000 procedures per year for the nontrained facilities. Moreover, results indicated that the mortality rates were equivalent for both groups, 14 per 1,000 procedures per year, at the end of the study. Additionally, propensity score matching illustrated that the decrease in the risk-adjusted mortality rate was approximately 50% greater in the trained facilities than in the nontrained facilities. A dose–response relationship for quarters of the MTT program resulted in a decrease of 0.5 deaths per 1,000 procedures for each additional quarter. Overall, the researchers concluded that enrollment in the VHA MTT program was related with lower surgical mortality.

Summary

Although evaluations do exist at this level, evidence is mixed and a clear picture of this level of training effectiveness is not achievable at this time. Although the results of most studies are encouraging, other studies have shown nonsignificant effects. For example, the MedTeams Labor and Delivery training resulted in no statistically significant differences between the intervention and control groups, or between any individual outcomes or most of the clinical process or outcome measures.[88] Overall, although few MTT evaluations have successfully assessed the impact of team training on organizational outcomes, the available evidence suggests that teamwork positively impacts patient outcomes. Nevertheless, better and more robust evaluations of MTT programs are required.

CONCLUDING REMARKS

In summary, few would argue the importance of teamwork in promoting safety and efficiency in healthcare. Moreover, the overall evidence that team training works and more specifically, it works in healthcare, is encouraging. Drawing from the available literature, team training is shown to be an effective instructional approach for improving teamwork in healthcare settings. In most cases, it evokes positive reactions, improves the knowledge, skills, and attitudes (KSAs) of its participants, improves behavior, and leads to positive organizational outcomes. The challenge to healthcare is to ensure training relevancy through careful design and development to create a proper learning environment for healthcare team members prior to selecting a training program. Moreover, training evaluation is a fundamental component in determining the effectiveness of team training interventions. In particular, multilevel evaluations help assess the impact of training programs on trainee reactions, learning, behavior, and on the impact to the organization. Within healthcare, multilevel evaluations can help shed light on how MTT programs impact patient safety. We commend those who take on this difficult but important task[63,70] and support future applications of multilevel evaluations. Although training evaluation measurement is often imperfect and even nonexistent in some cases, the data that exist are positive and should encourage further application of team training innovations in healthcare.

REFERENCES

1. Driskell, J. E., & Salas, E. (1992). Collective behavior and team performance. *Human Factors, 34,* 277–288.

2. Dyer, J. L. (1984). Team research and team training: A state-of-the-art review. In F. A. Muckler, A. S. Neal, & L. Strother (Eds.), *Human factors review* (pp. 285–323). Santa Monica, CA: Human Factors Society.

3. Hackman, J. R. (Ed.), (1990). *Groups that work (and those that don't): Creating conditions for effective teamwork.* San Francisco: Jossey-Bass.

4. Salas, E., Bowers, C. A., & Cannon-Bowers, J. A. (1995). Military team research: 10 years of progress. *Military Psychology, 7*(2), 55–75.

5. Salas, E., Rhodenizer, L., & Bowers, C. A. (2000). The design and delivery of crew resource

management training: Exploiting available resources. *Human Factors, 42,* 490–511.

6. Salas, E., Rozell, D., Mullen, B., & Driskell, J. E. (1999). The effect of team building on performance: An integration. *Small Group Research, 30,* 309–329.

7. Briggs, G. E., & Naylor, J. C. (1965). Team versus individual training, training task fidelity, and task organization effects on transfer performance by three-man teams. *Journal of Applied Psychology, 49,* 387–392.

8. Cannon-Bowers, J. A., & Salas, E. (Eds.), (1998). *Making decisions under stress: Implications for individual and team training.* Washington, DC: APA.

9. Salas, E., Burke, C. S., Bowers, C. A., & Wilson. K. A. (2001). Team training in the skies: Does crew resource management (CRM) training work? *Human Factors, 43,* 641–674.

10. Salas, E., Fowlkes, J. E., Stout, R. J., Milanovich, D. M., & Prince, C. (1999). Does CRM training improve teamwork skills in the cockpit? Two evaluation studies. *Human Factors, 41*(2), 326–343.

11. Arthur, W., Jr., Bennett, W., Jr., Edens, P. S., & Bell, S. T. (2003). Effectiveness of training in organizations: A metaanalysis of design and evaluation features. *Journal of Applied Psychology, 88,* 234–245.

12. George, G. C., Hannibal, M. J., & Hirsch, W. L. (2004). Building the brand through people. *World at Work Journal,* First Quarter, 39–45.

13. Noe, R. A. (2002). *Employee training and development.* Boston: McGraw-Hill.

14. Pfeffer, J., & Sutton, R. I. (2000). *The knowing-doing gap: How smart companies turn knowledge into action.* Boston: Harvard Business School Press.

15. Kohn, L. T., Corrigan, J. M., Donaldson, M. S. (1999). *To err is human: Building a safer health care system.* Washington DC: National Academy Press.

16. Miller, L. A. (2005). Patient safety and teamwork in perinatal care: Resources for clinicians. *Journal of Perinatal and Neonatal Nursing, 19*(1), 46–51.

17. Sorbero, M. E., Farley, D. O., Mattke, S., & Lovejoy, S. (2008). Outcome measures for effective teamwork in inpatient care (RAND technical report No: TR-462-AHRQ). Arlington, VA: RAND Corporation.

18. Kirkpatrick, D. L. (1976). Evaluation of training. In R. L. Craig (Ed.), *Training and development handbook: A guide to human resources development* (pp. 18.1–27). New York: McGraw-Hill.

19. Salas, E., Nichols, D. R., & Driskell, J. E. (2007). Testing three team training strategies in intact teams: A meta-analysis. *Small Group Research, 38,* 471–488.

20. Salas, E., DiazGranados, D., Klein, C., Burke, S., Stagl, K. C., Goodwin, G. F., Halpin, S. M. (2008). Does team training improve performance? A meta-analysis. *Human Factors, 50,* 903–933.

21. Cannon-Bowers, J. A., Salas, E., Blickensderfer, E., & Bowers, C. A. (1998). The impact of cross training and workload on team functioning: A replication and extension of initial findings. *Human Factors, 40,* 92–101.

22. Entin, E. E., & Serfaty, D. (1994). *Team adaptation and coordination training.* Unpublished technical report, Naval Air Warfare Center Training Systems Division, Orlando, FL.

23. Blickensderfer, E. L., Cannon-Bowers, J. A., & Salas, E. (1997). Theoretical bases for team self-corrections: Fostering shared mental models. In M. M. Beyerlein, D. A. Jackson, & S. T. Beyerlein (Eds.), *Advances in interdisciplinary studies of work teams,* 4th ed. (pp. 249–279). Greenwich, CT: JAI Press.

24. Burke, C. S., Stagl, K. C., Salas, E., Pierce, L., & Kendall, D. L. (2006). Understanding team adaptation: A conceptual analysis and model. *Journal of Applied Psychology, 91*(6), 1189–1207.

25. Salas, E., Dickenson, T. L., Converse, S. A., & Tannenbaum, S. I. (1992). Toward and understanding of team performance and training. In R. W. Swezey & E. Salas (Eds.), *Teams: Their training and performance* (pp. 3–29). Norwood, NJ: Ablex.

26. Hunter, J. E., & Schmidt, F. L. (1990). *Methods of meta-analysis: Correcting error and bias in research findings.* Newbury Park, CA: Sage.

27. Wiener, E. L., Kanki, B. G., & Helmreich, R. L. (Eds.), (1993). *Cockpit resource management.* CA: Academic Press.

28. Salas, E., Bowers, C. A., & Edens, E. (Eds.), (2001). *Improving teamwork in organizations: Applications of resource management training.* Hillsdale, NJ: LEA, Inc.

29. Helmreich, R. L., & Foushee, H. C. (1993). Why crew resource management? Empirical and theoretical bases of human factors in aviation. In E. L. Wiener, B. G. Kanki, & R. L. Helmreich (Eds.), *Cockpit resource management* (pp. 3–45). CA: Academic Press.

30. Helmreich, R. L., Merritt, A. C., Wilhelm, J. A. (1999). The evolution of crew resource management training in commercial aviation. *The International Journal of Aviation Psychology*, 9(1), 19–32.

31. Maurino, D. E. (1999). Safety prejudices, training practices, and CRM: A mid-point perspective. *International Journal of Aviation Psychology, 9*, 413–427.

32. Besco, R. O. (1997). The need for operational validation of human relations-centered CRM training assumptions. In R. S. Jensen & L. A. Rakovan (Eds.), *Proceedings of the 9th International Symposium on Aviation Psychology* (pp. 536–540). Columbus, OH: Ohio State University.

33. Simmon, D. A., Capt (Ret.) (1997). How to fix CRM. In R. S. Jensen & L. A. Rakovan, *Proceedings of the 9th International Symposium on Aviation Psychology* (pp. 550–553). Columbus, OH: Ohio State University.

34. Komich, J. (1997). CRM training: Which crossroads to take now? In R. S. Jensen & L. A. Rakovan (Eds.), *Proceedings of the 9th International Symposium on Aviation Psychology* (pp. 541–6). Columbus, OH: Ohio State University.

35. Salas, E., Wilson, K. A., Burke, C. S., & Wightman, D. (2006). Does CRM training work? An update, extension, and some critical needs. *Human Factors, 48*, 392–412.

36. Roberts, K. H. (1990). Some characteristics of one type of high reliability organization. *Organization Science, 1*(2), 160–177.

37. Driskell, J. E., & Johnston, J. H. (1998). Stress exposure training. In J. A. Cannon-Bowers & E. Salas (Eds.), *Making decisions under stress: Implications for individual and team training* (pp. 191–217). Washington, DC: American Psychological Association.

38. Saunders, T., Driskell, J. E., Johnston, J., & Salas, E. (1996). The effect of stress inoculation training on anxiety and performance. *Journal of Occupational Health Psychology, 1*, 170–186.

39. Schaafstal, A. M., Johnston, J. H., & Oser, R. L. (2001). Training teams for emergency management. *Computers in Human Behavior, 17*, 615–626.

40. Baker, D., Prince, C., Shrestha, L., Oser, R., & Salas, E. (1993). Aviation computer games for crew resource management training. *International Journal of Aviation Psychology, 3*, 143–156.

41. DeChurch, L. A., & Marks, M. A. (2003). *Teams leading teams: Examining the role of leadership in multi-team systems.* Unpublished doctoral dissertation. Florida International University: FL.

42. Entin, E. E., & Serfaty, D. (1999). Adaptive team coordination. *Human Factors, 41*, 312–325.

43. Marks, M. A., Sabella, M. J., Burke, C. S., & Zaccaro, S. J. (2002). The impact of cross-training on team effectiveness. *Journal of Applied Psychology, 87*, 3–13.

44. Smith-Jentsch, K. A., Salas, E., & Baker, D. P. (1996). Training team performance-related assertiveness. *Personnel Psychology, 49*, 909–936.

45. Barach, P., & Small, S. D. (2000). Reporting and preventing medical mishaps: Lessons from non-medical near miss reporting systems. *British Medical Journal, 320*, 759–763.

46. Barach, P., & Weinger, M. B. (2007). Trauma team performance. In W. C. Wilson, C. M. Grande & D. B. Hoyt (Eds.), *TRAUMA (Volume 1): Resuscitation, anesthesia and emergency surgery* (pp. 101–113). New York: Taylor & Francis.

47. Hamman, W. R. (2004). The complexity of team training: What we have learned from aviation and its applications to medicine. *Quality and Safety in Health Care, 13*, (Suppl. 1), i72–i79.

48. Leonard, M., Graham, S., & Bonacum, D. (2004). The human factor: The critical importance of effective teamwork and communication in providing safe care. *Quality & Safety in Health Care, 13*, i85–i90.

49. Leonard, M., & Tarrant, C. A. (2001). Culture, systems, and human factors—Two tales of patient safety: The KP Colorado region's experience. *The Permanente Journal, 5*, 46–49.

50. Weaver, S. J., Lyons, R., DiazGranados, D., Rosen, M., Salas, E., Oglesby, J., et al. (2010a). The anatomy of health care team training and the state of practice: A critical review. *Academic Medicine, 85*(11), 1746–1760.

51. Blum, R. H., Raemer, D. B., Carroll, J. S., Dufresnes, R. L., & Cooper, J. B. (2005). A method for measuring the effectiveness of simulation-based team training for improving communication skills. *Anesthesia & Analgesia, 100*, 1375–1380.

52. Cole, K. D., & Campbell, L. J. (1986). Interdisciplinary team training for occupational therapists. *Physical & Occupational Therapy in Geriatrics, 4*, 69–74.

53. Dunn, E. J., Mills, P. D., Neily, J., Crittenden, M. D., Carmack, A. L., & Bagian, J.P. (2007).

Medical team training: Applying crew resource management in the Veteran's Health Administration. *Joint Commission Journal on Quality and Patient Safety, 33,* 317–325.

54. Flanagan, B., Nestel, D., & Joseph, M. (2004). Making patient safety the focus: Crisis resource management in the undergraduate curriculum. *Medical Education, 38,* 56–66.

55. Flin, R., Yule, S., Paterson-Brown, S., Maran, N., Rowley, D., & Youngson, G. (2007). Teaching surgeons about non-technical skills. *The Surgeon, 5,* 86–89.

56. France, D. J., Stiles, R., Gaffney, F. A., Seddon, M. R., Grogan, E. L., Nixon, W. R., Jr., & Speroff, T. (2005). Crew resource management training— Clinicians' reactions and attitudes. *AORN Journal, 82,* 214–228.

57. Gaba, D. M., Howard, S. K., Flanagan, B., Smith, B. E., Fish, K. J., & Botney, R. (1998). Assessment of clinical performance during simulated crisis using both technical and behavioral ratings. *Anesthesiology, 89,* 3–18.

58. Grogan, E. L., Stiles, R. A., France, D. J., Speroff, T., Morris, J. A., Jr., Nixon, B., et al. (2004). The impact of aviation-based teamwork training on the attitudes of health-care professionals. *Journal of the American College of Surgeons, 199,* 843–848.

59. Haller, G., Garnerin, P., Morales, M. A., Pfister, R., Berner, M., Irion, O., et al. (2008). Effect of crew resource management training in a multidisciplinary obstetrical setting. *International Journal for Quality in Health Care, 20,* 254–263.

60. Haycock-Stuart, E. A., & Houston, N. M. (2005). Evaluation study of a resource for developing education, audit and teamwork in primary care. *Primary Health Care Research & Development, 6,* 251–268.

61. Le Blanc, P. M., Hox, J. J., Schaufeli, W. B., Taris, T. W., & Peeters, M. C. W. (2007). Take care! The evaluation of a team-based burnout intervention program for oncology care providers. *Journal of Applied Psychology, 92,* 213–227.

62. Moorthy, K., Munz, Y., Forrest, D., Pandey, V., Undre, S., Vincent, C., & Darzi, A. (2006). Surgical crisis management skill training and assessment: A simulation-based approach to enhancing operating room performance. *Annals of Surgery, 244,* 139–147.

63. Morey, J. C., Simon, R., Jay, G. D., Wears, R. L., Salisbury, M., Dukes, K. A., & Berns, S. D. (2002). Error reduction and performance improvement in the emergency department through formal teamwork training: Evaluation results of the MedTeams project. *Health Service Research, 37,* 1553–1581.

64. O'Donnell, J., Fletcher, J., Dixon, B., & Palmer, L. (1998). Planning and implementing an anesthesia crisis resource management training course for student nurse anesthetists. *CRNA, 9,* 50–58.

65. Østergaard, H. T., Østergaard, D., & Lippert, A. (2004). Implementation of team training in medical education in Denmark. *Quality & Safety in Health Care, 13*(Suppl 1), i91-i95.

66. Paige, J. T., Kozmenko, V., Yang, T., Gururaja, R. P., Hilton, C. W., Cohn, I., Jr., & Chauvin, S. W. (2009a). Attitudinal changes resulting from repetitive training of operating room personnel using of high-fidelity simulation at the point of care. *The American Journal of Surgery, 75,* 584–590.

67. Reznek, M., Smith-Coggins, R., Howard, S., Kiran, K., Harter, P., Sowb, Y., et al. (2003). Emergency medicine crisis resource management (EMCRM): A pilot study of a simulation-based crisis management course for emergency medicine. *Academic Emergency Medicine, 10*(4), 386–389.

68. Robertson, B., Schumacher, L., Gosman, G., Kanfer, R., Kelley, M., & DeVita, M. (2009). Simulation-based crisis team training for multidisciplinary obstetric providers. *Simulation in Healthcare, 4*(2), 77–83.

69. Sehgal, N. L., Fox, M., Vidyarthi, A. R., Sharpre, B. A., Gearhart, S., Bookwalter, T., et al. (2008). A multidisciplinary teamwork training program: The triad for optimal patient safety (TOPS) experience. *Journal of General Internal Medicine, 23*(12), 2053–2057.

70. Shapiro, M. J., Morey, J. C., Small, S. D., Langford, V., Kaylor, C. J., Jagminas, L., et al.,(2004). Simulation based teamwork training for emergency department staff: Does it improve clinical team performance when added to an existing didactic teamwork curriculum? *Quality & Safety in Health Care, 13*(6), 417–421.

71. Sica, G. T., Barron, D. M., Blum, R., Frenna, T. H., & Raemer, D. B. (1999). Computerized realistic simulation: A teaching module for crisis management in radiology. *AJR American Journal of Roentgenology, 172*(2), 301–304.

72. Stroller, J. K., Rose, M., Lee, R., Dolgan, C., & Hoogerf, B. J. (2004). Teambuilding and leadership training in an internal medicine

residency training program. *Journal of General Internal Medicine, 19*(6), 692–697.

73. Wallin, C. J., Meurling, L., Hedman, L., Hedegard, J., & Fellander-Tsai, L. (2007). Target-focused medical emergency team training using a human patient simulator: Effects on behaviour and attitude. *Medical Education, 41*(2), 173–180.

74. Weaver, S. J., Rosen, M. A., DiazGranados, D., Lazzara, E. H., Lyons, R., Salas, E., et al. (2010b). Does teamwork improve performance in the operating room? A multilevel evaluation. *The Joint Commission Journal on Quality and Patient Safety, 36*(3), 133–142.

75. Youngblood, P., Harter, P. M., Srivastava, S., Moffett, S., Heinrichs, W. L., & Dev, P. (2008). Design, development, and evaluation of an online virtual emergency department for training trauma teams. *Simulation in Healthcare, 3*(3), 154–160.

76. Ammentorp, J., Sabroe, S., Kofoed, P. E., & Mainz, J. (2007). The effect of training in communication skills on medical doctors' and nurses' self-efficacy. A randomized controlled trial. *Patient Education and Counseling, 66*, 270–277.

77. Gibson, C. B. (2001). Me and us: Differential relationships among goal-setting training, efficacy and effectiveness at the individual and team level. *Journal of Organizational Behavior, 22*, 789–808.

78. Pratt, S. D., Mann, S., Salisbury, M., Greenberg, P., Marcus, R., Stabile, B., et al. (2007). Impact of CRM-based training on obstetric outcomes and clinicians' patient safety attitudes. *Joint Commission Journal on Quality and Patient Safety, 33*(12), 720–725.

79. Sax, H. C., Browne, P., Mayewski, R. J., Panzer, R. J., Hittner, K. C., Burke, R. L., & Coletta, S. (2009). Can aviation-based team training elicit sustainable behavioral change? *Archives of Surgery, 144*(12), 1133–1137.

80. Awad, S. S., Fagan, S. P., Bellows, C., Albo, D., Green-Rashad, B., De La Garza, M., & Berger, D. H. (2005). Bridging the communication gap in the operating room with medical team training. *The American Journal of Surgery, 190*, 770–774.

81. Berkenstadt, H., Haviv, Y., Tuval, A., Shemesh, Y., Megrill, A., Perry, A., et al. (2008). Improving handoff communications in critical care: Utilizing simulation-based training toward process improvement in managing patient risk. *Chest, 134*, 158–162.

82. Cashman, S. B., Reidy, P., Cody, K., & Lemay, C. (2004). Developing and measuring progress toward collaborative, integrated, interdisciplinary health care teams. *Journal of Interprofessional Care, 18*,183–196.

83. Cooley, E. (1994). Training an interdisciplinary team in communication and decision-making skills. *Small Group Research, 25*, 5–25.

84. DeVita, M. A., Schaefer, J., Lutz, J., Wang, H., & Dongilli, T. (2005). Improving medical emergency team (MET) performance using a novel curriculum and a computerized human patient simulator. *Quality & Safety in Health Care, 14*, 326–331.

85. i Gardi, T., Christensen, U. C., Jacobsen, J., Jensen, P. F., & Ording, H. (2001). How do anaesthesiologists treat malignant hyperthermia in a full-scale anaesthesia simulator? *Acta Anaesthesiologica Scandinavica, 45*,1032–1035.

86. Jacobsen, J., Lindekaer, A. L., Østergaard, H. T., Nielson, K., Østergaard, D., Laub, M., et al. (2001). Management of anaphylactic shock evaluated using a full-scale anesthesia simulator. *Acta Anaesthesiologica Scandinavica, 45*(3), 315–319.

87. Murray, W. B., Jankouskas, T., Chasko-Bush, M., Liu, W., & Sinz, L. (2006). Crisis resource management: Anesthesia non-technical skills (ANTS) in pediatric nurses and residents. *Anesthesiology, 105*, A1325.

88. Nielsen, P. E., Goldman, M. B., Mann, S., Shapiro, D. E., Marcus, R. G., Pratt, S. D., et al. (2007). Effects of teamwork training on adverse outcomes and process of care in labor and delivery. *Obstetrics & Gynecology, 109*, 48–55.

89. Paull, D. E., Mazzia, L. M., Izu, B. S., Niely, J., Mills, P. D., & Bagian, J. P. (2009). Predictors of successful implementation of preoperative briefings and postoperative debriefings after medical team training. *The American Journal of Surgery, 198*(5), 675–678.

90. Taylor, C. R., Hepworth, J. T., Buerhaus, P. I., Dittus, R., & Speroff, T. (2007). Effect of crew resource management on diabetes care and patient outcomes in an innercity primary care clinic. *Quality & Safety in Health Care, 16*(4), 244–247.

91. Marshall, D. A., & Manus, D. A. (2007). A team training program using human factors to enhance patient safety. *AORN Journal, 86*, 994–1011.

92. Kraiger, K., Ford, K. J., & Salas, E. (1993). Application of cognitive, skill-based, and affective theories of learning outcomes to new

methods of training evaluation. *Journal of Applied Psychology, 78,* 311–328.

93. Salas, E., & Cannon-Bowers, J. A. (2001). The science of training: A decade of progress. *Annual Review of Psychology, 52,* 471–499.

94. Gaba, D. M., Howard, S. K., Fish, K. J., Smith, B. E. & Sowb, Y. A. (2001). Simulation based training in anesthesia crisis resource management (ACRM): A decade of experience. *Simulation & Gaming, 32,* 175–193.

95. Alonso, A., Baker, D. P., Holtzman, A., Day, R., King, H., Toomey, L., et al. (2006). Reducing medical error in the military health system: How can team training help? *Human Resource Management Review, 16,* 396–415.

96. Rivers, R. M., Swain, D., Nixon, W. R. (2003). Using aviation safety measures to enhance patient outcomes. *AORN Journal, 77,* 158.

97. Baker, D. P., Gustafson, S., Beaubien, J. M., Salas, E., & Barach, P. (2005). Medical team training programs in health care. In K. Henriksen, J. B. Battles, E. S. Marks, & D. I. Lewin (Eds.), *Advances in patient safety: From research to implementation,* Vols. 1–4. (pp. 253–267) AHRQ: Rockville MD.

98. Cannon-Bowers, J. A., Prince, C., Salas, E., Owens, J., Morgan, B., Jr., & Gonos, G. (1989). *Determining aircrew coordination training effectiveness.* Paper presented at the 11th Interservice/Industry Training Systems Conference, Fort Worth, TX.

99. Schaefer, H. G., & Helmreich, R. L. (1994). The importance of human factors in the operating room. *Anesthesiology, 80,* 479.

100. Tays, T. M. (2000). *Effect of anesthesia crisis resource management training on perceived self-efficacy.* Unpublished Manuscript, Pacific Graduate School of Psychology, Palo Alto, California.

101. Neily, J., Mills, P. D., Young-Xu, Y., Carney, B. T., West, P., Berger, D., et al. (2010). Association between implementation of a medical team training program and surgical mortality. *Journal of the American Medical Association, 304*(15), 1693–1700.

17

CONTRIBUTIONS OF SIMULATION-BASED TRAINING TO TEAMWORK

William C. McGaghie, Walter J. Eppich, and
Kevin J. O'Leary

INTRODUCTION

Healthcare team training grounded in simulation is judged in response to two questions. First, does team training work under controlled, laboratory conditions? Second, does team training pay off in busy, sometimes chaotic clinical settings? The first question addresses the *efficacy* of simulation-based (S-B) team training. Does it get results under ideal circumstances? The second question is about the *effectiveness* of S-B team training. Do laboratory outcomes yield measureable results that matter in situ?[1] Healthcare team training in any form needs to produce robust, reproducible results in laboratory and clinical settings to be taken seriously and warrant training resources. This chapter reviews evidence selectively and teaches today's "best practices" about using S-B team training to achieve efficacy and effectiveness goals.

The chapter has five sections. First it addresses S-B team-training goals, separating teamwork objectives from individual task work. This is about the team-training curriculum. It also treats curriculum inclusion and exclusion criteria and gives advice about preparing teams to benefit from S-B team training. Second, it covers S-B team-training methods—creating optimal conditions to produce intended outcomes. Here we emphasize powerful

educational interventions that engage learner teams in deliberate practice with rigorous measurement of skill acquisition and frequent feedback. The third focus is on measuring performance in S-B team training. Particular attention is given to indexes of data quality (reliability) and to rater training and calibration. Section four treats transfer of S-B team training results from laboratory to patient care settings. It reports how to establish better team-based approaches to healthcare delivery and presents evidence about better patient outcomes resulting from improved team-based care practices. The fifth section is a coda. It sets an agenda for future work; argues for greater standardization, reproducibility, and rigor in S-B teamwork training and research; and acknowledges the tradeoff between scientific reliability and clinical fidelity.

SIMULATION-BASED TEAM TRAINING GOALS

Effective application of instructional design principles is essential to create a curriculum of powerful S-B learning experiences for team training that focuses on relevant learning outcomes. Educators must consider in advance the specific knowledge, skills, and attitudes that are suited for this educational strategy to target the curriculum appropriately. Issenberg et al. reported that curriculum integration is one of the key features of S-B training that makes it effective.[2] Educators must also consider how to best prepare healthcare professionals to benefit from S-B team training activities by incorporating S-B events into a larger team-training curriculum. Prerequisite knowledge and skills may be acquired through pre-course readings, observing videos, and even participating in virtual simulations.[3] During S-B team training sessions, trainees can devote their attention to translating theory into practice with relevant contextual cues—both clinical and team-related—so that newly gained teamwork knowledge and skills can be transferred to real patient care settings. The goal is to create optimal training conditions related to intended learning outcomes.

Salas et al. present eight evidence-based principles for team training in general, but also provide useful guidance for creating S-B team training experiences set in the context of a larger team training initiative.[4] These eight principles, and relevant examples, are presented in Table 17.1.

Anderson et al.[12] outline the steps of the curriculum development process for simulation-based learning experiences. These steps include: (1) identify problems, learning needs, and targeted learners; (2) specify overarching goals and measureable learning objectives; (3) select curriculum content and educational strategies; and (4) assess learning outcomes, curriculum evaluation, and revision.

Although many team-related patient safety issues that serve as targets for S-B team training are reflected in the healthcare literature, such problems can also be revealed within institutions during retrospective

---

Table 17.1   Eight Evidence-Based Principles for Team Training

Principles	Examples
1. Identify teamwork competencies … use these as a focus for training content.	Use established crew resource management (CRM) principles and their derivatives for curriculum development.[4]
2. Emphasize teamwork over task work, design for teamwork to improve team processes.	Combat trauma teams undergo team training, not task training, at the US Army Ryder Trauma Training Center in Miami.[5]
3. One size does not fit all … let the team-based learning outcomes desired, and organizational resources, guide the process.	In situ simulation improves patient safety in a labor and delivery ward.[6]
4. Task exposure is not enough … provide guided, hands-on practice.	Internal medicine residents acquire ACLS skills to mastery standards from S-B team training with deliberate practice.[7]
5. The power of simulation … ensure training relevance to transfer environment.	S-B obstetrical team training on shoulder dystocia management transfers to actual clinical care and patient outcomes.[8]
6. Feedback matters … it must be descriptive, timely, and relevant.	Debriefing with good judgment is an essential feature of S-B healthcare education.[9]
7. Go beyond reaction data … evaluate clinical outcomes, learning, and behaviors on the job.	S-B team training on obstetrical emergencies improves neonatal Apgar scores and reduces neonatal brain injury.[10]
8. Reinforce desired teamwork behaviors … sustain through coaching and performance evaluation.	Interdisciplinary S-B in situ team training is an effective strategy to improve perinatal safety.[11]

Principles adapted from Salas, E., DiazGranados, D., Weaver, S. J., & King, H. (2008). Does team training work? Principles for health care. *Academic Emergency Medicine, 15*(11), 1002–1009.

evaluations of sentinel events (root cause analyses) or prospectively through critical incident reporting systems and even in situ simulations designed to uncover them.[13]

Once a detailed needs assessment has been completed, educators develop and express goals and specific learning objectives and link these to selection of course content for the S-B team-training intervention. Here curriculum planners make decisions about what content to include and what can be safely excluded as they determine specific areas of emphasis that can be trained using simulation. The focus should be on critical teamwork competencies and team processes (e.g., leadership, mutual performance monitoring, backup behavior, adaptability, team orientation) and not specific task work.[14] A local needs assessment can help curriculum planners prioritize the team competencies to be addressed with simulation. Such curricular decisions that focus the S-B training are essential because S-B team training is a resource-intensive endeavor. Multiple factors influence the design of the S-B team-training curriculum. These factors include but are not limited to specific educational goals, available resources, organizing the training from personnel and resource perspectives, and potential barriers to participation.

Once decisions are made about the intended learning outcomes for the S-B component of the curriculum, educators can create a comprehensive set of scenarios that address relevant team skills. For a single scenario it is best to focus on a subset of key teamwork competencies. The unit of instruction for planned S-B team-training experiences is the simulated scenario and subsequent debriefing.

In the scenario design process, it is helpful to consider what events in the simulation trigger behaviors related to specific team-related learning objectives. Anytime two or more healthcare providers participate in a simulation scenario, they exhibit team behaviors. For example, when a simulated patient's condition deteriorates slowly (e.g., falling heart rate, oxygen saturation), which requires initiation of basic and advanced life support measures, healthcare providers discuss the factors that could be contributing to the patient's declining status to develop a shared mental model of events. The providers may also call for help. When a senior clinician arrives to assist, the team needs to share relevant information such as events leading up to the deterioration. Thus some elements of teamwork and communication are inherent to most if not all simulation scenarios because multiple clinicians are working together.

In the context of the S-B team-training curriculum, however, educators deliberately design specific events for the scenario to produce standardized triggers addressing specific team skills.[6,15] Hamman et al. provide a roadmap for the scenario design process outlined by the Advanced Qualification Program.[6,13] As a simulation scenario unfolds, a series of event sets that comprise the problem situation are designed to trigger representative actions. These actions— or their absence—form the basis of performance ratings and shape discussion and reflection during debriefing.

Psychological fidelity is an essential element to enhance task demands that mimic real systems in scenarios that engage participants effectively.[16] Equipment and environmental fidelity in this model are managed according to the primary goals of the scenario and the stages of training. Instructional design decisions consider the technological features of the simulator (e.g., stationary versus portable) and the choice of venue for the training (e.g., simulation lab versus point of care or in situ simulations).[6,11,13,17–20] To illustrate, for providers early in training, simulation center-based training with technologically simple devices usually provides sufficient degrees of realism. Experienced clinicians, by contrast, may benefit from in situ simulations with more advanced simulators.

A good example of S-B curriculum development is provided by Adler et al.[21] These investigators developed and evaluated a simulation-based curriculum for pediatric emergency medicine. Although the curriculum did not emphasize team skills, the curriculum development process the authors used warrants emulation. The curriculum development team included pediatric emergency physicians, nurses, and educators. The team developed a content map to guide construction of cases that formed a comprehensive collection of simulation scenarios. The authors started by formulating and ranking curriculum objectives. Next, the objectives were cast as clinical problems and mapped to instruction and evaluation cases. In this way, the authors linked teaching with rigorous assessment to enable trainees to receive specific feedback about their performance. The team made a series of decisions during curriculum development:

which content areas to include and exclude; which clinical problems were most important and could be reproduced reliably in the simulation laboratory; and which outcomes could be assessed reliably. By creating the evaluation instruments in parallel with the teaching cases, the authors integrated triggers into the teaching scenarios that were linked to assessment. Adler et al.[21] also teach that when deciding on what to include or exclude in the S-B curriculum, educators need to choose content areas not well addressed with other educational strategies that can also be linked with robust modes of assessment.

SIMULATION-BASED TEAM TRAINING METHODS

Simulation-based team training has three key features: (1) orientation and preparation, (2) delivery of instruction by multiple methods with opportunities to practice key team skills and measure outcomes, and (3) debriefing which includes reviewing performance data, receiving feedback, and planning for future improvement.

Orientation and preparation are needed to familiarize trainees with the simulation laboratory setting; location, features, and operation of equipment; time allocations; and opportunity to get acquainted with other trainees ("ice breaker") if persons do not know each other. Orientation may include reading, observing video recordings, touring a facility, conversation with peers and training staff, and many other activities. Orientation also involves making sure trainees are clear about training objectives, procedures, the expected code of conduct (i.e., behavioral limits), and creating a psychologically safe learning environment.

There are many ways to deliver instruction in S-B team training. The list of options includes team activities addressing a shared objective, problem discernment and team response, serial management of problems embedded in a case by different team members, patient "handoffs" from one healthcare team to another, and many others. Of course, S-B curriculum objectives usually expressed as case scenarios dictate instructional delivery modes, settings, and duration.

A key principle of S-B team training, especially in laboratory settings, is that for maximum effectiveness educational experiences must be standardized, consistent, and powerful.[22] This means that teams, and individual team members, must work very hard during scenario sessions. Simulation-based team training should be relevant professionally, intellectually, and physically engaging, intense, and of sufficient duration to allow trainees and trainee teams to practice critical skills deliberately.

Deliberate practice (DP) is an instructional variable that originates from the research and writing of psychologist K. Anders Ericsson.[23,24] The DP model is grounded in information processing and behavioral theories of skill acquisition and maintenance. McGaghie et al. state, "Deliberate practice has at least nine features or requirements when used to achieve medical education goals. It relies on:

1. Highly motivated learners with good concentration (e.g., medical trainees);
2. Engagement with a well-defined learning objective or task, at an
3. Appropriate level of difficulty, with
4. Focused, repetitive practice, that leads to
5. Rigorous, precise measurements, that yield
6. Informative feedback [i.e., reliable data] from educational sources (e.g., simulator, teachers), and where
7. Trainees also monitor their learning experiences and correct strategies, errors and levels of understanding, engage in more DP, and continue with
8. Evaluation to reach a mastery standard, and then
9. Advance to another task or unit."[25]

Team and individual S-B educational interventions are too often disorganized, brief, or weak, lacking sufficient power (dose) to produce the intended learning outcome (response). This is seen in "negative" (no difference) comparative research studies and in studies that yield treatment by occasion statistical interactions where outcomes are delayed or weaker than expected.[21,26] By contrast, deliberate practice and mastery learning models that use rigorous assessment and establish minimum performance standards that must be achieved by all learners irrespective of time encourage S-B educators to focus on learning objectives during curriculum development and insist on uniformly high achievement among trainees.[7,27–30]

Debriefing is a critical component of S-B educational strategies[9,31-34] and specific evidence-based best practices for debriefing medical teams apply here.[35] Even before the simulation begins, instructors set the stage for an engaging learning context by making expectations clear and framing the activity to create a sense of psychological safety.[36] Effective debriefers have command of the learning objectives of the simulated case and how the event sets were designed to trigger key behaviors in the scenario. For example, conflicting information may be introduced during the course of a scenario. In high functioning teams this information will be shared and prompt a discussion that leads to actions that confirm or refute discrepant data. In the case of the conflicting information, observable team actions—acts of commission or omission in dealing with the data—form the basis of further inquiry.

Knowledge of the learning objectives for the case, the scenario design, and the actual performance by the team members allows debriefers to identify a series of performance gaps that are discussed and analyzed.[34] Rudolph et al.[34] outline performance gap focused analysis in the context of debriefings. Performance gaps are the differences between actual and desired team performance and may be above or below expectations among different team skills or even within the same skill set. For example, communication might be outstanding at one phase of a scenario but breaks down during a later phase. Using specific conversational methods to promote reflection, debriefers provide feedback to the team by sharing their interpretation of events and attempt to elicit reasons for the performance gap. By promoting a discussion that fosters reflective practice, an effective debriefer helps participants understand invisible drivers that contribute to the performance gap as well as the team or system factors that promote or inhibit optimal outcomes. Targeted teaching or facilitated discussion helps team members create new strategies for dealing with similar future situations or enact system improvements once the reasons for the performance gap are known. Healthcare organizations must create conditions that promote the transfer of new learning and insights from the simulation setting into actual clinical practice.[14]

MEASURING PERFORMANCE IN SIMULATION-BASED TEAM TRAINING

Measurement in S-B team training serves several purposes including formative and summative evaluation for teams and individual team members as well as an assessment of the effectiveness of S-B training. Measurement informs feedback and DP, essential components of a successful S-B training intervention. Tools should allow for evaluation of specific causes for effective and ineffective performance to facilitate directed feedback. Rosen et al. have described best practices in team performance measurement in S-B training.[5] They recommend that measures be grounded in scientifically based models of team performance and tightly linked to the specific competencies being trained.

Measures used for S-B team training and research must be rigorous and produce solid data. Rigorous measurement yields high-quality, reliable data (e.g., checklist recordings, rating scale numbers, time intervals, haptic pressure).[37] McGaghie asserts, "Reliable data have a high signal-to-noise ratio (more signal, less noise) like a 'loud and clear' radio reception versus one that is 'scratchy' and difficult to discern."[38] Reliable, trustworthy data are needed to give learners error-free feedback and as a foundation for rigorous quantitative research. Reliable data are essential to permit valid decisions or inferences about learners, either individuals or teams.[39,40]

The optimal approach to measuring team performance in S-B training includes multiple measures from different sources. This approach provides a comprehensive picture of team performance. Measures should be chosen to determine the origins of ineffective team performance, provide meaningful feedback to both the team and individual team members, and assess the success of S-B training.

TRANSFER OF SIMULATION-BASED TEAM TRAINING TO PATIENT CARE

The ultimate goal of S-B team training is to improve performance in the clinical setting. Though the literature supports the benefit of S-B training in improving team performance in the simulated environment, few studies have assessed the impact of S-B team training on clinical care. Team performance in the clinical setting can be measured by the same methods used in simulation exercises. Direct observation should be used to assess team-related behaviors. Complementing assessment of team performance, process and outcome measures should be used to assess clinical performance. Process measures reflect care delivered to the patient and may be collected by direct observation or medical record review. Outcome measures assess what happened to the patient and have high face validity. However, clinical outcomes are more difficult to affect because many variables influence patient outcomes, including comorbidity and latent errors, which may not be addressed in S-B team training.

Berkenstadt et al. used S-B training to improve a specific type of team-related behavior, nurse handoffs at shift change.[41] Direct observation was used to assess the intervention's impact on important components of the handoff. Several components, including communication about events that occurred during the preceding shift and treatment goals for the next shift, improved as a result of the intervention whereas others, including checking monitor alarms and the mechanical ventilator, did not.

Shapiro et al. conducted a study investigating whether S-B team training, when added to an existing didactic teamwork curriculum, improved observed teamwork in an emergency department.[42] The study used the Team Dimensions Rating Form and observers were blinded to the identity of the experimental and comparison groups. The experimental group showed a trend toward improvement in the quality of team behavior, whereas the comparison group did not change during two observation periods.

Draycott and other UK colleagues evaluated the benefit of S-B team training on outcomes in an obstetrical setting.[8,10,43] All obstetrical staff in their hospital are required to undergo an annual 1-day S-B obstetrical emergency team training session. The management of shoulder dystocia, umbilical cord prolapse, and obstetrical emergencies are among the scenarios used in the training. The investigators reviewed medical records before and after S-B team training and found a significant increase in the percentage of time recommended maneuvers for the resolution of shoulder dystocia. There was also a significant reduction in the proportion of babies born

with an obstetrical brachial palsy injury. Training also resulted in a significant reduction in the time from diagnosis of uterine cord prolapse to infant delivery. The research on obstetrical emergencies sought to reduce the incidence of infants born with low APGAR scores and also reduce the incidence of neonatal hypoxic-ischemic encephalopathy (HIE), a brain injury caused by lack of oxygen. Clinical research outcomes with actual patients showed that the number of infants with low 5-minute APGAR scores and the number of infants with HIE were both reduced significantly as a consequence of S-B team training.[10]

The team training research reported by Draycott and colleagues is important on educational and clinical grounds because it directly links educational interventions to improved patient care practices and better health outcomes among patients. Such clinical education research qualifies as "translational science" because the research endpoint stretches from the simulation laboratory to the bedside to improved patient and public health.[44]

Additional methods, not typically used to measure team performance in the simulation lab, may be useful in assessing the impact of S-B training in the clinical setting. For example, survey instruments designed to assess safety and team culture may be used in evaluating the impact of S-B team training.[45] In addition, multisource feedback, or 360-degree evaluation, may reinforce lessons learned in S-B team training.[46]

Although a small number of studies support the benefit of S-B training in improving team performance in the clinical setting, few evaluate the impact on clinical patient outcomes. The studies that include outcomes address very specific clinical scenarios (shoulder dystocia, umbilical cord prolapse, 5-minute APGAR scores, HIE). Future research should confirm the benefit of S-B training in improving team performance and evaluate whether it improves patient outcomes across a wide range of clinical situations and settings. Because of the complexity and large investment in resources required to implement S-B team training, future research should also evaluate whether S-B trained individuals have an effect on the teamwork skills of others and the culture of the institution. That is, can improved skills and attitudes diffuse through an organization if a critical mass of individuals undergoes successful team training?

Finally, studies should identify features that appear to be most important in applying skills learned in the simulated environment to the clinical setting.

CODA

This chapter has addressed S-B team training goals, S-B team training methods, measuring performance in S-B team training, and transfer of S-B team training to patient care. The chapter has reviewed evidence and argument selectively, not exhaustively, to provide ideas and guidance that begin to inform best practices about S-B team training. The knowledge base in this field has grown and matured over several decades. A recent research metaanalysis addressing the question, "Does team training improve performance?" concludes, "… team training interventions are a viable approach organizations can take in order to enhance team outcomes. They are useful for improving cognitive outcomes, affective outcomes, teamwork processes, and performance outcomes. Moreover, results suggest that training content, team membership, stability, and team size moderate the effectiveness of team training interventions."[47]

The research agenda for S-B training and its contribution to teamwork and patient safety is straightforward. There are two research priorities. First, work is needed to improve process and outcome measurement, a problem voiced more than 50 years ago that will not go away.[48] Current measures of team performance cover a very narrow bandwidth, whereas effective team performance in healthcare settings involves a broad and deep repertoire too complex to capture with today's evaluations. Second, S-B team research needs to be more intentional about establishing the *efficacy* of educational interventions in the controlled laboratory context and later demonstrating their in situ *effectiveness* in wards, clinics, EMS vehicles, and other community settings. Simulation-based team training research programs are most useful and informative when outcome studies are thematic, sustained, and cumulative.

In addition to increased standardization, reproducibility, and rigor in S-B team training research, there is growing awareness that science and professional practice are bounded by time and context. Pawson et al. argue that introduction of complex service interventions such as S-B team training into healthcare settings is rarely smooth or easy.[49,50] These scholars teach that such interventions have a variety of key elements including a long implementation chain, features that mutate as a result of refinement and adaptation to local circumstances, and

---

Table 17.2   Five Contributions of Simulation-Based Training to Teamwork

Contribution	Examples
1. Focused, standardized competency-based team training curriculum content grounded in patient care scenarios	Competency-based pediatric emergency medicine curriculum expressed as clinical scenarios for education and testing[21,29]
2. S-B team training methods—optimal conditions to yield intended learning outcomes: powerful interventions, engage learners in DP with feedback	Mastery learning of temporary hemodialysis catheter placement[27] and thoracentesis[30] skills via S-B training with DP
3. Rigorous measurement of behavioral processes and learning outcomes to produce reliable data that lead to valid decisions about trainees	Team performance measurement best practices[5] that yield reliable data[37] for valid personnel decision making[39,40]
4. Transfer of S-B team training results from laboratory to patient care settings. Better healthcare team training leads to improved patient outcomes.	S-B team training in obstetrical care and neonatal emergencies improves childbirth outcomes.[8,10,43]
5. Future S-B healthcare team education will be more standardized, reproducible, and rigorous. Strong research in health professions education qualifies as "translational science."	Research opportunities in simulation-based medical education with DP[38] that meets translational science standards[44] have been expressed.

represent open systems that feed back on themselves. "As interventions are implemented, they change the conditions that made them work in the first place."[50] The Greek philosopher Heraclitus had it right. "You cannot step twice into the same river."

Recall that a simulation is just that, a representation of reality. Simulation-based team training, like other applications of simulation technology in education, is limited because training exercises are always an approximation to the "real thing." Researchers and teachers need to acknowledge the tradeoff between scientific and educational reliability and clinical fidelity. Education, evaluation, and professional practice never match perfectly.

In conclusion, this chapter has addressed contributions of S-B training to teamwork. A summary of five contributions, each with cited examples, is given in Table 17.2. Education and research in the healthcare professions toward improved team practice and patient safety goals will be advanced from attention to these S-B principles.

REFERENCES

1. Fletcher, R. H., Fletcher, S. W., & Wagner, E. H. (1996). *Clinical epidemiology: The essentials.* Baltimore: Williams & Wilkins.

2. Issenberg, S. B., McGaghie, W. C., Petrusa, E. R., et al. (2005). Features and uses of high-fidelity medical simulations that lead to effective learning: A BEME systematic review. *Medical Teacher, 27,* 10–28.

3. Heinrichs, W. L., Youngblood, P., Harter, P. M., & Dev, P. (2008). Simulation for team training and assessment: case studies of online training with virtual worlds. *World Journal of Surgery, 32,* 161–70.

4. Salas, E., DiazGranados, D., Weaver, S. J., & King, H. (2008). Does team training work? Principles for health care. *Academic Emergency Medicine, 15*(11), 1002–9.

5. Rosen, M. A., Salas, E., Wilson, K. A., et al. (2008). Measuring team performance in simulation-based training: Adopting best practices for healthcare. *Simulation in Healthcare, 3*(1), 33–41.

6. Hamman, W. R., Beaudin-Seiler, B. M., Beaubien, J. M., et al. (2009). Using in situ simulation to identify and resolve latent environmental threats to patient safety: Case

study involving a labor and delivery ward. *Journal of Patient Safety, 5,* 184–7.

7. Wayne, D. B., Butter, J., Siddall, V. J., et al. (2006). Mastery learning of advanced cardiac life support skills by internal medicine residents using simulation technology and deliberate practice. *Journal of General Internal Medicine, 21,* 251–6.

8. Draycott, T. J., Crofts, J. F., Ash, J. P., et al. (2008). Improving neonatal outcome through practical shoulder dystocia training. *Obstetrics and Gynecology, 112,* 14–20.

9. Rudolph, J. W., Simon, R., Rivard, P., et al. (2007). Debriefing with good judgment: Combining rigorous feedback with genuine inquiry. *Anesthesiology Clinics, 25,* 361–76.

10. Draycott, T., Sibanda, T., Owen, L., et al. (2006). Does training in obstetric emergencies improve neonatal outcome? *British Journal of Obstetrics and Gynecology, 113,* 177–82.

11. Miller, K. K., Riley, W., Davis, S., & Hansen, H. E. (2008). In situ simulation: A method of experiential learning to promote safety and team behavior. *Journal of Perinatal and Neonatal Nursing, 22*(2), 105–13.

12. Anderson, J. M., Aylor, M. E., & Leonard, D. T. (2008). Instructional design dogma: Creating planned learning experiences in simulation. *Journal of Critical Care, 23,* 595–602.

13. Hamman, W. R., Beaudin-Seiler, B. M., & Beaubien, J. M. (2010). Understanding interdisciplinary health care teams: Using simulation design processes from the air carrier advanced qualification program to identify and train critical teamwork skills. *Journal of Patient Safety, 6,* 137–46.

14. Salas, E., Weaver, S. J., DiazGranados, D., et al. (2009). Sounding the call for team training in health care: Some insights and warnings. *Academic Medicine, 84*(10 Suppl), S128–31.

15. Shapiro, M. J., Gardner, R., Godwin, S. A., et al. (2008). Defining team performance for simulation-based training: Methodology, metrics and opportunities for emergency medicine. *Academic Emergency Medicine, 15,* 1088–97.

16. Beaubien, J. M., & Baker, D. P. (2004). The use of simulation for training teamwork skills in health care: How low can you go? *Quality and Safety in Health Care, 13*(Suppl 1), i51–6.

17. Kobayashi, L., Patterson, M. D., Overly, F. L., et al. (2008). Educational and research implications of portable human patient simulation in acute care medicine. *Academic Emergency Medicine, 15,* 1166–74.

18. DeVita, M. A., Schaefer, J., Lutz, J., et al. (2005). Improving medical emergency team (MET) performance using a novel curriculum and a computerized human patient simulator. *Quality and Safety in Health Care, 14,* 326–31.

19. Paige, J. Y., Kozmenko, V., Yang, T., et al. (2009). High-fidelity, simulation-based, interdisciplinary operating room team training at the point of care. *Surgery, 145,* 138–46.

20. Weinstock, P. H., Kappus, L. J., Gardon, A., & Burns, J. P. (2009). Simulation at the point of care: reduced-cost, in situ training via a mobile cart. *Pediatric Critical Care Medcine, 10,* 176–81.

21. Adler, M. D., Vozenilek, J. A., Trainor, J. L., et al. (2009).Development and evaluation of a simulation-based pediatric emergency medicine curriculum. *Academic Medicine, 84,* 935–41.

22. Cordray, D. S., & Pion, G. M. (2006). Treatment strength and integrity. In R. R. Bootzin, & P. E. McKnight (Eds.), *Strengthening research methodology: Psychological measurement and evaluation.* (pp. 103–24). Washington, DC: American Psychological Association.

23. Ericsson, K. A. (2004). Deliberate practice and the acquisition and maintenance of expert performance in medicine and related domains. *Academic Medicine, 79*(10 Suppl), S70–81.

24. Ericsson, K. A., Krampe, R. T., & Tesch-Römer, C. (1993). The role of deliberate practice in the acquisition of expert performance. *Psychological Review, 100,* 363–406.

25. McGaghie, W. C., Issenberg, S. B., Petrusa, E. R., & Scalese, R. J. (2010). A critical review of simulation-based medical education (SBME) research: 2003–2009. *Medical Education, 44,* 50–63.

26. Butter, J., Grant, T. H., Egan, M., et al. (2007). Does ultrasound training boost year 1 medical student competence and confidence when learning abdominal examination? *Medical Education, 41,* 843–8.

27. Barsuk, J. H., Ahya, S. N., Cohen, E. R., et al. (2009). Mastery learning of temporary hemodialysis catheter insertion skills by nephrology fellows using simulation technology and deliberate practice. *American Journal of Kidney Diseases, 54,* 70–6.

28. Barsuk, J. H., McGaghie, W. C., Cohen, E. R., et al. (2009). Use of simulation-based mastery learning to improve the quality of central venous catheter placement in a medical intensive care unit. *Journal of Hospital Medicine, 4,* 397–403.

29. McGaghie, W. C., Miller, G. E., Sajid, A., & Telder, T. V. (1978). *Competency-based curriculum development in medical education: An introduction.* Public Health Paper No. 68. Geneva, Switzerland: World Health Organization.

30. Wayne, D. B., Barsuk, J. H., O'Leary, K. J., et al. (2008). Mastery learning of thoracentesis skills by internal medicine residents using simulation technology and deliberate practice. *Journal of Hospital Medicine, 3,* 48–54.

31. Steinwachs, B. (1992). How to facilitate debriefing. *Simulation and Gaming, 23,* 186–95.

32. Fanning, R. M., & Gaba, D. M. (2007). The role of debriefing in simulation-based learning. *Simulation and Healthcare, 2,* 115–25.

33. Rudolph, J. W., Simon, R., Dufresne, R. L., & Raemer, D. B. (2006). There's no such thing as "nonjudgmental" debriefing: A theory and method for debriefing with good judgment. *Simulation and Healthcare 1,* 49–55.

34. Rudolph, J. W., Simon, R., Raemer, D. B., & Eppich, W. J. (2008). Debriefing as formative assessment: Closing performance gaps in medical education. *Academic Emergency Medicine, 15,* 1010–6.

35. Salas, E., Klein, M. S., King, H., et al. (2008). Debriefing medical teams: 12 evidence-based best practices and tips. *Joint Commission Journal on Quality and Patient Safety, 34,* 518–27.

36. Simon, R., Rudolph, J. W., & Raemer, D. B. (2009). *Debriefing assessment for simulation in healthcare.* Cambridge, MA: Center for Medical Simulation.

37. Downing, S. M. (2004). Reliability: On the reproducibility of assessment data. *Medical Education, 38,* 1006–12.

38. McGaghie, W. C. (2008). Research opportunities in simulation-based medical education using deliberate practice. *Academic Emergency Medicine, 15,* 995–1001.

39. Downing, S. M. (2003). Validation: On the meaningful interpretation of assessment data. *Medical Education, 37,* 830–7.

40. Kane, M. T. (2006). Validation. In R. L. Brennan (Ed.), *Educational measurement.* 4th ed. (pp. 17–64). Westport, CT: American Council on Education and Praeger Publishers.

41. Berkenstadt, H., Haviv, Y., & Tuval, A., et al. (2008). Improving handoff communications in critical care: Utilizing simulation-based training toward process improvement in managing patient risk. *CHEST 134,* 158–62.

42. Shapiro, M. J., Morey, J. C., Small, S. D., et al. (2004). Simulation based teamwork training for emergency department staff: Does it improve clinical team performance when added to an existing didactic teamwork curriculum? *Quality and Safety in Health Care, 13,* 417–21.

43. Siassakos, D., Hasafa, Z., Sibanda, T., et al. (2009). Retrospective cohort study of diagnosis-delivery interval with umbilical cord prolapse: The effect of team training. *British Journal of Obstetrics and Gynecology, 116,* 1089–96.

44. McGaghie, W. C. (2010). Medical education research as translational science. *Science Translational Medicine, 2,* 19cm8.

45. Sexton, J. B., Helmreich, R. L., Neilands, T. B., et al. (2006). The safety attitudes questionnaire: Psychometric properties, benchmarking data, and emerging research. *BMC Health Services Research, 6,* 44.

46. Higgins, R. S., Bridges, J., Burke, J. M., et al. (2004). Implementing the ACGME general competencies in a cardiothoracic surgery residency program using 360-degree feedback. *Annals of Thoracic Surgery, 77,* 12–7.

47. Salas, E., DiazGranados, D., Klein, C., et al. (2008). Does team training improve team performance? A meta-analysis. *Human Factors, 50,* 903–33.

48. Gagne, R. M. (1954). Training devices and simulations: Some research issues. *American Psychologist, 9,* 95–107.

49. Pawson, R. (2006). Evidence-based policy: A realist perspective. Thousand Oaks, CA: Sage.

50. Pawson, R., Greenhalgh, T., Harvey, G., & Walshe, K. (2005). Realist review: A new method of systematic review designed for complex policy interventions. *Journal of Health Services Research & Policy, 10*(Suppl 1), 21–34.

PART FIVE
COMMENTARIES

18

A US FEDERAL AGENCY'S ROLE IN TEAMWORK RESEARCH AND IMPLEMENTATION: A COMMENTARY

James B. Battles

The Agency for Healthcare Research and Quality (AHRQ) is a part of the U.S. Department of Health and Human Services (DHHS). Congress, in its reauthorization of AHRQ in 1999, stated that the director of AHRQ shall conduct and support research and build private-public partnerships to identify the causes of preventable health care errors and patient injury in health care delivery; develop, demonstrate, and evaluate strategies for reducing error and improving patient safety; and disseminate such effective strategies throughout the healthcare industry.[1] Since then, AHRQ has pursued a robust patient safety agenda of research and implementation to deal with all issues of patient safety, including identifying risks and hazards as well as promoting safe practices designed to eliminate or mitigate harm.

One of the leading contributing factors to events leading to harm to patients is poor communication and lack of teamwork among health providiers.[2] The Institute of Medicine (IOM), in its publication *To Err Is Human*, stated that healthcare organizations and health professional academic programs "establish interdisciplinary team training programs, such as simulation, that incorporate proven methods for team management."[3] As Paul M. Schyve, MD, senior vice president of The Joint Commission, has observed, "Our challenge ... is not whether we will deliver care in teams but rather how well we will

deliver care in teams."[4] Recent evidence from the Veteran's Administration, has shown that improved teamwork through team training has had a positive impact on suicidal mortality.[5] Teamwork saves lives and is now one of the safe practices listed by the National Quality Forum (NQF).[6]

But it currently takes 17 years to turn 14% of original research into beneficial, patient care.[7] This lag time from original research to adoption of care "based on the best scientific knowledge and the care we have, lies not just a gap, but a chasm."[8] On average, patients receive only about 55% of the available best or safe practices for which they would have likely benefited.[9] There is a growing consensus that United States healthcare is neither safe nor consistent in quality. American healthcare is also the most expensive care in the industrialized world. Compounding the quality and safety problem is the fact nearly 13% to 15% of patients who receive hospitalized care are harmed by the structure and process of care they recieive.[10,11] Recognizing the need for healthcare reform, Congress passed the Patient Protection and Affordable Care Act (ACA) in spring of 2010.[12]

Why does it take so long for research to be adopted in healthcare? One answer to the question is the fact that an infrastructure to promote the adoption of new safe practices does not exist within healthcare. In the healthcare and biomedical research enterprise there has been the traditional attitude of publish it and practitioners will adopt the research and evidence findings.[13] In the past, AHRQ and other healthcare research agencies have pursued this more passive role in the implementation and adoption process. Placing a list of tools and resources on a web site has proved to be insufficient. A much more aggressive implementation strategy is required if indeed we are to improve healthcare for all Americans as stated in AHRQ's mission statement.

To meet this challenge of accelerating healthcare reform, AHRQ has focused on developing tools and resources to facilitate implementation and adoption of safe practices. In partnership with the U.S. Department of Defense (DoD), AHRQ has developed the TeamSTEPPS® resource kit for improving teamwork and is actively supporting its implementation and adoption.[14]

AHRQ recognized the need to create an infrastructure to facilitate the adoption and implementation of TeamSTEPPS®. AHRQ in cooperation with the DoD developed and funded a national implementation effort to aggressively promote and facilitate the adoption and use of teamwork improvement strategies using TeamSTEPPS®. A key component of AHRQ's teamwork improvement strategy has been in training Master Team Trainers/Change Agents to facilitate the adoption of teamwork improvement activities within healthcare provider organizations at the system and individual institution level. In addition to the support of provider organizations, AHRQ is partnering with other organizations such as the Association of American Medical Colleges (AAMC) and Accreditation Council for Graduate Medical Education (ACGME) to promote the adoption of improved teamwork in health professional schools and residency training programs. AHRQ has also worked with others agencies within the DHHS to integrate teamwork improvement into other quality improvement efforts. Working with the Centers for Medicare and Medicaid Services (CMS), TeamSTEPPS® was included as part of the 9th Scope of Work for its Quality Improvement Organizations (QIOs). All QIOs in the country were trained in the use of TeamSTEPPS®. AHRQ is also working with state-based quality improvement efforts to promote more effective teamwork.

Poor teamwork can kill or severely harm patients, whereas good teamwork improves care. Effective team work is a cornerstone for quality improvement and patient safety within healthcare. We know how to measure the outcomes for effective teamwork in inpatient care.[15] Teamwork and coordination of care among health professionals is a key component of the patient's experience of care as measured by Hospital Consumer Assessment of Healthcare Providers and Systems (HCAHPS).[16] It has been said that the best way to improve an organization's patient satisfaction is to improve teamwork among the physicians and nurses who provide care to patients. Teamwork is also fundamental to a culture of safety as measured by the Hospital Survey on Patient Safety Culture (HSOPS).[17]

Whether effective teamwork is present or not is best measured by direct observation. The tools for measuring teamwork exist. Because teamwork is essential to the delivery of safe, reliable, and effective healthcare, it is not inconceivable that in the near future healthcare organizations seeking accreditation will be required to demonstrate effective teamwork during site visits by organizations such as the Joint Commission or the CMS Survey and Certification Group.

As the acceleration of healthcare reform takes place over the next few years, AHRQ will accelerate its efforts to promote improved teamwork as a cornerstone of quality and safety of care.

REFERENCES

1.   Healthcare Research and Quality Act of 1999 Title IX of the Public Health Service Act (42 U.S.C. 299 1).

2.   Joint Commission. Sentinel Event Statistics Data—Updated through December 31, 2010. http://www.jointcommission.org/sentinel_event_statistics_quarterly/.

3.   Kohn, L. T., Corrigan, J. M., Donaldson, M. S.(Eds.). (2000). *To Err Is Human: Building a Safer Health System*. Washington, DC: National Academy Press.

4.   Schyve, P. M. (2005). Editorial: The changing nature of professional competence. *Joint Commission Journal of Quality and Patient Safety, 31*, 185–202.

5. Neily, J., Mills, P. D., Young-Xu, Y., et al. (2010). Association between implementation of a medical team training program and surgical mortality. *Journal of the American Medical Association, 304*(15), 1693–1700.

6. National Quality Forum. (2010). *Safe Practices for Better Healthcare 2010 Update.* Washington, DC: National Quality Forum.

7. Balas, E. A., Boren, S. A. (2000). Managing clinical knowledge for heath care improvement. In Bemmel J, McCray A.T (Eds.), *Yearbook of Medical Informatics 2000: Patient-centered Systems* (pp. 65–70). Stuttgart: Schattauer.

8. Corrigan, J. M., Donaldson, M. S., Kohn, L. T., Magure, S. K., Pike, K . C., (Eds.). (2001). *Crossing the Quality Chasm: A New Health System for the 21st Century.* Washington, DC: National Academy Press.

9. McGlynn, E. A., Asch, S. M., Adams, J., Keesey, J., Hicks, J., DeCristofaro, A., et al. (2003). The quality of health care delivered to adults in the United States. *New England Journal of Medicine, 348*(26), 2635–45.

10. Levinson, R. D. (2010). *Adverse Events in Hospitals: National Incidence Among Medicare Beneficiaries:* (OEI-06-09-00090) Washington, DC: Office of the Inspector General, Department of Health Service.

11. U.S. Agency for Healthcare Research and Quality. (2009). *The National Healthcare Quality Report 2008.* Rockville, MD: U.S. Agency for Healthcare Research and Quality.

12. Green, L. W. (2008). Making research relevant: if it is an evidence-based practice, where's the practice-based evidence? *Family Practice, 25*(Supple1), i20–4.

13. Patient Protection and Affordable Care Act (PPACA) (Public Law 111–148, 124 Stat. 119, to be codified as amended to sections of 42 U.S. Code. March 30, 2010.

14. Clancy, C. M., Tornberg, D. N. (2007). TeamSTEPPS: assuring optimal teamwork in Clinical settings. *American Journal of Quality, 22*(3), 214–7.

15. Sorbero, M. E., Farley, D. O., Mattke, S., Lovejoy, S. L. (2008). *Outcome Measures for Effective Teamwork in Inpatient Care.* Santa Monica: RAND.

16. Agency for Healthcare Research and Quality (AHRQ). *Hospital Consumer Assessment of Healthcare Providers and Systems (HCAHPS).* http://www.hcahpsonline.org/home.aspx.

17. Agency for Healthcare Research and Quality (AHRQ). (2004). *Hospital Survey on Patient Safety Culture.* Rockville, MD: AHRQ.

19

MEASURING AND DIAGNOSING TEAM PERFORMANCE

David P. Baker and Jonathan Gallo

As demonstrated throughout this book, training is the key to improving teamwork. Nurses, physicians, pharmacists, and other ancillary healthcare professionals must work together to deliver safe, efficient, high-quality care. To demonstrate the importance of improved teamwork in healthcare, this chapter examines the potential impact using the reported Institute of Medicine statistics from 1999 (98,000 lives and 17 billion dollars per year). A 5% performance improvement in teamwork could potentially yield approximate 5,000 lives saved and more than 800 million dollars. The authors know from the meta-analytic studies conducted by Ed Salas and his colleagues that such a goal is attainable. The potential value of team training for improving team performance in the delivery of quality care cannot be dismissed.

However, team training programs cannot be effective without reliable and valid measures. Measurement is extremely important because it allows trainers to identify and diagnose the deficiencies in a team's performance. It is only through measurement and diagnosis that training interventions can be prescribed. Moreover, measurement is critical in the development of team skills in which feedback and debriefing lead to learning.

WHAT TO MEASURE

The central theme of our argument is that training is required to improve team performance, and effective training relies on measurement and diagnosis. Before one can determine what intervention is required, the breakdowns in teamwork must be identified. Importantly, diagnosis cannot occur if measures just focus on team outcomes (e.g., the patient lived or died; the patient did or did not acquire a healthcare-associated infection); team process also must be assessed. In other words, one cannot simply assess whether or not the team made the right decision; it is also important to understand if the decision was made correctly.

Measuring both team processes and outcomes is especially important in training environments in which feedback and remediation are used to improve team performance. Naturally, outcome measures must be collected for trainers to determine the degree to which trainees have successfully accomplished their objectives. However, outcome measures alone do not have the ability to convey why teams were successful or how one should go about training less effective teams to perform like more effective ones. Outcome measures alone are not diagnostic. They do not identify the particular aspects of performance that may be deficient. Moreover, it has been suggested that providing trainees with only outcome-based performance feedback actually may hamper the learning process. Consider a situation in which a team makes an accurate decision to provide a specific method of care using flawed processes. Unless process measures are in place, this flawed process may go uncorrected and could result in an undesirable outcome in a future performance situation. Thus, to correctly identify specific performance deficiencies and make recommendations for follow-up training, process measures must be collected in addition to outcomes. This will help ensure that trainees are not only achieving the desired outcomes, but also that they are using the right approach in doing so.

The collection of process and outcome measures also serves other purposes. Specifically, the collection of processes and outcomes is critical if one wishes to determine which processes are associated with (or predictive of) effective performance in a given domain. Data collected on a variety of processes can be regressed on critical outcomes to determine the processes that contribute to team outcomes. It is these unique processes that would then serve as objectives during training. Such an effort was undertaken in a study conducted by Smith-Jentsch et al.[1] Videotaped performance during 30-minute training scenarios involving combat information center teams was analyzed. Data were collected on four teamwork processes (i.e., communication, information exchange, leadership, and supporting behavior) as well as on two critical team outcomes (i.e., decision accuracy and latency). Results from the multiple regression analysis indicated that variation in three teamwork processes predicted team outcomes. Specifically, teams that made accurate decisions at key scenario events also received higher ratings on communication, information exchange, and leadership. However, the fourth teamwork process (i.e., supporting behavior) did not account for a significant portion of variance in decision accuracy. It was suggested that this might have been because the opportunities to provide supporting behavior were not as well controlled during the scenarios as other teamwork processes.

Based on the discussion thus far, the authors recommend that when measuring team performance *measure both outcomes and team process.* However, because organizations are likely to be concerned with more than one performance outcome, it can be difficult to determine which outcome(s) to measure during a given training episode. To answer this question, the authors suggest that trainers carefully examine the learning objectives that they have identified as targets for training. If written correctly, learning objectives will naturally lead one to select one outcome over others. For instance, a learning objective for a medical resident might be to diagnose each patient's symptoms without error. This objective clearly indicates the need to employ a measure of accuracy (i.e., one type of outcome) as opposed to productivity (e.g., how many patients the resident sees per day; an alternative outcome). Because it is also important to collect process measures, trainers should then generate a list of tasks that the resident would need to accomplish so as to make an accurate diagnosis (e.g., taking a patient's medical history, asking probing question about the patient's symptoms, examining the patient, ordering necessary tests). Such tasks can then be used to develop appropriate tools for measuring processes.

In addition to measuring processes and outcomes, the authors recommend that when measuring team performance, *measure both taskwork and teamwork processes, when appropriate.* In this way, one can determine if a problem stems from an individual's inability to perform his or her individual task responsibilities (i.e., taskwork), the individual is having trouble coordinating his or her efforts with others (teamwork), or both are problematic to some degree. This type of in-depth diagnosis is necessary if effective recommendations regarding remediation and follow-up training are to be made.

Although the importance of teamwork and taskwork has been stressed in the literature, few studies have collected data on both types of processes simultaneously, and the authors know of none in healthcare. In a rare study, Stout et al.[2] investigated the impact of individual task proficiency (i.e., taskwork) and teamwork on team performance during a low-fidelity flight simulation involving two-person teams. Taskwork was measured by observer ratings of the pilot's ability to maneuver the joystick (e.g., to keep targets centered on the screen) and the copilot's ability to use the keyboard (e.g., to stabilize the aircraft's altitude). Stout et al. reported that teamwork ratings predicted variance in team performance above and beyond that explained by taskwork ratings.[2] Thus, it was concluded that although it is important for team members to possess individual task competence, taskwork or technical skills alone do not determine whether teams will be successful. Teamwork is also a significant contributor.

Although the authors have attempted to make a case for measuring both taskwork and teamwork in addition to measuring critical task outcomes, the authors acknowledge that this can be labor intensive and perhaps a bit overwhelming. Further, just as there is a danger in employing too few measures, the same danger exists for attempting to measure too much. That is, both situations potentially can result in the loss of valuable data. Although there has been little research to suggest the optimum number of measures that instructors are able to reliably complete, *the authors recommend that each trainer try to limit their assessments to one or two critical outcomes and two to three process measures related to each of the selected learning objectives.*

HOW TO MEASURE

It has been said that when it comes to measuring team performance, there is no escaping observation. Within healthcare, the use of observation as a method for assessing team performance has grown significantly over the past 10 years. Most of the available tools specify a set of team performance dimensions, and these dimensions are defined by subsets of behavioral markers; observable behaviors that contribute to superior or substandard team performance. In addition to providing a tool for assessing an aspect of performance traditionally judged through gut feeling, behavioral marker systems supply a common language for discussing team skills and can function as frameworks to structure teaching and debriefing. As with any assessment system, the behavior observation and rating tool needs to be explicit, transparent, reliable, and valid for effective assessment of teamwork. In addition, the observation tool must be underpinned by properly developed models of teamwork. Ideally, one would first identify the core teamwork skills required for a specific job (and operational environment) using appropriate task

analysis techniques. However, in the absence of this information, models of team performance, which now exist in healthcare, could be used. For example, the teamwork framework that is the basis for the Agency for Healthcare Research and Quality's Team Strategies and Tools to Enhance Performance and Patient Safety (TeamSTEPPS®) curriculum is an excellent starting point.

A major challenge with observation is the limited capacity of human cognition. Although some researchers have attempted to train individuals to observe and evaluate as many as seven different teamwork processes within a single study, research has found that it is difficult for observers to distinguish more than four distinct teamwork processes at any given time. Smith-Jentsch et al.[3] found that subject matter experts could reliably discriminate among the following four higher-level teamwork dimensions: communication, information exchange, leadership, and supporting behavior.

STANDARDS FOR MEASUREMENT

In addition to the need to develop measures to support team training initiatives, the authors cannot overemphasize enough to the medical community that measures must be developed systematically and meet certain standards; measures must be reliable and valid.

First measures designed for assessing teamwork skills in healthcare need to be face valid. *Face validity*, a nonstatistical form of validity, is the realism that a measurement tool projects to the team being evaluated and the observer conducting the evaluation. It is the laymen's way of being able to see how this measure relates to the construct being assessed. Face validity is important because it helps the team know that the assessment will be a good representation of their performance, which will in turn elicit the most desirable response possible. In the context of healthcare, face validity is established by designing tools that have been contextualized to the healthcare environment, as opposed to using tools from other environments.

Second, *content validity* describes the systematic examination of the measurement tool's content to determine whether it covers a representative sample of the behavior domain to be measured. In other words, it is the extent to which a measure represents all parts of a construct, in this case teamwork. Content validity implies that new measures of healthcare team performance should be based on theoretically derived and validated models of teamwork and seeks to assess those knowledge and/or skills represented in the model.

When observers evaluate team performance, they must demonstrate reasonable levels of *interrater reliability* (IRR). High levels of IRR mean that those who observe and evaluate team performance are interchangeable; scores on the scale are a function of the team's performance and not the individual observer making the judgment. Interrater reliability is typically measured using Cohen's Kappa, where 0.21–0.40 is considered fair agreement, 0.41–0.60 is considered a moderate level of agreement, and 0.61–0.80 is considered a substantial level of agreement.

Construct validity involves the extent to which the tool may be said to measure a theoretical construct or trait. Construct validity is often examined by assessing convergent and discriminant validity. Convergent validity is the degree to which scales measuring the same construct are related, whereas discriminant validity is the degree to which scales measuring different constructs are unrelated.

Finally, *criterion-related validity* addresses how well a particular tool predicts current (concurrent validity) or future performance (predictive validity) on a job or some other form of independent criterion measure. Criterion validity is usually measured by correlating measures on the assessment tool with measures on the criterion to establish a significant relation.

SUMMARY AND CONCLUSIONS

The three factors presented here—what to measure, how to measure, and standards for measurement—are guiding issues for developing team performance measures that are critical for successful training. Healthcare must know that these programs work, how they work, and how to improve them; without measurement none of this possible.

Therefore, in closing, four guiding principles for healthcare and health services research are summarized for your consideration.

Principle 1: Align Measures of Team Performance with Current Models of Teamwork

It is only within the last 5 years that research has blossomed regarding the core competencies of healthcare teams. As noted, uniformed set of knowledge, skill, and attitude competencies that are related to most healthcare teams have been established in team training programs specifically designed for healthcare such as TeamSTEPPS®. Nonetheless, the extent to which these competencies are generic and apply to all healthcare teams needs to be tested. Moreover, regarding measurement, the authors are uncertain as to whether generic teamwork measures are sufficient for healthcare or tools must be contextualized to the specific team being measured.

Therefore, the authors believe strongly that research must validate models like the one presented in TeamSTEPPS® within care and across different healthcare teams to establish it robustness. Ironically, measures will have to be developed to accomplish such validation; therefore, this reciprocal process will push both measurement and theory development forward simultaneously.

Principle 2: Measure Both Process and Outcomes When Assessing Team Performance

In addition to developing valid measures of healthcare teamwork based on prevailing theory, future research must define and build valid measures of relevant outcomes. The low base rate of serious errors such as sentinel events potentially precludes this "ultimate criterion" from serving as a viable outcome construct. Given the vast number of medical procedures conducted each day, applying this "ultimate criterion" to the team performance in healthcare is impractical to say the least, despite the prevalence of errors cited in the IOM report, *To Err is Human*.

In an effort to resolve the base rate issue, the authors believe that healthcare should define and develop both process and outcome measures from a more theoretically focused perspective. For example, the TeamSTEPPS® model specifies knowledge, attitudinal, and performance outcomes and suggests that high levels of teamwork lead to team members holding more accurate shared mental models (i.e., knowledge) and more positive attitudes toward teamwork (i.e., mutual trust, belief in the importance of teamwork). Moreover, although not sequential, when these outcomes occur, performance should improve. Performance examples might include the time taken to execute the initial decision in an emergency-medicine unit, the time it takes to intubate a patient who has stopped breathing, or the reduction of health-acquired infections in a given intensive care unit.

Another important outcome that healthcare practitioners should consider is tapping voluntary event-reporting systems that capture "near misses." Such events can be viewed as a proxy criterion for error. The Patient Safety and Quality Improvement Act of 2005 (Patient Safety Act), which authorized the creation of patient safety organizations, provides a significant resource for such investigations. The Patient Safety Act encourages clinicians and healthcare organizations to voluntarily report and share quality and patient safety information without fear of legal discovery.

Principle 3. New Measures Must Be Developed and Tested

Our basic conclusion is that research on measurement and the development of measures to assess team performance must catch up with the deployment of interventions to improve quality in healthcare. Since the IOM report more than 10 years ago, there has been an explosion of tools and strategies, but not measures. For example, the Agency for Healthcare Research and Quality supports the national deployment of TeamSTEPPS®, but few tools are available to assess the impact of TeamSTEPPS training. Lacking these metrics it will be difficult for organizations consuming these patient safety interventions to know *if* and *how* they worked. This is critical in healthcare, in which financial resources are extremely limited. Therefore, researchers must focus not only on how to improve quality, team performance, and safety, but also concurrently develop measurement tools so that the effects of these interventions can be established.

Principle 4. The Psychometric Properties of New Measures Must Be Established

To date, limited information exists on the psychometric qualities of tools designed to measure team performance in healthcare. Such data are critical if we are to know that the measures we have developed actually work. In particular, these studies must examine multiple facets of reliability (i.e., internal consistency, rater agreement) and validity (convergent and discriminant, criterion-related). This work is extremely challenging because it requires access to healthcare teams on which to test new measures. Second, how to train staff to use these metrics is another question that must be explored. The combination of effectively designed team performance measures and adequately trained raters yields the highest-quality information for debriefing a team performance episode. Finally, healthcare practitioners should consider the role of simulation in these activities. Properly designed simulation scenarios are critical for stimulating the team behaviors that one is trying to measure and diagnose.

In closing, the authors believe that significant progress has been made, although significant work remains to be done. Measuring and diagnosing team performance is the key to performance improvement, and healthcare must continue to develop, test, and publish new measures as it seeks to improve care coordination. It will only be through proper measurement and diagnosis that true improvements in the delivery of care by highly trained teams will be realized.

REFERENCES

1. Smith-Jentsch, K. A., Johnston, J. H., & Payne, S. C. (1998). Measuring team-related expertise in complex environments. In J. A. Cannon-Bowers, & E. Salas (Eds.), *Making decisions under stress: Implications for individual and team training* (pp. 61–87). Washington, DC: American Psychological Association.

2. Stout, R. J., Salas, E., & Carson, R. (1994). Individual task proficiency and team process behavior: What's important for team functioning? *Military Psychology, 6*(3), 177–92.

3. Smith-Jentsch, K. A., Zeisig, R. L., Acton, B. & McPherson, J. A. (1998). Team dimensional. In J. A. Cannon-Bowers, & E. Salas (Eds.), *Making decisions under stress: Implications for individual and team training* (pp. 271–297). Washington, DC: American Psychological Association.

20

TEAMWORK IN HEALTHCARE: FROM TRAINING PROGRAMS TO INTEGRATED SYSTEMS OF DEVELOPMENT

Michael A. Rosen and Peter J. Pronovost

Healthcare has benefited from the hard-won lessons of other safety-critical industries. One of the most critical lessons learned has been the need for effective teamwork and systematic methods for developing and maintaining it. Military organizations know that good communication and teamwork are essential for avoiding incidents of combat misidentification and fratricide, such as the ones leading to the death of Pat Tillman and so many others. The aviation industry knows that a culture promoting assertiveness and deference to expertise, not authority, is essential to avoiding disasters such as the collision on Tenerife in 1977, which took 583 lives.

Increasingly, the healthcare industry is becoming aware of the teamwork and communication failures that pervade care delivery systems and the preventable harm these failures cause. Although teamwork failures in healthcare have been known for a long time, only recently has healthcare developed a detailed and theory-driven understanding of the nature of teamwork and communication failures as well as effective programs to reduce them. We know that mortality and complication rates increase when surgical teams fail to communicate intraoperatively and during briefings and handoffs.[1] We know that lack of or low-quality communication between nurses and physicians accounts for approximately 37% of errors in intensive care units.[2] We know that staff perceptions of handoff quality accounts for 25% of the variance in administratively coded patient safety indicators.[3] We know that members of care teams frequently have dangerously inconsistent conceptualizations of patient goals, and that simple communication interventions can address this problem.[4]

HOW FAR HAVE WE COME?

Although initial efforts to directly apply aviation-based models of team training to healthcare in an unaltered manner met with some resistance and were ultimately less than effective, the science and practice of team training in healthcare has evolved. The industry is beginning to adapt the training content, delivery methods, and process of implementation to its own needs, context, and constraints. Healthcare team training is maturing, and emerging evidence suggests that it is not only effective at improving teamwork behaviors, but also clinical processes and outcomes. Team training saves lives, yet it is still not broadly implemented in healthcare.

The number of team training programs and evaluation studies has grown dramatically in recent years.[5] The Agency for Healthcare Research and Quality (AHRQ) and Department of Defense funded Team Strategies and Tools to Enhance Performance and Patient Safety (TeamSTEPPS®) has been widely implemented in the military healthcare system as well as some civilian systems. This program is rooted in the theory and science of teams and focuses on building leadership, communication, mutual support, situation monitoring, and team structure (e.g., role clarity) competencies.

The US Department of Veterans Affairs has implemented a similar program, coupled with coaching and operating room checklists systemwide in its surgical services and found significant decreases in mortality rates, as well as a dose-response relationship such that greater use of teamwork was associated with greater reductions in mortality rates.[6] This large and well-designed study provides strong evidence that team training is a method for improving safety and quality, reducing preventable harm, and saving lives.

Although team training is effective and programs such as TeamSTEPPS® are broadly available, healthcare has not yet widely implemented team training into its educational and training systems or routine practice. Although some health systems have implemented team training programs, few if any have implemented a comprehensive system of selecting, developing, evaluating, and remediating teamwork competencies throughout the careers of healthcare workers. Few medical schools and residency programs include teamwork as a routine part of curricula. Unlike some airlines, medical schools, residency programs, and hospital appointment committees generally do not include predictors of team effectiveness such as collective orientation in their selection processes. In fact, these issues are often overlooked in admission and hiring even when someone may have a known and documented difficulty working in teams. Accrediting and licensing bodies do not consider teamwork or other nontechnical competencies. Given the magnitude of preventable harm caused by poor teamwork and the availability and evidence supporting team training, it is unclear why healthcare has not more broadly created systems to ensure teamwork competencies.

WHAT ARE THE BARRIERS TO BROAD ADOPTION OF TEAMWORK PRINCIPLES IN HEALTHCARE?

The obstacles to truly integrating principles of effective teamwork and communication into care delivery processes are numerous, and rooted in medical culture and the nature of teamwork failures in healthcare, the history and culture of medicine, the capabilities and capacities of educational institutions, and the regulatory structures of the industry.

First, *teamwork and communication failures are invisible.* They are only attended to when they result in errors of clinical processes and adverse outcomes, and then the clinical error is usually at the forefront. Even when teamwork errors result in harm, many of those investigating events in healthcare lack the "lenses" to see teamwork problems or the deep understanding of teamwork to diagnose the specific teamwork error and recommend effective interventions. Root cause analyses increasingly recognize communication errors, but this is largely an undifferentiated catchall category insufficient for guiding learning and correction. There are no diagnostic tools that link events to underlying causes, corrective interventions, and strategies to evaluate whether or not problems have been addressed. Unlike the examples from military and aviation domains introduced in the preceding, breakdowns in healthcare do not usually result in immediate and apparent catastrophe. Results can be far removed in time from their causal factors (e.g., a missed diagnosis resulting from inaccurate communication can take years to surface), which complicates the process of team members learning from experience and improving their teamwork skills. Methods and tools of evaluation-driven feedback for developing team competencies are few in number, and the ones that do exist are not widely accessible to providers.

Second, *social norms and expectations are still a problem.* Healthcare education and training, particularly for physicians, still emphasizes autonomy and promotes the mythology of a heroic provider, single-handedly caring for patients. Individual accountability and a drive for personal excellence are core values of the field, as they should be. However, when these values are enacted outside of an understanding that translating individual expertise into effective care is dependent on interactions with others, the result can be counterproductive. These expectations and values are not incompatible, but they have yet to be integrated and adopted wholeheartedly into healthcare.

Medicine has largely labeled patient harm from poor teamwork as "forgivable" and largely inevitable. In his elegant book, *Forgive and Remember*, the medical sociologist Charles Bosk[7] reports on 6 months spent following surgical teams at an academic medical center, trying to understand how these doctors dealt with error. He found that errors that resulted from lack of effort or withholding or providing inaccurate information were unforgivable, and errors that resulted from a sincere effort to provide care were forgiven. Such an individualistic ethic makes it difficult to address errors that result from the complex interplay of multiple factors or people.

Third, *those in educational and mentoring roles were not formally educated in teamwork competencies*. Healthcare educational institutions do not have ready access to qualified educators with expertise in teamwork. Even when the need for team-based educational activities is recognized, the capacity to execute often lags behind. There is an emphasis on developing professionalism and interpersonal communication, but exposure to these concepts frequently is limited to discussions of theory and values. Practical behavioral strategies for improving performance are rarely addressed.

Fourth, *teamwork competence is neither incentivized nor regulated*. Healthcare as a whole has not signified the importance of these concepts to providers, and has provided no compelling reasons to change how providers practice. Teamwork is not a part of licensing or accreditation processes. There is no binding regulatory requirement to engage in training, develop skills, or demonstrate competency in teamwork. Although communication errors frequently surface in malpractice claims, this is a blunt and indirect tool, ineffective for guiding the needed changes.

Fifth, *funding for advancing teamwork training and development in healthcare is insufficient*. There is an existing science of teams, and it has informed the development of interventions in healthcare to date. However, there are unanswered questions, and funding to support the needed research is limited. Specifically, high need areas include: developing an understanding of the specificity or generalizability of different teamwork behaviors across different clinical domains, team types, and task situations (e.g., is teamwork in obstetrics the same as in the intensive care unit? are teamwork skills during rounds the same as those needed during a code?); developing practical, valid, and reliable methods of assessing teamwork and diagnosing underlying issues (e.g., are observed problems to the result of skill deficiencies, work structure, or process issues?); and the development of effective feedback strategies to drive improvements over time.

WHAT IS THE WAY FORWARD?

The described barriers are significant, and only a subset of the challenges has been faced; however, initial efforts are promising. The road ahead involves scaling up from the demonstrated successes achieved through training programs and moving toward integrated systems of development. Training programs have an impermanent connotation. They are ephemeral, coming and going in organizations all the time, and as such, alone they are unlikely to ensure competency in teamwork. Although training will be a part of the ultimate solution, an integrated approach involves the alignment of factors in healthcare facilities, educational institutions, and regulatory bodies. This concerted effort is needed to drive widespread and lasting change. Several of the essential requirements are described in the following.

First, *ensure that all clinicians receive training and are competent in teamwork behaviors*. Most frequently, teamwork training is delivered after people have completed the bulk of their formal education or have been practicing for years. An integrated system of development would include coordinated efforts across formal educational activities as well as routine practices in healthcare systems. First, teamwork concepts need to be integrated throughout the continuum of healthcare education, from undergraduate medical and nursing programs, to residency programs, and lifelong continuing education. Innovation is happening in this area with interprofessional education and team-based learning initiatives, but these efforts remain nascent, isolated, and uncommon. Second, healthcare systems must reinforce this training through ongoing coaching, feedback, and opportunities to practice and develop teamwork behaviors in safe and structured environments.

Second, *create the infrastructure necessary to train teamwork*. Addressing the preceding need is beyond the current capacities of healthcare systems and educational institutions. Most academic medical centers and teaching hospitals lack sufficient numbers of skilled trainers and educators needed to ensure competency in teamwork. To address this, medical colleges can hire psychologists to develop and evaluate educational and training activities. The attributes of effective clinical teamwork trainers need to be determined. Train the trainer programs need to be evaluated more rigorously (i.e., are they producing competent trainers capable of and comfortable with delivering teamwork training?) and ultimately expanded.

Third, *support ongoing long-term development with tools to evaluate, provide feedback, and coach teamwork behaviors on the job*. It is probably unrealistic to believe that teamwork competency develops after a single or even several training sessions. Clinicians' diagnostic and treatment skills are honed over years, often over a decade of formal education and apprenticeship during residency and fellowship. Teamwork skills likely mature over time. Given the challenge of transferring teamwork behaviors from training to the clinical context as well as the practical constraints of scheduling dedicated training time for providers, evaluation of teamwork behaviors during actual care delivery will need to drive feedback and coaching processes. We need to develop the tools and the human capital necessary to make this a reality.

Fourth, *strengthen incentives for ensuring competency in teamwork*. This must occur on several levels. Selection processes for hiring clinicians, especially physicians, can include behavioral interviewing not unlike some assessment centers in the corporate world. Board certification can include teamwork competencies assessed through multiple means, including simulation, 360-degree evaluations, and observation. Licensing boards can evaluate teamwork, and continuing education in the health professions can require participation and training in teamwork. Some incentives have been put in place by malpractice insurers who reduce the premiums of physicians who engage in simulation or teamwork training. This model needs to be explored further and expanded where appropriate.

Fifth, *continue to advance the science of teamwork*. We know a good deal about what makes teams effective, but we need a deeper and more detailed understanding of teamwork in the broad variety of healthcare contexts. For example, to effectively integrate teamwork in the continuum of healthcare education, we need to know which teamwork competencies are generalizable across clinical areas and which are context-, team-, or task-specific. We need research on the most effective methods for training teamwork to get the most out of limited time resources. We need practical measurement systems and behavioral markers that can drive improvement, as well as an understanding of which feedback strategies are most effective.

Teamwork and communication failures contribute to a large proportion of alarmingly high number of patients harmed in healthcare systems today. Given the availability of proven methods, and the demonstrated benefits of teamwork training and coaching, the time has come to ensure care providers are competent team members. Patients deserve nothing less.

REFERENCES

1. Mazzocco, K., Petitti, D. B., Fong, K. T., Bonacum, D., Brookey, J., Graham, S., et al. (2009). Surgical team behaviors and patient outcomes. *American Journal of Surgery, 197,* 678–85.

2. Donchin, Y., Gopher, D., Olin, M., Badihi, Y., Biesky, M., Sprung, C. L., et al. (1995). A look into the nature and causes of human errors in the intensive care unit. *Critical Care Medicine, 23,* 294–300.

3. Mardon, R. E., Khanna, K., Sorra, J., Dyer, N., & Famolaro, T. (2010). Exploring relationships between hospital patient safety culture and adverse events. *Journal of Patient Safety, 6,* 226–32.

4. Pronovost, P., Berenholtz, S., Dorman, T., Lipsett, P. A., Simmonds, T., & Haraden, C. (2003). Improving communication in the ICU using daily goals. *Journal of Critical Care, 18*(2), 71–5.

5. Weaver, S. L., Lyons, R., DiazGranados, D., Rosen, M. A., Salas, E., Oglesby, J., et al. (2010). The anatomy of health care team training and

the state of practice: a critical review. *Academic Medicine, 85,* 1746–60.

6. Neily, J., Mills, P. D., Young-Xu, Y., Carney, B. T., West, P., Berger, D. H., et al. (2010). Association between implementation of a medical team training program and surgical mortality. *Journal of the American Medical Association, 304,* 1693–700.

7. Bosk, C. L. (2003). *Forgive and remember: Managing medical failure,* 2nd ed. Chicago: University of Chicago Press.

21

LESSONS LEARNED FROM THE VETERANS HEALTH ADMINISTRATION MEDICAL TEAM TRAINING PROGRAM

Douglas E. Paull and Lisa M. Mazzia

The Veterans Health Administration (VA) is the nationwide healthcare provider network for Veterans. It includes primary care, specialty care, behavioral health, and geriatrics. Healthcare is administered within 21 Veterans Integrated Service Networks (VISNs) at 153 hospitals, 773 community-based outpatient clinics (CBOCs), 135 community living centers, 47 residential rehabilitation programs, and 260 readjustment counseling centers. The VA National Center for Patient Safety (NCPS) developed, piloted, and rolled out a national medical team training (MTT) program in 2006. The purpose of this chapter is to share the lessons learned from the MTT program.

ENGAGE LEADERSHIP AND LOCAL CHAMPIONS

A leadership conference call occurs before MTT preparation and planning and the learning session.[1] The purpose of the call serves to explain the goals of MTT, crew resource management (CRM) principles, the results of MTT thus far, and expectations. Facility and clinical area leadership are strongly encouraged to attend the MTT learning session and give opening remarks.

Leadership involvement at the time of the MTT learning session is associated with a greater chance of success of the patient safety initiative checklist-guided preoperative briefings and postoperative debriefings in the operating room.[2] Facilities with superior leadership were four times more likely to conduct checklist-guided briefings for all cases on all services 1 year after MTT compared with other facilities.

Likewise, MTT program leadership (senior NCPS physicians and nurses) are present on leadership calls, preparation and planning calls, at learning sessions, and on follow-up interviews. The positive effect of leadership on the outcomes of a broad range of VA patient safety initiatives has been previously reported.[3]

We have also examined the beneficial consequence of local champions for MTT projects. Operating room nurse manager engagement in the MTT preparation and planning conference calls was significantly associated with measured briefing success in the operating room 1 year later.[4] These data have important ramifications for the structure and leadership of change teams implementing patient safety initiatives.

IMPLEMENT MEDICAL TEAM TRAINING IN CLINICAL MICROSYSTEMS

Patient safety improvement initiatives are developed and implemented by frontline staff and champions ("the sharp end of healthcare").[5] Clinical microsystems represent a core group of healthcare workers caring for a particular population of patients.[6] Successful microsystems can be characterized as having constancy of purpose, integration of information, interdependence of care team, and measurement of results. Microsystems concerned with patient safety share features of high reliability organizations such as a preoccupation with failure (e.g., learning from near misses) and deference to expertise (rather than hierarchy).[6]

The MTT program works with microsystems (e.g., surgery, intensive care unit, emergency room, floor, catheterization laboratory, interventional radiology). Local champions and implementation teams brainstorm patient safety vulnerabilities within their respective microsystems. A patient safety project is developed (e.g., checklist-guided preoperative briefings and postoperative debriefings in the operating room). Process and outcome measurements and targets are developed.

The MTT learning session is protected time for teams to gain knowledge, practice new skills in a safe environment, and reflect on their patient safety processes. Following the learning session, the patient safety improvement plan is implemented. Follow-up with quarterly conference calls allows troubleshooting and further refinements. National Center for Patient Safety faculty serve as facilitators linking facility microsystems (e.g., structured handoffs between emergency room and intensive care unit).

An example of this one step at a time approach involves checklist-guided preoperative briefings and postoperative debriefings in the operating room. One hundred twenty-nine facilities underwent MTT. Each surgical team developed their own checklist, implementation plan, and measurements. The microsystem approach led to remarkable patient safety improvements for the entire organization. Studies demonstrated improved antibiotic and deep venous thrombosis prophylaxis compliance rates and decreased surgical mortality following MTT.[7,8]

MASS CUSTOMIZATION

Mass customization was popularized by the automotive industry.[9] In-depth consumer focus group studies led to the development of "packages" of options for automobiles that appealed to large groups of the population. Instead of making individually customized cars for each customer, cars with standard features and available option packages were designed. This same concept was useful for rolling MTT out to many clinical areas at multiple facilities.

All operating room teams were required to implement checklist-guided preoperative briefings and postoperative debriefings as a patient safety initiative. Teams could choose additional projects from a list including: interdisciplinary patient-centered rounds, structured patient handoffs (e.g., Situation-Background-Assessment-Recommendation), interdisciplinary administrative briefings, code debriefings, or fatigue management.[1]

Implementation teams often had a patient safety issue (e.g., miscommunication of information regarding patients being admitted to floor from the emergency room) identified at the time of the first preparation and planning conference call 8 weeks before the MTT learning session. Frequently, the team would choose one of the readily available suggested projects (e.g., structured handoffs between emergency room and floor). The team would then select champions, process and outcome measures, and target dates for improvement.

SIMULATION

Simulation is a highly effective modality in the demonstration and acquisition of CRM teamwork and communication techniques.[10] Specific CRM behaviors can be elicited within simulation scenarios. With simulation, interprofessional teams can practice CRM techniques in a safe environment.[11] Self-reflection of the shared simulation experience during the debriefing is an important component of the learning process.[12]

The VA MTT program has used in situ, point of care simulation-based training. Participant self-report of attitudes and observational scores of teamwork and communication skills improve significantly following training.[13] Several important questions remain; however, including the sustainability of CRM skills following training and whether simulation-demonstrated skills translate to improved clinical care.

We have recently demonstrated significant improvement of CRM skills following observational learning (staff watching colleagues in a live simulation).[14] Instructional features included didactic lecture, a live simulation projected onto a screen, audience participation using an observational tool, and the entire audience participating in a facilitated debriefing.[15] Such an observational learning platform would allow for CRM training for a larger number of participants in a shorter time period at less cost.

BUILD IN A 360-DEGREE ASSESSMENT OF THE MEDICAL TEAM TRAINING PROGRAM

The framework for evaluation of teamwork training in aviation and healthcare consists of four levels of information:[16–18] trainees' attitudes toward the program; trainees' understanding of the principles and skills addressed in the training; demonstration of behaviors in the job or in simulation that are consistent with the training; and organizational impact such as improved outcomes.

Such a 360-degree assessment was built into the VA NCPS MTT program from the beginning.[19]

Initial data demonstrating success was useful in securing "buy in" for the national roll out. The MTT mission of improving patient outcomes and staff morale, and positively changing the culture of patient safety within the organization was fulfilled as supported by the results from a variety of survey, observational, and administrative tools and databases.

Safety attitude questionnaire (SAQ) survey results, including the safety and teamwork domains, significantly improved at 9 to 12 months after MTT as compared with baseline (Fig. 21.1).[20] Important patient safety behaviors such as compliance with antibiotic and deep venous thrombosis prophylaxis guidelines improved (Fig. 21.2).[7] There was an association between reduced adjusted surgical morbidity and mortality and the implementation of the MTT program (including checklist-guided preoperative briefings and postoperative debriefings).[8,21] Sites that had yet to have MTT had higher surgical mortality than comparable sites undergoing the training. There was improved mortality at sites following MTT.

COMMON THEME: COMMUNICATION THROUGH CONVERSATION

All clinical areas receiving MTT are required to select at least one project (or design their own) to implement. The project activity or intervention—preoperative briefings guided by a checklist, interdisciplinary

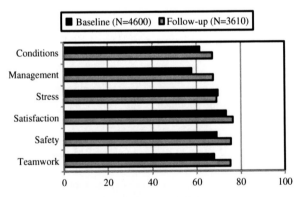

Figure 21.1
Safety Attitudes Questionnaire (SAQ) Data. SAQ scores for each of six domains before and 9 to 12 months following medical team training, p < 0.05, all pre vs. post comparisons except for 'stress'.
Reprinted from Neily, J., Mills, P. Lee, P., et al. (2010). Medical team training and coaching in the VA: Assessment and impact of the first 32 facilities in the program. *Quality and Safety in Health Care, 19,* 360–364, with permission from BMJ Publishing Group Ltd.[20]

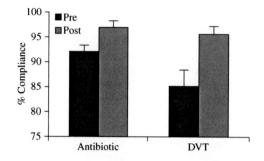

Figure 21.2
Antibiotic and deep venous thrombosis prophylaxis. Compliance rates before and 12 months following medical team training and implementation of check-list-guided preoperative briefings and postoperative debriefings, $p < 0.05$ both pre vs. post comparisons. Reprinted from: Paull, D. E., Mazzia, L. M., Wood, S. D., Theis, M. S., Robinson, L. D., Carney, B., et al. (2010). Briefing guide study: preoperative briefing and postoperative debriefing checklists in the Veterans Administration medical team training program. *American Journal of Surgery,* 200, 620–3.[7]

administrative briefings, or something else—provides a platform for direct conversation among team members. The focus of the conversation is how to achieve an agreed-on patient-centered outcome with all team members having the opportunity to share information, voice concerns and suggest solutions. Provonost has suggested that it is the conversation itself, rather than the checking of items on a check-list, that may be the essential factor in the results that have been obtained.[22]

SUSTAINABILITY

Many change programs are initially successful, yet implementation of the intervention decreases over time. Factors that determine what causes a program to be effective several months or years after implementation have yet to be determined. It is our expectation that serial monitoring of checklist-guided briefing rates, SAQ scores, and mortality data will lead to questions concerning sustainability to be formulated and, hopefully, answered.

REFERENCES

1. Dunn, E. J., Mills, P. D., Neily, J., Crittenden, M. D., Carmack, A. L., & Bagian, J. P. (2007). Medical team training: applying crew resource management in the Veterans Health Administration. *J Qual Patient Safe, 33,* 317–25.

2. Paull, D. E., Mazzia, L. M., Izu B. S., Neily, J., Mills, P. D., & Bagian, J. P. (2009). Predictors of successful implementation of preoperative and postoperative debriefings after medical team training. *American Journal of Surgery, 198,* 675–8.

3. Mills, P. D., & Weeks, W. B. (2004). Characteristics of successful quality improvement teams: Lessons from five collaborative projects in the VA. *Joint Commission Journal on Quality and Patient Safety, 30,* 152–62.

4. Robinson, L., Paull, D. E., Mazzia, L., Hay, J., Neilly, J., Mills, P., et al. (2010). Role of the operating room nurse manager in success of preoperative briefings and postoperative debriefings during medical team training. *Journal of PeriAnesthesia Nursing, 25,*302–6.

5. Dekker, S. (2010). *The Field Guide to Understanding Human Error* Burlington, VT: Ashgate Publishing.

6. Mohr, J. J., Batalden, P., & Barach, P. (2004). Integrating patient safety into the clinical microsystem. *Quality and Safety in Health Care, 13*(Suppl II), ii34–8.

7. Paull, D. E., Mazzia, L. M., Wood, S. D., Theis, M. S., Robinson, L. D., Carney, B., et al. (2010). Briefing guide study: preoperative briefing and postoperative debriefing checklists in the Veterans Health Administration medical team training program. *American Journal of Surgery, 200,* 620–3.

8. Neily, J., Mills, P. D., Young-Xu, Y., Carney, B. T., West, P., Berger, D. H., et al. (2010). Association between implementation of a medical team training program and surgical mortality. *Journal of the American Medical Association, 304,* 1693–700.

9. Hart, C. W. L. (1995). Mass customization: conceptual underpinnings, opportunities and limits. *International Journal of Service Industry Management, 6,* 36–45.

10. Gaba, D. M. (2004). The future vision of simulation in health care. *Quality and Safety in Health Care, 13*(Suppl 1), i2–10.

11. Fox-Robichaud, A. E., & Nimmo, G. R. (2007). Education and simulation techniques for improving reliability of care. *Current Opinions in Critical Care, 13,* 737–41.

12. Rosen, M. A., Salas, E., Wilson, K. A., King, H. B., Salisbury, M., Augenstein, J. S., et al. (2008). Measuring team performance in simulation-based training: Adopting best practices for healthcare. *Sim Healthcare, 3*, 33–41.

13. Wolk, S., Paull, D. E., Mazzia, L. M., Robinson, L. D., Hatwood, C., Paige, J. T., et al. (2011). *Team training simulation pilot for VHA surgical services.* Abstract, Association of VA Surgeons Meeting, Irvine, CA.

14. Paull, D. E., Williams, L., Hoeksema, L. J., Friedlander, A. H. (2011). Simulation-based medical team training utilizing an observational-experiential learning model. *Association of American Medical Colleges,* June 9–10, Chicago.

15. Rosen, M. A., Salas, E., Pavlas, D., Jensen, R., Fu, D., & Lampton, D. (2010). Demonstration-based training: A review of instructional features. *Human Factors, 52,* 596–609.

16. Sorbero, M. E., Farley, D. O., Mattke, S., & Lovejoy, S. (2008). *Outcome measures for effective teamwork in inpatient care.* Final report. Agency for Healthcare Research and Quality. Santa Monica, CA: Rand Health.

17. Salas, E., Burke, C. S., Bowers, C. A. et al. (2001). Team training in the skies: Does crew resource management (CRM) training work? *Human Factors, 43,* 641–74.

18. Salas, E., Almeida, S. A., Salisbury, M., King, H., Lazzara, E.H., Lyons, R., et al. (2009). What are the critical success factors for team training in health care? *Joint Commission Journal on Quality and Patient Safety, 35,* 398–405.

19. Dunn, E. J. Medical Team Training in the Veterans Health Administration. (2011). White Paper. Retrieved from: http://www.patientsafety.gov/MTT/WhitePaper.pdf

20. Neily, J., Mills, P., Lee, P., Carney, B., West, P., Percarpio, K., et al. (2010). Medical team training and coaching in the VA: Assessment and impact of the first 32 facilities in the program. *Quality and Safety in Health Care, 19,* 360–4.

21. Young-Xu, Y., Neily, J., Mills, P. D., Carney, B. T., West, P., Berger, D. H., et al. (2011). Association between implementation of a medical team training program and surgical morbidity. *Archives of Surgery, 146,* 1368–73.

22. Pronovost, P. J., & Freischlag, J. A. (2010). Improving teamwork to reduce surgical mortality. *Journal of the American Medical Association, 304,* 1721–22.

22

MEDICAL TEAM DEBRIEFS: SIMPLE, POWERFUL, UNDERUTILIZED

Scott I. Tannenbaum and Sara N. Goldhaber-Fiebert

There can be little doubt that teamwork and coordination are crucial for patient safety. In addition to clinical expertise, healthcare professionals must possess teamwork competencies to perform their routine duties safely and to effectively manage crisis situations (e.g., crisis resource management or CRM).[1] The healthcare field must continually seek and apply techniques that will enhance team coordination, communication, and competency. One such technique worthy of greater attention is team debriefing.

During a team debrief, team members reflect on a recent experience, discuss what went well, and identify opportunities for improvement. To be effective, these discussions should focus on practitioner actions, communications, and underlying mindsets. Team debriefs can be relatively inexpensive to conduct and may be used during planned team training activities or as a way to learn from "on-the-job" experiences. Research supports the contention that well-conducted debriefs work[2] with a recent meta-analysis of prior empirical studies revealing average improvements of 20 to 25%.[3] Given their benefits, we would hope to see them deeply embedded in medical education, training, and practice.

Unfortunately, debriefs are underutilized in healthcare, and when they are used, they are not always conducted in an optimal manner. A few highly skilled, extensively trained facilitators lead debriefs in many institutions and interest in team debriefing is rising as evidenced by the many presentations on the topic at recent medical simulation and education conferences. However, it is also clear that there are too many missed opportunities to deploy effective, structured team debriefs and to embed them into standard medical practice.

This commentary is a call to increase the use and quality of debriefing to enhance teamwork skills throughout the healthcare field. To support this, we highlight why debriefs work, discuss a few myths about debriefing, and offer recommendations for embedding debriefs into medical education, training, and practice.

TEAM DEBRIEFS: WHY DO THEY WORK?

A team debrief is conducted after a training event (e.g., a simulation), work experience (e.g., treating a patient), or time period (e.g., end of a shift). The person leading the debrief may be a medical content expert, trained facilitator, or both.

The intent of a team debrief is to ensure that the right learning occurs from an experience. For example, after treating a trauma patient or performing a surgery, in either a real or a simulated setting, what did the team take away from the experience? If the patient survived, does that mean the team did everything correctly? Not necessarily.

Reasonable questions include: Did the team communicate effectively? Who was the leader? Were handoffs and briefings successful? Did people feel comfortable speaking up? Were the right equipment and personnel available? Did everyone know and maintain the "big picture?" What triggered a call for help and was this the appropriate time? Would the team do anything differently in the future?

Team debriefs explicitly examine teamwork and coordination, so they often uncover and correct knowledge gaps or misconceptions that could lead to future problems. Fortunately, a teamwork deficiency doesn't always cause patient harm. Teams "get away" with suboptimal coordination at times. But left unexamined, underlying teamwork problems are likely to harm a future patient. Individuals may incorrectly assume that the situation was handled appropriately (e.g., "I guess that handoff was okay"), even if another team member such as the receiver of the handoff knows otherwise. Without an explicit debrief, a valuable learning opportunity may be missed and next time an inappropriate handoff might cause a serious patient safety problem that could have been averted.

Debriefs are based on sound scientific principles. The type of information sharing, feedback, discussion, and action planning that occur during a well-designed debrief prepares teams to perform more effectively. For example, a meta-analysis of over 70 studies showed how information sharing is essential for team performance and cohesion.[4] It also revealed that not all teams naturally share information adequately. One reason debriefs work is that they foster the type of information sharing and feedback that does not occur naturally in many settings, including some training environments.

Debriefs also help teams form shared mental models. Team members are said to have a shared mental model when they possess a clear, common understanding, for example of a patient's status in ventricular fibrillation and who should do what to treat it quickly. A meta-analysis of over 20 empirical studies reveals that teams with shared mental models consistently perform better than other teams.[5] Debriefs are effective, in part, because they help teams establish shared mental models.

Finally, team debriefs work because they reinforce the importance of teamwork. Periodically asking a few questions about how the team worked together is a reminder that coordination is an integral part of good medical practice. If teamwork is never discussed, it sends the opposite signal. When used in conjunction with CRM and team training, a brief effective clinical team debrief reinforces the competencies that were taught during training.

DEBRIEF MYTHS

Several myths exist that can contribute to sub-optimal debriefing practices. Given that research has disproven each of these, it is important to be aware of them and take actions to overcome them.

Myth 1: He is good with people, so he'll be a good debrief facilitator. It is logical to believe that a person with good interpersonal skills will be an effective debrief facilitator. Good interpersonal skills may be necessary but are not sufficient to lead effective debriefs. Additional preparation is needed.

Myth 2: I'm an expert, so I'm an effective debriefer. Facilitators with technical competence do not necessarily conduct effective debriefs. In fact, experts often talk too much and fail to involve the team adequately. Because even an expert can't know what team members were thinking, some key points may not surface. Equally important, people are far more likely to "own" and change behaviors when they are involved in uncovering the problem. So having an expert tell the team what to do is unlikely to produce the desired results. Experts need guidance to lead a debrief properly.

Myth 3: Simply working together will build teamwork. Each of us has probably been on a team that did not improve or even became less effective over time. Simply spending time together provides no assurance that teamwork will ensue. Over the years, the military has learned that "free-play" or allowing teams to practice together without structured debriefing, even when conducted in very realistic high-fidelity simulation environments, does not work and can sometimes teach the wrong lessons. Learning together from experience is highly desirable, but working together is not enough. Good, structured, debriefing is needed.

Myth 4: Any discussion is a team debrief. Although discussing a case is useful, how it is discussed, what is discussed, and who participates in the discussion matter. Most team leaders were promoted because of their professional expertise, so they are often more comfortable discussing taskwork than teamwork. An engineering team leader is apt to guide her team to discuss tensile strength and a doctor is likely to focus on diagnosis or treatment. Both are less likely to ask questions about teamwork.

Not all discussions are equivalent. A conversation among doctors is helpful, but won't improve coordination with nurses and technicians. If teamwork is a goal, then a debrief process can be structured to ensure that happens, but not just any type of discussion will suffice.

These myths partly explain why effective team debriefs are not deeply embedded into medical education and practice. For us to make progress, there is a need to scale up the number of people who can facilitate them effectively, including medical school professors, hospital trainers, and medical team leaders. We need to encourage them to conduct team debriefs, find opportunities to educate them about the value and ease of debriefing, and provide them with the necessary tools, processes, and skills for doing so. Without guidance, these leaders are less likely to conduct debriefs and the ones they do may be perceived as a waste of time, which discourages the use of future debriefs.

RECOMMENDATIONS FOR EMBEDDING TEAM DEBRIEFING INTO MEDICAL EDUCATION AND PRACTICE

If we view the ongoing effort to encourage teamwork in healthcare as a large-scale culture change effort, then we can examine another similar change for lessons learned. The aviation community underwent a similar culture change effort to enhance teamwork and increase safety. Although the fields have important differences, a few key insights emerged from the aviation experience that are equally relevant in healthcare:

• **Teach teamwork to people early in their educational experience.** This is when early habits

are formed. If aviators are not introduced to teamwork when they are first learning how to fly, they will not view it as standard operating procedure when they are subsequently asked to fly real missions. This analogy holds for medical education.

• **Early exposure is not enough—address teamwork in subsequent training programs.** Training should continue to build teamwork competencies after early education is complete. Repeat exposure is needed. This is particularly important in the early stages of a culture change, because most people who are currently working were not exposed to teamwork competencies during their education. For them, training in the field may be their first concentrated exposure to teamwork practices.

• **Reinforce teamwork on-the-job.** Research has shown that less than 10% of learning in organizations occurs in formal training environments, so on-the-job learning is critical.[6] In any significant change effort, we need to find ways to regularly reinforce key messages. Ideally, teamwork gets integrated into the job and becomes "the way we perform our jobs," rather than an additional responsibility.

Team debriefing has a role to play in promoting teamwork and building CRM skills during medical education, subsequent training, and on-the-job. Below we provide a few recommendations for each of these three opportunities.

DEBRIEFING DURING MEDICAL EDUCATION

Medical education is the foundation point when teamwork competency building and awareness begins. Building periodic team debriefs into the curriculum helps set the stage.

Prepare professors. Professors send the earliest signals to students about the relative importance of teamwork, so they are a key leverage point. When professors conduct team debriefs they send a powerful message about the importance of teamwork. But we must be careful not to assume that because professors are educators with deep medical knowledge that they will naturally be good team debrief facilitators. If we do not ensure that they have a working knowledge of teamwork skills and prepare them to conduct team debriefs, they will be unlikely to conduct them or may do so ineffectively. In contrast, when they are well prepared they can model correct debriefing behaviors for all of their students to emulate.

Teach future doctors to be medical team leaders. To what extent do doctors in training view themselves as future leaders? When doctors perceive themselves as medical leaders, rather than strictly as individual experts, they are more likely to take actions that help ensure their teams are effective. Look for opportunities to convey this message during their education, and teach them to use debriefs as a leadership tool that promotes effective patient care.

Use interprofessional training. Healthcare teams are made up of individuals from different disciplines. Yet they are often educated independently, with limited training interaction. When possible, identify opportunities to bring together student doctors, nurses, and other healthcare professionals as part of their education. Conduct training exercises or simulations and use team debriefs to initiate conversations about inter-profession collaboration. Create an early understanding that the healthcare team includes everyone who supports the care of the patient.

RESIDENCY AND BEYOND: SIMULATION TRAINING

The most extensive use of debriefing has been in medical simulation training, often focusing on residency training in a particular specialty. Most residents are now exposed to some simulation training with debriefing as part of their program, several medical boards are now requiring simulation with debriefing as part of recertification, and at least one malpractice carrier has incentivized departments to require attending physicians to do simulation training with debriefing. These programs all expose more people to the concepts and vocabulary of team training and CRM principles, so that they are more likely to be reinforced in the workplace. Without a multiprong effort, it is unrealistic to expect students or residents to integrate these behaviors if they are not modeled

and reinforced in the workplace. As hospitals continue to add simulation capabilities, the opportunities to use debriefing to build team competencies will continue to grow.

Prepare for and build in team debriefing opportunities during team training. Consider the role of debriefing when designing team training. For example, develop scenarios that create the need for teamwork and then use debrief questions that examine whether key behaviors were exhibited. Do not expect "free play" to work. Also, be sure to allocate sufficient time to conduct a thorough team debrief. Otherwise, a potentially useful simulation experience won't produce the desired results.

Conduct team debriefs even when the primary focus is not on teamwork. When the primary training objective is to build team competencies, it is logical to include a team debrief, but how about when training a team to perform a new medical technique? Consider whether it would be valuable to ask a couple of debrief questions about how the team worked together, and not simply whether the technique worked as planned.

Prepare facilitators to lead effective debriefs. Be sure the people who are conducting training or simulation exercises in your facility are very comfortable leading team debriefs and be alert to the common pitfalls noted earlier. Provide facilitator training that includes advice for leading a debrief and handling common challenges.

DEBRIEFING ON-THE-JOB

Debriefing in situ, whether in hospitals or other healthcare environments, is significantly more challenging than in educational or training environments, but has tremendous potential. The biggest challenges to debriefing on-the-job are time constraints and focus, given the clinical demands for team members. For these reasons, we need to acknowledge the value of peoples' time and recognize that not all clinical teams can conduct debriefs. Carefully choose where and when to introduce them, keep them simple, and provide just enough structure to make them valuable.

Consider scheduling periodic debriefs. In some settings, it may be possible to schedule periodic team debriefs. For example, perhaps once per month an operating room team could plan to stay a few extra minutes after a surgery to conduct a team debrief.

Consider conducting quick end of shift debriefs. Sometimes the right time to conduct a debrief is not after a case but at the end of a shift. Because different shifts often don't overlap for long, it is not possible to conduct thorough debriefs each day. However, it may be possible to periodically schedule a time when two shifts will overlap a little longer than usual and conduct a structured debrief about handoffs and cross-shift coordination. To be successful, this increase in overlap time would need to be valued by the institution given the current pressure to get one shift in and the other out promptly.

Rounds. As more people see the patient safety benefits of better communication, rounds in settings like ICU and Labor and Delivery floors are becoming more interdisciplinary. Periodically, a short team debrief as part of interdisciplinary rounds would be helpful, focusing on teamwork, handoffs, interdisciplinary coordination, etc. The exact composition of these teams changes several times a day, but many of the players will subsequently participate in similar teams whose patients would benefit from any lessons learned during prior rounds.

Teach medical team leaders how to conduct a 5-minute debrief. Although a team debrief in a training environment could last 15 to 45 minutes, in a clinical setting, it can be hard to find even a few minutes. Teach team leaders how to lead a quick, targeted 5-minute debrief. Sometimes, these debriefs can focus on systems issues which were identified as a concern during prior training or patient care.

Find a few champions and share success stories. A key to gaining traction is to find a few team leaders who are willing and prepared to conduct periodic team debriefs, equip them with what they need, and then capture and share their success stories to gain momentum.

Team debriefs are a simple, inexpensive, scientifically sound method for building teamwork competencies and team effectiveness. Hopefully the ideas advocated in this commentary can stimulate greater use of effective debriefing techniques in medical education, training, and practice, and help advance the culture of teamwork in healthcare.

REFERENCES

1. Gaba, D. M., Howard, S. K., Fish, K. J., Smith, B. E., & Sowb, Y. A. (2001). Simulation-based training in anesthesia crisis resource management (ACRM): A decade of experience. *Simulation & Gaming, 32*(2), 175–93.

2. Smith-Jentsch, K. A., Cannon-Bowers, J. A., Tannenbaum, S. I., & Salas, E. (2008). Guided team self-correction: Impacts on team mental models, processes, and effectiveness. *Journal of Small Group Research, 39*, 303–27.

3. Tannenbaum, S.I. & Cerasoli, C.P. (in press). Do team and individual debriefs enhance performance? A meta-analysis. Human Factors: *The Journal of Human Factors and Ergonomics Society.*

4. Mesmer-Magnus, J. R. & DeChurch, L. A. (2009). Information sharing and team performance: A meta-analysis. *Journal of Applied Psychology, 94*, 535–46.

5. DeChurch, L. A. & Mesmer-Magnus, J. R. (2010). Measuring shared team mental models: A meta-analysis. *Group Dynamics, 14*, 1–14.

6. Tannenbaum, S. I. (1997). Enhancing continuous learning: Diagnostic findings from multiple companies. *Human Resource Management, 36*, 437–52.

PART SIX

SUMMARY

23

USING THE SCIENCE OF TEAMWORK TO TRANSFORM HEALTHCARE: THEMES AND WHAT'S NEXT

Eduardo Salas and Michael A. Rosen

Teamwork training took center stage as a healthcare safety and quality improvement initiative in 2000 with a strong endorsement from the Institute of Medicine. The seminal report, *To Err is Human*, advocated teamwork training as a means for protecting against what seemed to be a pervasive communication problem in care delivery systems. At the time, the evidence surrounding the exact nature of the problem (e.g., what specifically is a communication error, and what causes them?) as well as the efficacy of teamwork training as a means to combat these errors in healthcare was not convincing to many stakeholders. There were strong indications that teamwork training would be an effective strategy, and a very logical case to be made; however, studies linking teamwork to clinical processes and patient outcomes were limited and contentious. Consequently, the early implementations of teamwork training programs met with resistance from various communities and facilities. There were those fundamentally opposed to the concept as well as those delaying action based on very practical concerns: Implementing teamwork training would be culturally challenging, costly in terms of staff time, and the guarantee of results had yet to be demonstrated.

However, a decade later, the story is changing. Evidence continues to emerge at an increasing rate, and the preponderance of this evidence indicates that *teamwork training works*: it can improve the teamwork behaviors of staff members in a variety of domains;[1,2] it can improve clinical processes and safety;[3–5] and it can improve patient outcomes and quality of care.[6,7] It is a concept whose time has come and an imperative for the thousands of patients experiencing preventable harm each year.

Significant advancements have been made in recent years, including the adaptation of proven methods, tools, and strategies applied successfully in other domains, as well as the development of new approaches to meeting the unique demands of a complex industry. The chapters in this volume attest to this progress. They detail a deep knowledge-base and a rich set of practical tools for improving teamwork and saving patients' lives through more effective communication, coordination, and collaboration.

This chapter summarizes the state of healthcare team training and highlights some critical gaps and future directions for the field. To that end, 10 themes that cut across the chapters in this volume are presented.

1. ALL TEAMS ARE NOT CREATED EQUAL.

Healthcare is an incredibly varied field, and there are important differences in the structure, composition, and tasks of healthcare teams working in different clinical areas. Teams in ambulatory care clinics neither look nor function like surgical teams. An intensive care unit team does not interact in the same way as an emergency department team. This variability in the nature of the teams and the work they do requires different approaches to building and managing teamwork. There is no one-size-fits-all solution to training teamwork in healthcare. From a science of teams perspective, this means that we must understand which teamwork competencies or forms of those competencies apply in which contexts (e.g., leadership will most likely be important in all circumstances, but the specific types of leadership behaviors may be more or less important in different contexts). From a practical perspective, we need to understand how teamwork concepts can be integrated with clinical work in different domains. Many accomplishments in this area have already been achieved, as illustrated by the diversity of domains represented in this volume: labor and delivery (Mann and Pratt), the emergency department (Perry, Wears, and McDonald), the intensive care unit (Marsteller, Thompson, Pennathur, and Pronovost), trauma (Stahl, Garcia, Birnbach, and Augenstein), surgical recovery rooms (Anders, France, and Weinger), and pediatrics (Coleman, Lambert, and Slonim).

2. IT IS ALL ABOUT THE ORGANIZATION.

Teamwork is situated within complex care delivery systems, and building effective teamwork means addressing the interconnectedness of staff behaviors with organizational culture, history, regulatory concerns, policies, procedures, and a host of other contextual issues. The preexisting context within which a team training program is implemented exerts great influence on the ultimate outcomes. This is not unique to teamwork training programs, but is a consistent finding across all quality and safety improvement initiatives. Alignment of organizational goals and the objectives of the team training program as well as engagement of leadership at all levels are two of the most frequently cited critical success factors. Although training is the method of change, efforts to improve teamwork behaviors are also organizational and culture change initiatives. Managing this change effectively means looking far beyond what happens in the training sessions.

In her chapter on implementation, Salisbury provides numerous examples of how challenging the process of navigating an organizational context can be during a team training implementation as well as insightful lessons learned for maximizing any potential gains in behavior change. Equally important, King and Harden discuss how organizational culture and context drive the long-term sustainment of any improvement in teamwork behaviors resulting from training. These factors are supremely important, and the next frontier in truly understanding how to improve teamwork in healthcare.

3. PRACTICE MATTERS, BUT SOUND INSTRUCTIONAL DESIGN TRUMPS TECHNOLOGY.

Changing teamwork behaviors means changing patterns of communication and interaction among staff members. These behaviors are rooted not only in knowledge, skill, and attitude competencies, but in social norms and expectations reinforced during education and experiences working in an industry with a largely hierarchical culture that does not always reinforce open and assertive communication. Repeated practice and feedback (i.e., simulation-based teamwork training) is a powerful tool for building and reinforcing new teamwork behaviors, but simulation is defined as an instructional strategy or a method, and not by the specific technology used to implement that strategy. The fundamentals of competency and learning objective driven curriculum and scenario design, team performance measurement, and effective feedback matter more than the physical fidelity of the simulator used. McGaghie, Eppich, and O'Leary give a state of the science and practice review on the methods, concepts, and tools used for simulation-based team training, and codify methods for the gold standard method of team training delivery.

4.YOU HAVE TO KNOW WHERE YOU'RE AT TO GET WHERE YOU WANT TO GO: MEASURE AND EVALUATE TO DRIVE CHANGE.

Measurement and evaluation systems are critical at several levels: as input for systematic feedback processes to maximize learning, evaluating the effectiveness of training programs, and understanding teamwork and safety issues on a unit in a diagnostic manner. Unfortunately, valid, reliable, and practical methods for measuring team performance throughout the implementation process (i.e., during initial assessment, training, transfer, and sustainment) has been a challenge because of a relatively small set of existing tools accompanied by validity evidence. Additionally, just as there is no one-size-fits-all team training solution, team performance measures are often tied to specific clinical domains or task situations. However, Rosen and colleagues describe a decision-point framework for developing team performance measures that can simplify the process of adapting or creating new team performance measures for a given team training need.

5.LEADERS AT ALL LEVELS MUST EMBODY THE CHANGES DESIRED. THEY MUST SET AND CONTINUOUSLY REINFORCE A VISION AND VALUES CONSISTENT WITH TEAMWORK.

In many ways, leaders are an embodiment of organizational values and visions. Staff members take cues from leaders on the organization's priorities and act accordingly. From executive leadership to front-line leaders and champions on the units, staff members must receive a clear and consistent message that teamwork matters and is an integral component of how work is done at their facility. Leaders can achieve this in multiple ways, by assuring that staff time and other needed resources are available for teamwork training, recognizing outstanding team players, attending training sessions, putting measurement and incentive systems in place for improving teamwork on the units, acting to hold disruptive and noncompliant staff members accountable, or being vocal supporters of teamwork

training initiatives, for example. Leonard, Frankel, and Knight cogently describe the role of leaders in building and maintaining a climate that fosters effective teamwork.

6.BUILDING EFFECTIVE TEAMWORK IS A LONG-TERM ENDEAVOR.

Single training sessions have been shown to have demonstrable effects. They can produce learning and change behaviors. However, just as clinical skills are developed over the course of many years and continue to mature throughout a provider's career, building teamwork is not a "one shot deal." A single training session, or even a series of sessions, will not likely be sufficient to ensure high levels of team performance. Organizations must ensure that team competencies remain high in the face of skill decay over time as well as high staff turnover rates. Again, King and Harden provide valuable lessons for long-term sustainment.

7.THE INDUSTRY HAS A ROLE IN ENSURING TEAMWORK COMPETENCE.

For long-term change to take place, teamwork training concepts must be integrated throughout all aspects of the healthcare industry, including the full continuum of healthcare education, from basic to ongoing and continuing education programs. Frush, Sherwood, Wright, and Segall discuss the issue of teamwork training in healthcare education. This is a necessary step for truly integrating teamwork into the culture of the industry. Additionally, teamwork concepts must move from training and education programs and into licensing, certification, and accreditation. Team competence must be regulated and incentivized to ensure that providers and health systems are accountable for ensuring these critical skills are in place. Frush, Maynard, Koeble, and Schwendimann discuss how models and processes from the aviation domain can help to inform healthcare's journey toward a comprehensive industry and governmental system for regulating teamwork competence.

8. THERE IS A SCIENCE OF TEAMS... FOLLOW IT.

We know a lot about the factors that drive effective team performance. This scientific knowledge-base has been developed across many domains, contributed to by many scientific disciplines, and grown over decades of systematic research. Weaver and colleagues provide a comprehensive review of the theory and extensive findings produced by this multidisciplinary research community, and Driskell and colleagues provide a synthesis of the evidence on team training effectiveness. Unfortunately, we know less about healthcare teams specifically, than we know about teams in other domains (e.g., aviation crews, military teams, project management teams). However, as discussed by Alonso and Dunleavy, the scientific knowledge-base of teams in healthcare is growing rapidly. This literature base is rigorous and theoretical, but also extremely practice-oriented. It can and has driven the development of effective teamwork improvement projects, and can be used to guide decisions in healthcare.

9. THE SCIENCE ISN'T COMPLETE... WE NEED TO KNOW MORE.

Healthcare's teamwork journey is still in the earliest stages. Amazing progress has been made, valuable lessons have been learned, but so much more remains to be done. As an industry priding itself on a connection to evidence, the teamwork journey in healthcare must continue coupled with rigorous evaluation of innovations and continuous accumulation of scientific knowledge.

10. THE NEED TO MOVE BEYOND A TEAM TRAINING "PROGRAM".

Changing the culture of healthcare will take time. And although progress has been made, of course more is needed. What is also needed is the move against seeing team training as a "program" in which one goes to learn about teamwork for a few hours. What is needed is a mental model from the top-down that values and reinforces teamwork in the healthcare system. Teamwork must be part of the DNA of healthcare, not a place or a program.

REFERENCES

1. Rabol, L. I., Ostergaard, D., & Mogensen, T. (2010). Outcomes of classroom-based team training interventions for multiprofessional hospital staff: A systematic review. *Quality and Safety in Health Care, 19,* 1–11.

2. Weaver, S. L., Lyons, R., DiazGranados, D., Rosen, M. A., Salas, E., Oglesby, J., et al. (2010). The anatomy of health care team training and the state of practice: A critical review. *Academic Medicine, 85,* 1746–60.

3. Deering, S., Rosen, M. A., Ludi, V., Munroe, M., Pocrnich, A., Leaky, C., et al. (2011). On the front lines of patient safety: Implementation and evaluation of team training in Iraq. *Joint Commission Journal on Quality and Patient Safety, 37*(8), 350–6.

4. Capella, J., Smith, S., Philp, A., Putnam, T., Glibert, C., Fry, W., et al. (2010). Teamwork training improves the clinical care of trauma patients. *Journal of Surgical Education, 6,* 439–43.

5. Siassakos, D., Hasafa, Z., Sibanda, T., Fox, R., Donald, F., Winter, C., et al. (2009). Retrospective cohort study of diagnosis-delivery interval with umbilical cord prolapse: The effect of team training. *British Journal of Obstetrics and Gynaecology, 116,* 1089–96.

6. Neily, J., Mills, P. D., Young-Xu, Y., Carney, B. T., West, P., Berger, D. H., et al. (2010). Association between implementation of a medical team training program and surgical mortality. *Journal of the American Medical Association, 304,* 1693–700.

7. Strasser, D. C., Falconer, J. A., Stevens, A. B., Uomoto, J. M., Herrin, J., Bowen, S. E., et al. (2008). Team training and stroke rehabilitation outcomes: A cluster randomized trial. *Archives of Physical Medicine and Rehabilitation, 89,* 10–5.

INDEX

Lightning Source UK Ltd.
Milton Keynes UK
UKOW020013290413

209914UK00003B/19/P